Principles of Pediatric Neurosurgery

Series Editor: Anthony J. Raimondi

Principles of Pediatric Neurosurgery

Head Injuries in the Newborn and Infant
Edited by Anthony J. Raimondi, Maurice Choux,
and Concezio Di Rocco

Head Injuries in the Newborn and Infant

Edited by Anthony J. Raimondi, Maurice Choux, and Concezio Di Rocco

With 108 Figures

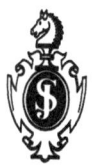

Springer Verlag
New York Berlin Heidelberg
London Paris Tokyo

Anthony J. Raimondi, M.D., Division of Pediatric Neurology, Children's Memorial Hospital, Northwestern University Medical School, Chicago, Illinois, 60614, U.S.A.

Maurice Choux, M.D., Hôpital des Infantes de la Timone, Rue Saint Pierre, 13005 Marseille, France

Concezio Di Rocco, M.D., Instituto di Neurochirurgia, Università Cattolica del Sacro Cuore, Largo Gemelli 8, 00168 Rome, Italy

Library of Congress Cataloging in Publication Data
Main entry under title:
Head injuries in the newborn and infant.
  (Principles of pediatric neurosurgery)
  Includes bibliographies and index.
  1. Brain—Wounds and injuries. 2. Head—Wounds and
injuries. 3. Infants (Newborn)—Wounds and injuries.
4. Infants—Wounds and injuries. I. Raimondi, Anthony J.,
1928–   II. Choux, M. (Maurice) III. Di Rocco, C.
(Concezio) IV. Series. [DNLM: 1. Brain Injuries—in
infancy & childhood. 2. Head Injuries—in infancy &
childhood. WE 706 H307]
RD594.H39   1985   617′.51044   85-26191

Typeset by Bi-Comp, Inc., York, Pennsylvania.

9 8 7 6 5 4 3 2 1

ISBN 978-1-4615-7185-8   ISBN 978-1-4615-7183-4 (eBook)
DOI 10.1007/978-1-4615-7183-4

Series Preface

It is estimated that the functionally significant body of knowledge for a given medical specialty changes radically every 8 years. New specialties and "sub-specialization" are occurring at approximately an equal rate. Historically, established journals have not been able either to absorb this increase in publishable material or to extend their readership to the new specialists. International and national meetings, symposia and seminars, workshops and newsletters, successfully bring to the attention of physicians within developing specialties what is occurring, but generally only in demonstration form without providing historical perspective, patho-anatomical correlates, or extensive discussion. Page and time limitations oblige the authors to present only the essence of their material.

Pediatric neurosurgery is an example of a specialty that has developed during the past 15 years and over this period, neurosurgeons have obtained special training in pediatric neurosurgery and then dedicated themselves primarily to its practice. Centers, Chairs, and educational programs have been established as groups of neurosurgeons in different countries throughout the world organized themselves respectively into national and international societies for pediatric neurosurgery. These events were both preceded and followed by specialized courses, national and international journals, and ever-increasing clinical and investigative studies into all aspects of surgically treatable diseases of the child's nervous system.

Principles of Pediatric Neurosurgery is an ongoing series of publications, each dedicated exclusively to a particular subject, a subject which is currently timely either because of an extensive amount of work occurring in it, or because it has been neglected. The two first subjects, "Head Injuries in the Newborn and Infant" and "The Pediatric Spine," are expressive of those extremes.

Volumes will be published continuously, as the subjects are dealt with, rather than on an annual basis, since our goal is to make this information available to the specialist when it is new and informative. If a volume becomes obsolete because of newer methods of treatment and concepts, we shall publish a new edition.

The chapters are selected and arranged to provide the reader, in each instance, with embryological, developmental, epidemiological, clinical, therapeutic, and psychosocial aspects of each subject, thusly permitting each specialist to learn what is most current in his field and to familiarize himself with sister fields of the same subject. Each chapter is organized along classical lines, progressing from introduction through symptoms and treatment, to prognosis for clinical material; and introduction through history and data, to results and discussion for experimental material.

Contents

Contributors

L. BASAURI
Professor of Neurosurgery
Instituto de Neurocirugia e
  Investigaciones Cerebrales
Santiago, Chile

DEREK A. BRUCE
Division of Neurological Surgery
The Children's Hospital of
  Philadelphia
Philadelphia, Pennsylvania, U.S.A.

N. CHIOFALO
Centro de Exporacion Funcional del
  Cerebro
Profidencia, Santiago, Chile

MAURICE CHOUX
Hôpital des Enfantes de la Timone
Marseille, France

CONCEZIO DI ROCCO
Instituto di Neurochirurgia
Università Cattolica del Sacro Cuore
Rome, Italy

I. FANKHAUSER
Department of Pediatric Surgery
University Children's Hospital
Bern, Switzerland

LORENZO GENITORI
Department of Pediatric Neurosurgery
Hôpital des Enfants de la Timone
Marseille, France

JENS HAASE
Department of Neurosurgery
Aalborg, Sygehus Syd
Aalborg, Denmark

JEFFREY HIRSCHAUER
Division of Pediatric Neurology
Children's Memorial Hospital
Northwestern University Medical
  School
Chicago, Illinois, U.S.A.

HAROLD J. HOFFMAN
Professor of Surgery
University of Toronto
The Hospital for Sick Children
Toronto, Ontario, Canada

KARL H. HOVIND
Department of Neurosurgery
National Hospital of Norway
Oslo, Norway

G. KAISER
Department of Pediatric Surgery
University Children's Hospital
Bern, Switzerland

MARIANNE LARSEN
Division of Pediatric Neurology
Children's Memorial Hospital
Northwestern University Medical
  School
Chicago, Illinois, U.S.A.

GABRIEL LENA
Department of Pediatric Neurosurgery
Hôpital des Enfants de la Timone
Marseille, France

THOMAS G. LUERSSEN
Division of Neurological Surgery
The Children's Hospital of
   Philadelphia
Philadelphia, Pennsylvania, U.S.A.

J. MADSEN
Professor of Neuropediatry
Centre de Exploracion Funcional del
   Cerebro
Santiago, Chile

ROBERT L. MCLAURIN
Departments of Neurosurgery and
   Radiology
Children's Hospital Medical Center
Cincinnati, Ohio, U.S.A.

DAVID G. MCLONE
Children's Memorial Hospital
Chicago, Illinois, U.S.A.

SHIZUO OI
Department of Neurosurgery
National Kagawa Children's Hospital
Kagawa, Japan

KUNIHIKO OSAKA
Kobe University School of Medicine
Kobe, Japan

WARWICK J. PEACOCK
Associate Professor of Surgery
UCLA School of Medicine
Los Angeles, California U.S.A.

ANTHONY J. RAIMONDI
Professor of Surgery (Neurosurgery)
Professor of Anatomy and Cell
   Biology
Children's Memorial Hospital
Northwestern University Medical
   School
Chicago, Illinois, U.S.A.

A. RÜDEBERG
Department of Pediatric Surgery
University Children's Hospital
Bern, Switzerland

OSAMU SATO
Department of Neurosurgery
Tokai University Medical School
Bohseidai, Japan

LUIS SCHUT
Division of Neurological Surgery
The Children's Hospital of
   Philadelphia
Philadelphia, Pennsylvania, U.S.A.

NIELS SÖRENSEN
Professor of Neurosurgery
University Hospital of Neurosurgery
University of Würzburg
Federal Republic of Germany

BRUCE B. STORRS
Primary Children's Medical Center
Salt Lake City, Utah, U.S.A.

LESLIE N. SUTTON
Division of Neurological Surgery
The Children's Hospital of
   Philadelphia
Philadelphia, Pennsylvania, U.S.A.

CHOPEOW TAECHOLARN
Division of Neurosurgery
University of Toronto
The Hospital for Sick Children
Toronto, Ontario, Canada

RICHARD TOWBIN
Department of Radiology
Children's Hospital Medical Center
Cincinnati, Ohio, U.S.A.

FRANCESCO VELARDI
Institute of Neurosurgery
Catholic University
Rome, Italy

MARION L. WALKER
Primary Children's Medical Center
Salt Lake City, Utah, U.S.A.

ISAO YAMAMOTO
Department of Neurosurgery
Tokai University Medical School
Bohseidai, Japan

C. ZÜMBUHL
Department of Pediatric Surgery
University Children's Hospital
Bern, Switzerland

CHAPTER 1

Intrauterine Development of the Skull

Isao Yamamoto and Osamu Sato

Introduction

Depressed skull fracture may occur in utero[1,2] as well as during the process of delivery. The mechanism of these depressions is not entirely clear. Even in the newborn and infant, roentgenographic diagnosis of linear skull fracture is sometimes ambiguous because numerous accessory sutures may be present.[3] To understand depressed skull fracture, more details about the normal developmental anatomy of the skull in utero are needed. There have been a great number of extensive studies regarding the embryology of the human skull,[4-11] but much of the information is not practical for neurosurgeons to utilize.

Development of the Fetal Skull

The earliest noticeable cranial element in the human embryo first appears as a mesenchymal condensation about the notochord at the level underlying the hindbrain. The mesenchyme develops at the end of the first month and the beginning of the second month of gestation. It may convert into two components: the primordial cartilaginous cranium (chondrocranium) and the primordial membranous cranium (desmocranium or blastemal skull). The components usually undergo endochondral ossification, but in some regions persist through life.

In general, the chondrocranium first appears early in the second month. It is limited to the base of the skull, where it forms the clivus and the dorsum sellae and then the nasal capsules rostrally and the otic capsules on the farther sides caudally. The base of the skull is primarily chondrified in three regions: the occipital around the foramen magnum (basal plate or parachondral cartilage), the sphenoid beneath the hypophyseal region (prechordal or trabecular region), and the ethmoid beneath the rostral part of the telencephalon (Fig. 1.1). The body of the sphenoid sends an extension forward on each side to surround the craniopharyngeal canal, and

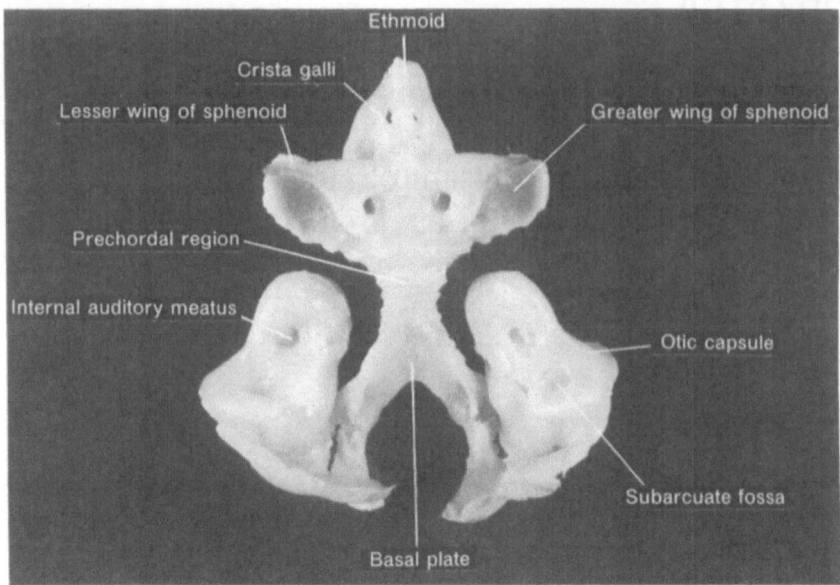

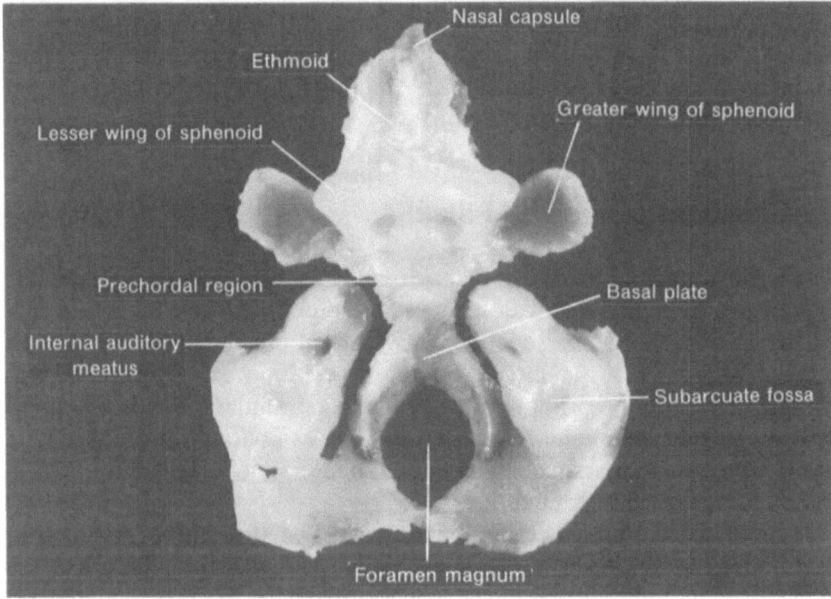

Figure 1.1. The chondrocranium of a human embryo in the 11th week: crown-rump (CR) length of 68 mm (**A**); and the 14th week: CR length of 105 mm (**B**), of life (viewed from above).

these extensions join to form the rostral part of the body of the sphenoid (presphenoid). This craniopharyngeal canal is usually occluded during the third month of fetal life.[12] The cartilaginous nasal capsule is preformed by the presphenoid, the ethmoid bone, and the inferior nasal chonchae. The two otocysts (auditory or otic vesicles) are surrounded by mesoderm, which becomes chondrified to form the mesenchymal otic capsule. In this capsule the petromastoid part of the temporal bone is developed in cartilage. Each otic capsule becomes fused with the lateral margin of the basal plate, but this fusion is not complete and in subsequent development forms the jugular foramen between the posterior extremity of the otic capsule and the basal plate. The roof and parts of the base of the skull, such as the frontal, parietal, squamous, and tympanic parts of the temporal bone, as well as parts of the sphenoid and the occipital bone, are formed by the membranous bone. The maxillary, zygomatic, lacrimal, nasal, palatine, and vomerine bones are also formed directly from the mesenchymal membrane of the nasal capsule and the face. In addition, the mandible is developed in membrane from the first branchial or pharyngeal arch. Finally, the cartilaginous and membranous parts of the skull develop together and complement each other in forming the osseous cranium.

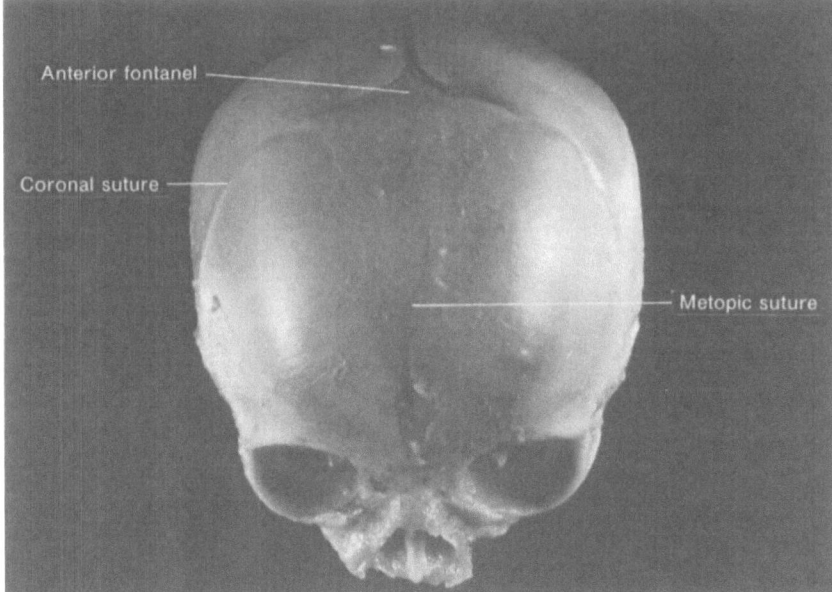

A

Figure 1.2. The skull in the eighteenth week of fetal life: crown-rump (CR) length of 160 mm. (**A**) Anterosuperior aspect, (**B**) lateral aspect, and (**C**) superior aspect. (Fetuses courtesy of Dr Hiroshi Osakabe.)

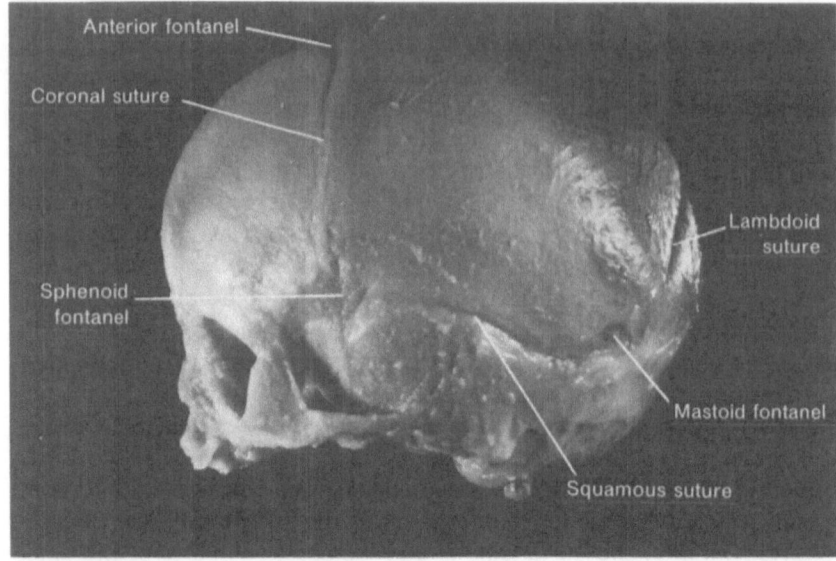

B

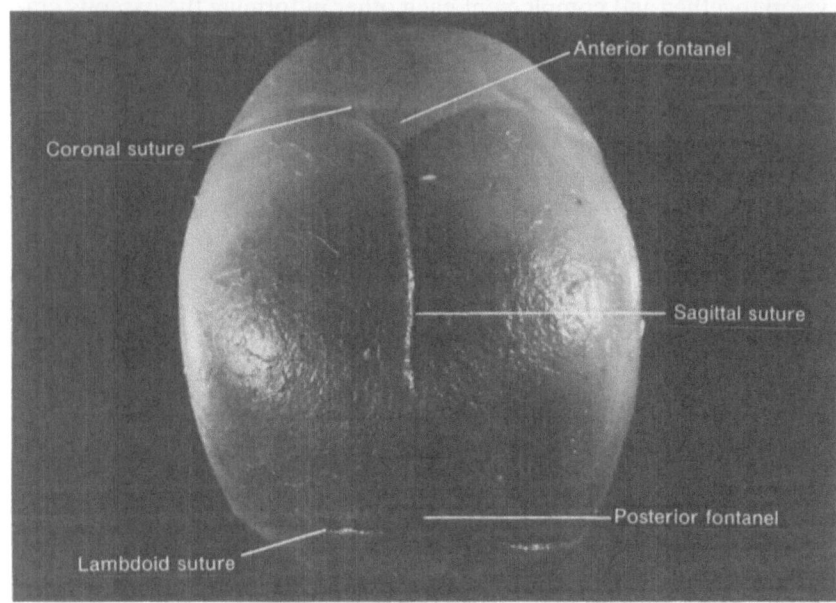

C

Figure 1.2 *Continued*

At the time of birth, ossification is not complete, and the bones forming the sides and roof of the skull are still united by membrane; some of those of the base of the skull are united by cartilage. The frontal and parietal bones are separated from each other by a rhomboid spot, the anterior fontanel (bregma). The anterior fontanel may contain a separate ossicle,[13] which is uncommon and occurs mostly in males. Posterior, there is a median gap in the angle between the two parietal bones and the occipital one at the sagittal suture, known as the posterior fontanel (lambda). On the sides of the cranium, there are two unclosed areas: the anterolateral area in the angle between the sphenoid, parietal, and frontal bones, in which the sphenoid fontanel (pterion) is formed; and the posterolateral area between the parietal, temporal, and occipital bones, in which the mastoid fontanel (asterion) is formed (Fig. 1.2A, B, and C).

Development of the Individual Bones

Frontal Bone

The frontal bone (Fig. 1.3) has no cartilaginous precursor and at first develops within the outermost layer of the membranous covering of the brain (dura mater). In the eighth or ninth week of fetal life, it begins to ossify from two primary centers. There is one chief center for each frontal tuber; secondary centers for smaller parts of the frontal bone appear later. From these centers, ossification extends upward to form the corresponding half of the bone, backward to form the orbital plate, and downward to form the nasal part of the frontal bone.

During fetal development the frontal suture exists between the two halves of the frontal bone as a metopic suture. Berry[14] reported that the

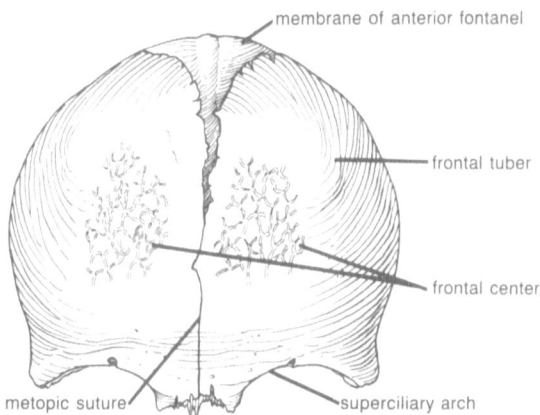

Figure 1.3. Location of ossification centers in the frontal bone (anterior aspect) of the skull. Intramembranous ossification centers and endochondral ossification are shown. (Drawings modified from Reference 10.)

incidence of metopism remaining in adults was 0% to 7.4% in individuals in various racial groups.

Parietal Bone

The parietal bone (Fig. 1.4) appears at first as a membranous neurocranium. It begins to ossify in the seventh or tenth week of intrauterine life from two centers that appear one above the other at the parietal tuber. These centers then unite in the fourth month, and ossification gradually extends toward the margins of the bone in a centrifugal manner. Even at the time of birth, however, the parietal bone may occasionally be divided into two components by an anteroposterior suture.[15]

Occipital Bone

The fetal occipital bone (Fig. 1.5) exhibits four enchondral ossification centers and paired intermembranous centers. Basioccipital, supraoccipital, and two exoccipital centers are of cartilaginous origin. The squamous (interparietal) part above the superior nuchal line is of membranous origin. In about the sixth week of intrauterine life, the ossification center in the basioccipitals appears. Each supraoccipital center in the squamous part of the superior nuchal line usually begins to ossify in about the seventh week of gestation; these centers soon unite to form a single piece. Each exoccipital then ossifies from a single center that appears during the eight week. In the third month of gestation, the upper and lower portion of the squamous part unite, but this may be incomplete at birth. The four main components are united by cartilage until after birth. The basioccipi-

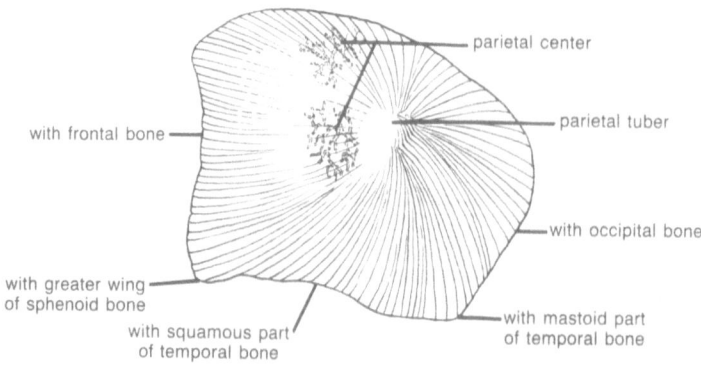

Figure 1.4. Location of ossification centers in the parietal bone (external surface) of the skull. Intramembranous ossification centers and endochondral ossification centers are shown. (Drawings modified from Reference 10.)

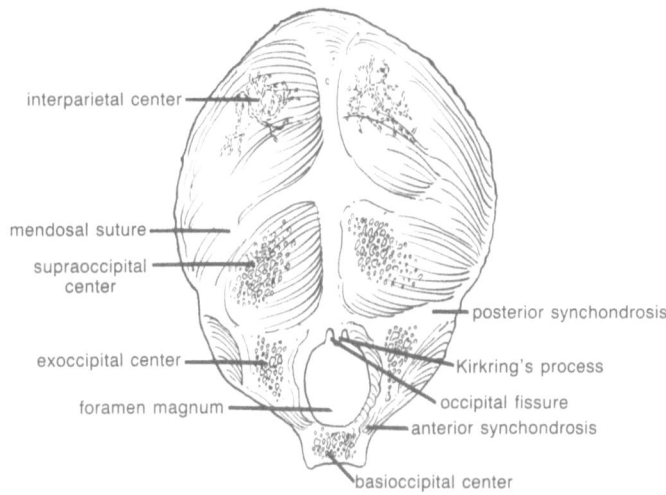

interparietal center

mendosal suture

supraoccipital
center

exoccipital center

foramen magnum

posterior synchondrosis

Kirkring's process

occipital fissure

anterior synchondrosis

basioccipital center

Figure 1.5. Location of ossification centers in the occipital bone (external surface) of the skull. Intramembranous ossification centers and endochondral ossification centers are shown. (Drawings modified from Reference 10.)

tal and exoccipital bones are separated by two anterior synchondroses, and the exoccipital and supraoccipital bones are separated by two posterior synchondroses.

There are many arguments about the number of ossification centers in the squamous portion of the occipital bone. This question is significant because roentgenological diagnosis of skull fracture in an infant is sometimes made difficult by the numerous accessory sutures simulating fracture lines around the foramen magnum. Srivastava[16] has reported a complex developmental anatomy of the ossification centers in the squamous portion. The interparietal portion develops from three pairs of ossification centers: one pair for the lateral plates, one pair for the central piece, and the third pair representing the preinterparietals. The supraoccipital portion develops from five ossification centers, two centers for each lateral segment and a single center for the central segment. Franken,[3] however, mentions that the supraoccipital bone forms from a single center that is arranged around the dorsal surface of the original foramen magnum, the occipital fissure. This fissure closes in a complicated fashion, with descent of a median process (Kirkring's process) and apposition of the lateral margins of the fissure. Anomalous sutures corresponding to this area are found in the infant, but they should extend no farther dorsally than the original occipital fissure. Hence almost all midline linear fissures extending the entire length of the supraoccipital bone are to be recognized as fracture.

Temporal Bone

The temporal bone (Fig. 1.6) is composed of four parts: the squamous, the tympanic, the petromastoid, and the styloid process. The squamous and tympanic parts develop in membrane, the petromastoid and the styloid process develop in cartilage. The squamous portion is ossified from a single center that appears in the region of the roots of the zygomatic process in about the seventh or eighth week of fetal development. Another intramembranous ossification of the tympanic portion begins to occur in the lateral wall of the tympanum during the ninth to tenth week and forms a curved tympanic ring. After birth, the ossification of this tympanic ring spreads to form the tympanic plate.

The petromastoid part is ossified from as many as 14 centers that appear in the cartilaginous otic capsule in the fifth month of fetal development. The first ossification center appears around the cochlea during the 16th week of fetal life. The last center appears around the semicircular canal at about the 20th week. The inner portion of the bony otic capsule develops into the perilymph structures that surround the membranous labyrnth. The whole otic capsule is more or less fused by the end of the sixth month of gestation, and the inner ear changes little in structure or growth into adult life. The styloid process ossifies from two centers in the cranial end of cartilage of the second pharyngeal arch: one for the proximal part of the process (tympanohyal), and the other for the distal part of the process (stylohyal).

Sphenoid Bone

The sphenoid bone (Fig. 1.7) is of mixed cartilaginous and membranous origin. A pair in the lesser wings (orbitosphenoid), a pair in the greater

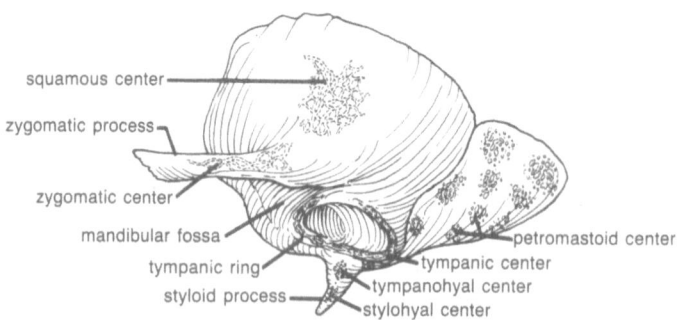

Figure 1.6. Location of ossification centers in the temporal bone (external aspect) of the skull. Intramembranous ossification centers and endochondral ossification centers are shown. (Drawings modified from Reference 10.)

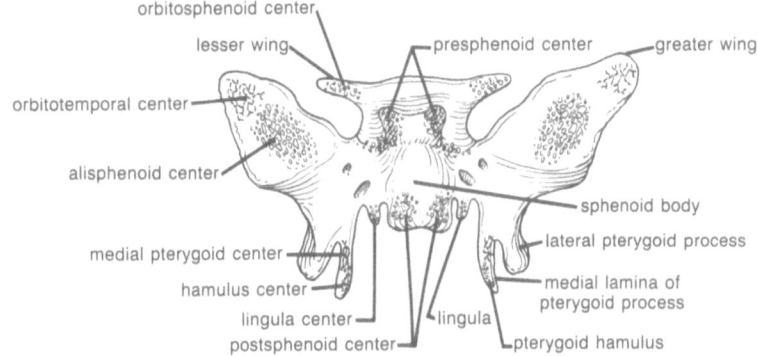

Figure 1.7. Location of ossification centers in the sphenoid bone (posterior aspect) of the skull. Intramembranous ossification centers and endochondral ossification centers are shown. (Drawings modified from Reference 10.)

wings (alisphenoid), a pair in the rostral part of the body of the sphenoid (presphenoid), a pair in the caudal part of the body of the sphenoid (postsphenoid), and a pair in the lingulae are cartilaginous in origin. A pair in the lateral part of the greater wing (orbitotemporal) and a pair in the medial lamina of the pterygoid process, except for the hamulus, are membranous in origin.

There are 18 separate ossification centers in the sphenoid anlage. The first ossification center is that of the greater wing. In about the eighth week of intrauterine life, an alisphenoid center begins to ossify in cartilage, and two orbitotemporal centers are ossified in membrane. In about the ninth fetal week an orbitosphenoid center appears; shortly thereafter, two centers in the presphenoid part of the body ossify. In about the ninth or tenth week of gestation, a pair in the medial lamina of the pterygoid process begins to ossify. During the third month, the hamulus is chondrified. In about the fourth month, one ossification center appears for each lingula, and two centers appear in the postsphenoid part of the body, one on each side of the sella turcica; these soon fuse. The presphenoid and the postsphenoid parts fuse to form the body of the sphenoid in about the eighth month of intrauterine life. But even at the time of birth, the sphenoid bone is still in three parts: a central part consisting of a body and a lesser wing, and two lateral parts, each comprising a greater wing and the pterygoid process. The superior surface of the body of the sphenoid consists of three parts at birth: the ossifying dorsum sellae; the ossified postsphenoid (sellar floor), and the ossified presphenoid, which forms the anterosuperior wall of the sella and develops anteriorly toward the cribriform plate. Although the tuberculum sellae is present at birth, the planum sphenoidale is not yet formed.[17] Ratner and Quencer[18] describe three cases of failure of fusion of the presphenoid ossification center in which a skull base density was initially interpreted as an anterior clinoid meningioma.

Prior to the 12th week of gestation, three principal fenestrations through which cranial nerves and blood vessels pass are present at the base of the skull. They are the foramen lacerum anterius, foramen lacerum medium, and foramen lacerum posterius.[19] The foramen lacerum anterius is the hiatus between the orbitosphenoid and alisphenoid. By the 12th to 16th week of fetal life, this foramen has completely separated to form two discrete orifices, the superior orbital fissure and the foramen rotundum. The foramen lacerum medium is the hiatus between the basisphenoid and periotic capsule, which persists as a foramen lacerum. The foramen lacerum posterius, the space between the basiocciput and the otic capsule, persists as the jugular foramen.

The optic foramen is at first formed by the cartilaginous lesser wing (orbitosphenoid) to outline the anterosuperior and lateral margins of the foramen during the third month of fetal life.[20] The presphenoid center then enlarges to form the medial border of the foramen. During the fifth month the bony optic foramen resembles a keyhole in appearance. The optic strut extends medially from the lesser sphenoid wing to join the presphenoid center, which consists of two separate segments, transitory foramina. This foramen gradually becomes obliterated by the fusion of the two segments into a single strut during the last two months of fetal life.

Ethmoid Bone

The ethmoid bone (Fig. 1.8) is cartilaginous in origin, and the cartilaginous nasal capsule is well developed by the end of the third month. It consists of a medial and two lateral parts. Between the fourth and fifth months of intrauterine life, three ossification centers appear in the cartilaginous nasal capsule, one for the medial perpendicular plate and one for each lateral labyrnth. The medial portion (mesethmoid) extends to the tip

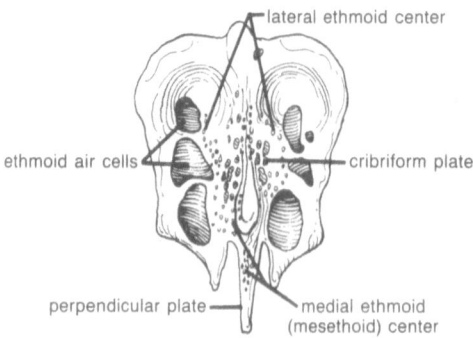

Figure 1.8. Location of ossification centers in the ethmoid bone (superior aspect) of the skull. Intramembranous ossification centers and endochondral ossification centers are shown. (Drawings modified from Reference 10.)

Figure 1.9. Location of ossification centers in the lacrimal bone (lateral surface) of the skull. Intramembranous ossification centers and endochondral ossification centers are shown. (Drawings modified from Reference 10.)

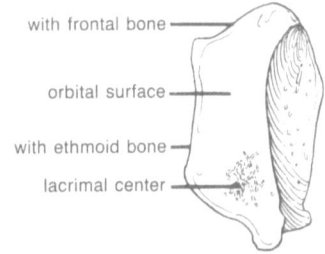

of the developing nose. Its more rostral part persists with little alteration as the cartilaginous part of the nasal septum. During the 12th week of fetal life the crista galli begins to ossify in the cartilage of the nasal capsule for the perpendicular plate and projects medially above the cranial floor. During the fourth and fifth months, the lateral part of the nasal capsule becomes ossified as the ethmoid labyrnth. The medial and lateral ethmoid cartilages are at first not fused with each other; gradually, the space between the medial and lateral cartilages is replaced by bone. This region, where the olfactory nerves go through many small foramina, is known as the cribriform plate.

Lacrimal Bone

Each lacrimal bone (Fig. 1.9) is of membranous origin and begins to ossify from a single center in the mesenchyme around the cartilaginous nasal capsule in about the 12th week of intrauterine life.

Vomerine Bone

The vomer (Fig. 1.10) is ossified in membrane from two centers appearing in the eighth week of intrauterine life on either side of the posteroinferior part of the septal cartilage. These two centers then fuse with each other along their lower edges in the third month of fetal life.

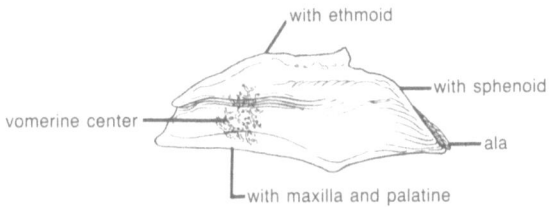

Figure 1.10. Location of ossification centers in the vomerine bone (left lateral aspect) of the skull. Intramembranous ossification centers and endochondral ossification centers are shown. (Drawings modified from Reference 10.)

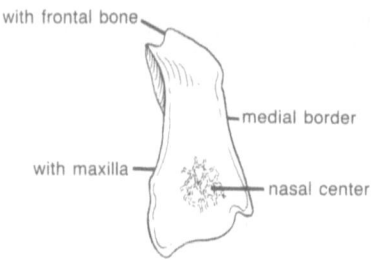

Figure 1.11. Location of ossification centers in the nasal bone (outer aspect) of the skull. Intramembranous ossification centers and endochondral ossification centers are shown. (Drawings modified from Reference 10.)

Nasal Bone

Each nasal bone (Fig. 1.11) ossifies at the end of the second or the beginning of the third month of fetal life from a single center in the membrane on the outside of the nasal capsule.

Maxillae

Three ossification centers have been described for the maxilla (Fig. 1.12), which is of membranous origin. One, for the main mass of the bone, appears in the wall of the oral cavity above the germ of the canine tooth in the sixth week of intrauterine life; two are for the premaxillary part of the bone (os incisivum). The first of the two ossification centers of the premaxilla appears above the incisor tooth germs in the sixth week to form most of the premaxilla; the second appears in the 12th week to form the wall of the incisive canal. The maxillary sinus first appears as a shallow groove on the medial side of the bone in about the fourth month of intrauterine life.

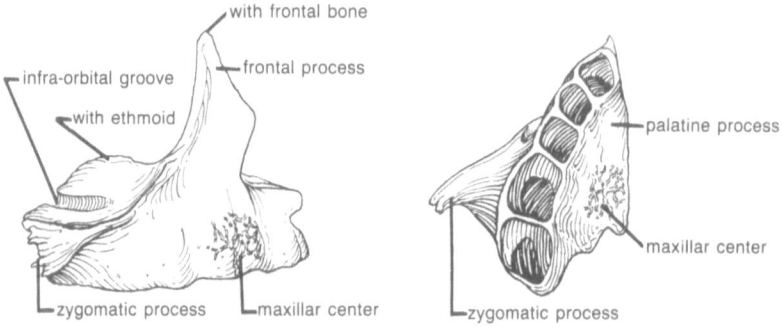

Figure 1.12. Location of ossification centers in the maxilla (left: lateral aspect; right: inferior aspect) of the skull. Intramembranous ossification centers and endochondral ossification centers are shown. (Drawings modified from Reference 10.)

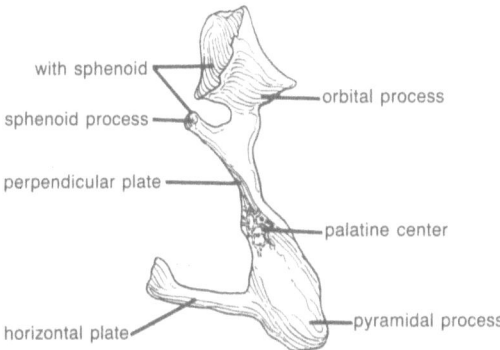

Figure 1.13. Location of ossification centers in the palatine bone (posterior aspect) of the skull. Intramembranous ossification centers and endochondral ossification centers are shown. (Drawings modified from Reference 10.)

Palatine Bone

The palatine bone (Fig. 1.13) is of membranous origin and ossifies from one center in the perpendicular plate during the eighth week of intrauterine life. From this center, ossification spreads upward into the orbital and sphenoid proceses, medially into the horizontal plate, and downward into the pyramidal process.

Zygomatic Bone

The zygomatic bone (Fig. 1.14) ossifies in membrane from one ossification center appearing between the eighth and tenth weeks of intrauterine life.

Mandible

Each half of the mandible (Fig. 1.15) is ossified from one membranous center that appears near the mental foramen during the sixth week of

Figure 1.14. Location of ossification centers in the zygomatic bone (lateral surface) of the skull. Intramembranous ossification centers and endochondral ossification centers are shown. (Drawings modified from Reference 10.)

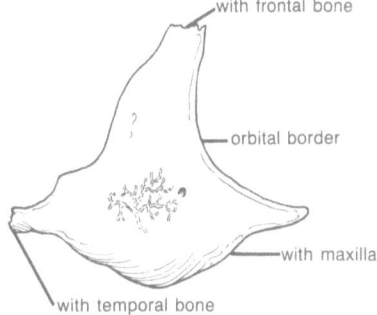

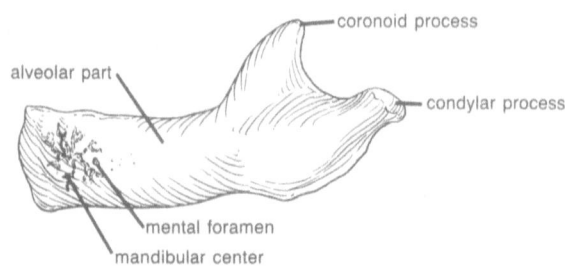

Figure 1.15. Location of ossification centers in the mandible (lateral aspect) of the skull. Intramembranous ossification centers and endochondral ossification centers are shown. (Drawings modified from Reference 10.)

intrauterine life. From this center, the ossification spreads to form the body and ramus of the mandible.

Roentgenological Observation on the Development of the Fetal Skull

Although incomplete ossification begins to appear in the second month of gestation, as may be illustrated with histological staining, radiograms do not show any evidence of ossification in the head of the human em-

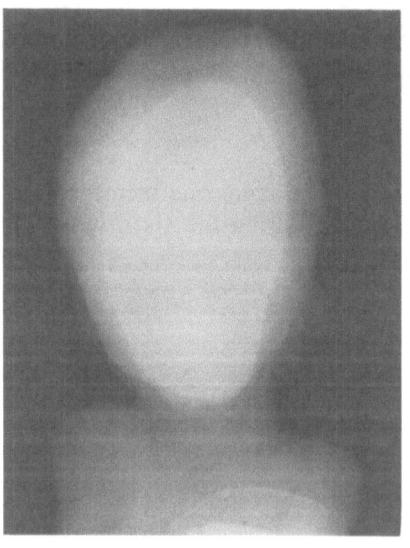

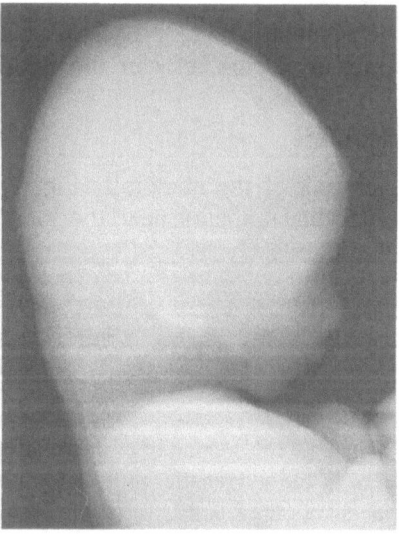

A   B

Figure 1.16. Anteroposterior (left) and lateral (right) skull radiographs of a fetus in the 11th week of development (CR length: 68 mm) reveal incomplete evidence of ossification. (Fetuses courtesy of Dr. Hiroshi Osakabe.)

bryo.[21,22] Even in the 11th week of fetal life, evidence of ossification is incomplete (Fig. 1.16A and B).

In the 14th week of intrauterine life, when crown-rump (CR) length is about 105 mm, part of the skull may be outlined in radiograms taken with the soft radiation technique. The lateral view reveals formations of the occipital squama and the supraciliary arch of the frontal bone as well as the ossification of the facial skeleton in the vicinity of the mandible and maxilla. The clivus is also recognizable as a pole-like bony segment. The sphenoid bone begins to appear, although the typical structures of the mature sphenoid bone are still missing (Fig. 1.17A). The mandibular and the maxillar ossifications, as well as the frontal bone, are better defined in the anteroposterior projection than in the lateral projection (Fig. 1.17B).

Ossification of the skull progresses further in the fourth and fifth months. Solitary centers of ossification are seen with more complete clarity after CR length has reached about 130 mm, at around the 16th week of development. In particular, the pattern of bone deposition in the

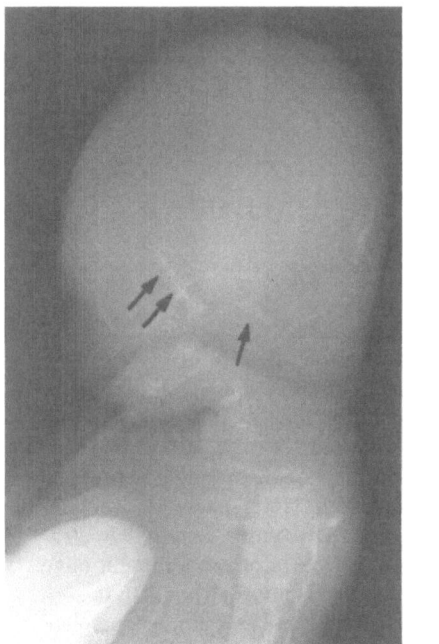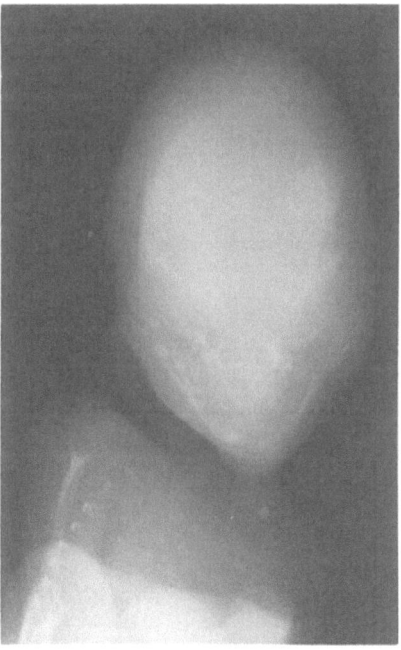

A   B

Figure 1.17. (**A**) Lateral skull radiograph of a fetus in the 14th week of development (CR length: 105 mm) shows the ossification of the occipital squama, frontal bone, and facial skeleton, such as the maxilla and mandible. The clivus (↑) and the sphenoid bone (↑↑) also begin to appear. (**B**) In the anteroposterior view, the mandible is clearly visible, and the maxilla, sphenoid, and exoccipital portion of the occipital bone are also recognizable. (Fetuses courtesy of Dr. Hiroshi Osakabe.)

vicinity of the sphenoid and petrous temporal bones may be identified. In the 18th week of fetal life, at a CR length of about 160 mm, various structures are apparent in the lateral view. The ossification center for the body of the sphenoid bone is now readily visible, but the space between the pre- and postsphenoids remains patent as an intersphenoid synchondrosis. The areas of calcification around the semicircular canals overlying the clivus and the supraoccipital and interparietal parts of the occipital bone are also well defined in the lateral projection.

In the facial skeleton, the mandible and maxilla are well defined, and the nasal bone appears as a characteristically fine linear structure of ossifi-

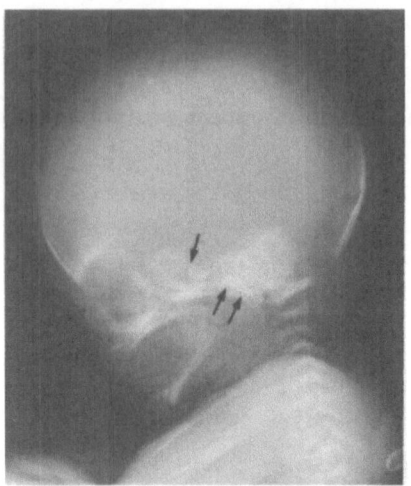

A

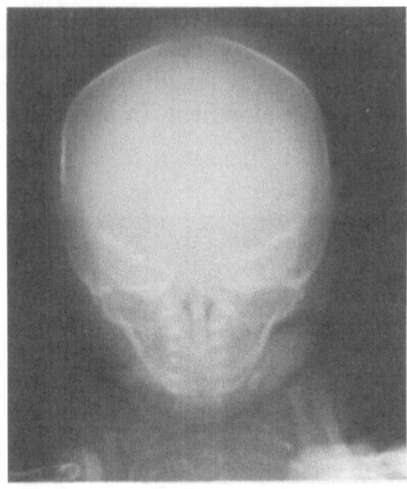

B

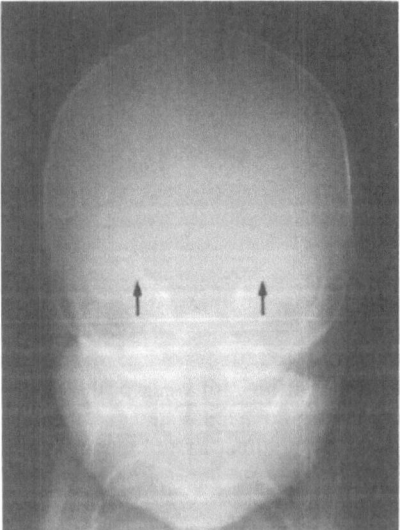

C

Figure 1.18. (**A**) In the lateral skull radiograph of a fetus in the 11th week of development (CR length: 106 mm), the separate centers of the ossification of the sphenoid bone are clearly shown. A single arrow ($\downarrow$) shows the intersphenoid synchondrosis. The tympanic and the petromastoid parts of the temporal bone overlie the clivus ($\uparrow\uparrow$). (**B**) In the anteroposterior view, almost complete ossification of the cranium is defined. (**C**) In the Towne projection, the basioccipital part of the occipital bone is readily visible. The outlines of the internal auditory canal ($\uparrow$) begin to be recognizable. (Fetuses courtesy of Dr. Hiroshi Osakabe.)

cation (Fig. 1.18A). In the anteroposterior projection of the skull, the outline of the cranium is almost completely defined. The greater wing of the sphenoid bone is clearly visible, but the bone still remains separate. The semicircular canals in the temporal bones appear as comparatively large structures with narrow rims of calcification (Fig. 1.18B). In the Towne projection, the basioccipital part of the occipital bone is easily seen, but the posterolateral boundaries of the foramen magnum cannot yet be well distinguished. The ossification of the petrous temporal bones and the tympanic rings are defined, and the outlines of the internal auditory canals begin to be recognizable (Fig. 1.18C). Usually about two or three weeks later, all three middle-ear ossicles may be recognized, and details of the semicircular canals are better defined.

References

1. Alexander E, Davis CH: Intra-uterine fracture of the infant's skull. *J Neurosurg* 1969;30:446–454.
2. Guha-Ray DK: Intrauterine spontaneous depression of fetal skull: A case report and review of literature. *J Reproduct Med* 1976;16:321–324.
3. Franken ED: The midline occipital fissure: Diagnosis of fracture versus anatomic variants. *Radiology* 1969;93:1043–1046.
4. Allen FD: *Essentials of Human Embryology*, ed 2. New York, Oxford University Press, 1969.
5. Hamilton WJ, Mossman HW: *Human Embryology: Prenatal Development of Form and Function*, ed 4. Baltimore, The Williams & Wilkins Co, 1972.
6. Harwood-Nash DC, Fitz CR: *Neuroradiology in Infants and Children*. St. Louis, The CV Mosby Co, 1976, vol 1.
7. Hollinshead WH: *Textbook of Anatomy*, ed 3. Philadelphia, JB Lippincott Co, 1974.
8. Langman J: *Medical Embryology: Human Development—Normal and Abnormal*, ed 2. Baltimore, The Williams & Wilkins Co, 1969.
9. Lockhart RD, Hamilton GF, Fyfe FW: *Anatomy of the Human Body*. London: Farber & Farber Limited, 1969.
10. Patten BM: *Human Embryology*, ed 3. New York: McGraw-Hill Book Co, 1968.
11. Romanes GJ: Cunningham's Textbook of Anatomy, ed 12. New York: Oxford University Press, 1981.
12. Newton TH, Potts DG: *Radiology of the Skull and Brain*. St. Louis, The CV Mosby Co, 1971, vol 1, book 1.
13. Girdany WJ, Mossman HW: Anterior fontanel bones. *Am J Roentgen* 1965;95:148–153.
14. Berry AC: Factors affecting the incidence of non-metrical skeletal variants. *J Anat* 1975;120:519–535.
15. Williams PL, Warwick R (eds): *Gray's Anatomy*, ed 36. New York, Churchill Livingstone, 1980.
16. Srivastava HC: Development of ossification centers in the squamous portion of the occipital bone in man. *J Anat* 1977;124:634–649.

17. Kier EL: The infantile sella turcica: New roentgenologic and anatomic concepts based on a developmental study of the sphenoid bone. *Am J Roentgen* 1968;102:747–767.
18. Ratner LM, Quencer RM: Nonunited ossification center of the presphenoid bone. *Am J Roentgen* 1983;141:503–506.
19. Shapiro R, Robinson F: The foramina of the middle fossa; A phylogenetic anatomic and pathologic study. *Am J Roentgen* 1967;101:779–794.
20. Kier EL: Embryology of the normal optic canal and its anomalies, an anatomic and roentgenographic study. *Invest Radiol* 1966;1:346–362.
21. Berkvens T: Radiology of the fetal skull. *Acta Radiol* 1950;34:250–252.
22. Decker K, Backmund H: *Paediatric Neuroradiology*. New York, Thieme-Edition/Publishing Sciences Group Inc, 1975.

CHAPTER 2

Embryological Concepts for Head Injury in the Newborn and Infant

Kunihiko Osaka and Shizuo Oi

Introduction

To participate in the treatment of head injury in infants and young children, one must be familiar with the overall development of the nervous system, including the cerebrospinal fluid (CSF) pathway. In addition to grasping the functional and structural organization of the nervous system, one must also understand the development of neurons, neural tracts, and the structure for brain protection as they relate to the unique clinical features of head injuries in infants and young children. This chapter focuses on the development of (1) neurons and neural tracts and (2) the subarachnoid space, and the arachnoid membrane.

Development of Neurons and Neural Tracts

Although both the nerve cell formation in cerebral cortex and the formation of the CSF pathway start in the embryonal stage, development of the synapses and myelination of the nerve tracts begin at a much later stage in the fetus. The spinal anterior root is one of the nerve structures that begins to be myelinated at the earliest stage—at around 16 weeks of fetal life—whereas the pyramidal tract begins to be myelinated just before birth and is completed at around 2 years of age. Appearance of the muscle tonus of the body and pathological reflexes are observed as the myelination processes develop. The different stages of these processes are shown in Figure 2.1.

Neurulation

The first phase of caudal neural tube formation in the embryo—from Carnegie stages 8 to 12, when the crown-rump (CR) length is approximately 1 to 4.5 mm—is called neurulation.[18] During stages 8 and 9, the neural folds are formed and the neural groove created. The anterior neu-

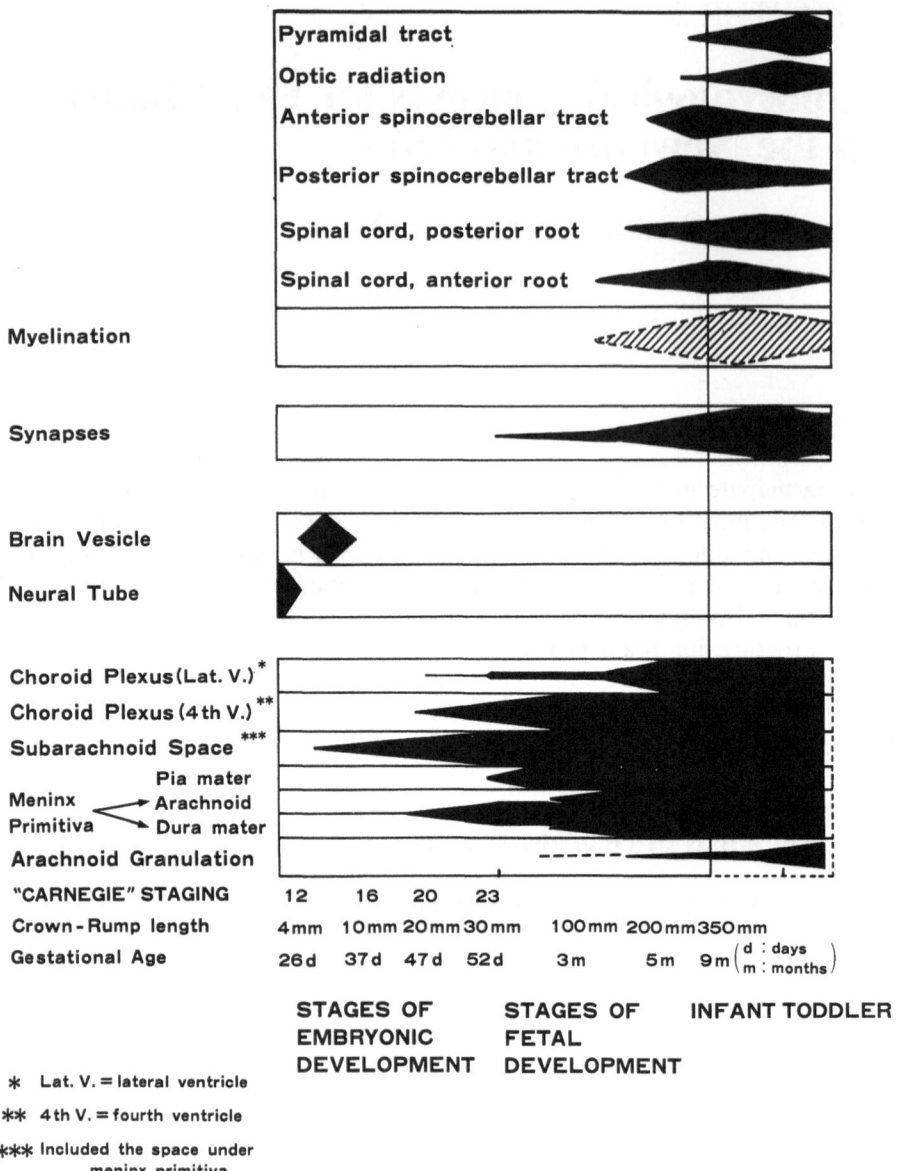

Figure 2.1. Stages of myelination processes.

ropore closes at this stage, when there are between 13 and 20 somites, and the posterior neuropore closes at stage 12, when the embryo has between 21 and 29 somites and is about 26 days old. According to the classical *Keimzellentheorie* of William His,[16] the neural tube in the early stages of embryonal development consists of two main cells, *Keimzellen* and *Spongioblasten*. The former was thought to originate in the neuroblast and the latter in the neuroglia. Bailey and Cushing[2] added the intermediate cell as "medulloblast," but essentially accepted His' theory. Although this theory is still debated in discussions of the early developmental process of the neuronal cell,[24] investigators have generally agreed that in the later stage of intrauterine life the neural tube develops three layers in an inside-out fashion: the matrix, mantle, and marginal layers. The innermost structure, the matrix layer, is when cells proliferate; the intermediate or mantle layer is important for cell migration; and the outer or marginal layer plays a role in connective system formation. Differentiation of a neuron is completed in the matrix layer, the marginal layer receives the axon.

Canalization/Retrogressive Differentiation in the Caudal Neural Tube; Development of Neurons in the Rostral Nervous System

The second phase of caudal neural tube formation in the embryo—from Carnegie stages 13 to 20, when the embryo is from 28 to 47 days old and has a CR length of approximately 4 to 30 mm—is called canalization. The third phase is known as retrogressive differentiation.[18] In these periods, production of neurons becomes very active both in the rostral and caudal neural tubes; however, it differs depending upon the site of the neural tube and the stage of development. The change of thickness of the matrix layer is called matrixphase[17] and is mainly responsible for the development of morphological appearances in each stage of neural tube formation (Fig. 2.2). In the spinal tube, differentiation of the neuron begins and ends

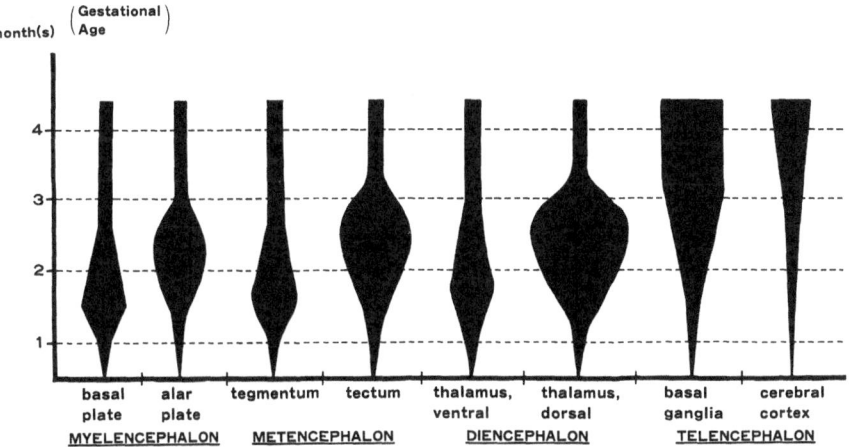

Figure 2.2. Thickness of the matrix (germinal) layer in the human embryo.

sooner in the ventral half than in the dorsal half. Neuronal development is delayed in the dorsal half, but the matrix layer becomes much thicker. These areas are separated by a horizontal line, the sulcus limitans. The ventral part (basal plate) develops neurons in the anterior funiculus and intermediate gray areas, and the dorsal part (alar plate) develops neurons in the posterior funiculus. Thus, somatic/visceral sensory or afferent areas develop from the dorsal half, and somatic/visceral motor or efferent areas are formed from the ventral half.

The development of neurons in the metencephalon is little different from that in the myelencephalon described above. First, the basal and alar plates are oriented to one another horizontally; the basal plate medial to the alar plate. The matrix layer in the basal plate in the metencephalon produces neurons of hypoglossal, vagal, and ambiguous nuclei, whereas that in the alar plate delivers spinal trigeminal and solitary nuclei. Second, the metencephalon has an extra center for neural differentiation, the rhombic lip, which is located next to the alar plate and produces the cerebellum and neurons of the olive and pons. Neurons of the cerebellum develop not only from its matrix layer but also from the secondary matrix layer, the so-called external granular layer. Purkinje and Golgi neurones are derived from the former, molecular and granular layers from the latter.

From the midbrain, the alar plate produces neurons of the superior and inferior colliculi, and the basal plate produces (one of) the reticular oculomotors and trochlear nuclei. The reticular formation of the brain stem develops mainly from the basal plate.

In the prosencephalon, the matrix layer of diencephalon develops various neurons of the epithalamus, thalamus, hypothalamus, and subthalamus. The ventral portion of the telencephalon becomes very active in the early stages, colliculus ganglionaris, and neurons of the striatum and insula develop from the matrix layer in this region. The dorsal portion of the telencephalon remains thin, but plays an important role in the formation of the neurons in the frontal, parietal, temporal, and occipital lobes.

Development of Neurons/Neural Tracts and Clinical Traumatology of the Immature Brain

When neural tube formation is completed, the neuroepithelial cells change to neuroblasts, which no longer perform the activity of DNA synthesis. The neuroblasts grow from the inside out, extending their axons and forming the mantle and marginal layers. The speed of axon growth in tissue culture is approximately 1 μm/min. The axon is guided in the direction of this growth by the neuroblast's specific control, which is called chemotaxis. Axon formation and myelination processes are completed over a long period during and after the embryonic stages.

The types of traumatic lesions characteristic of newborn or infants

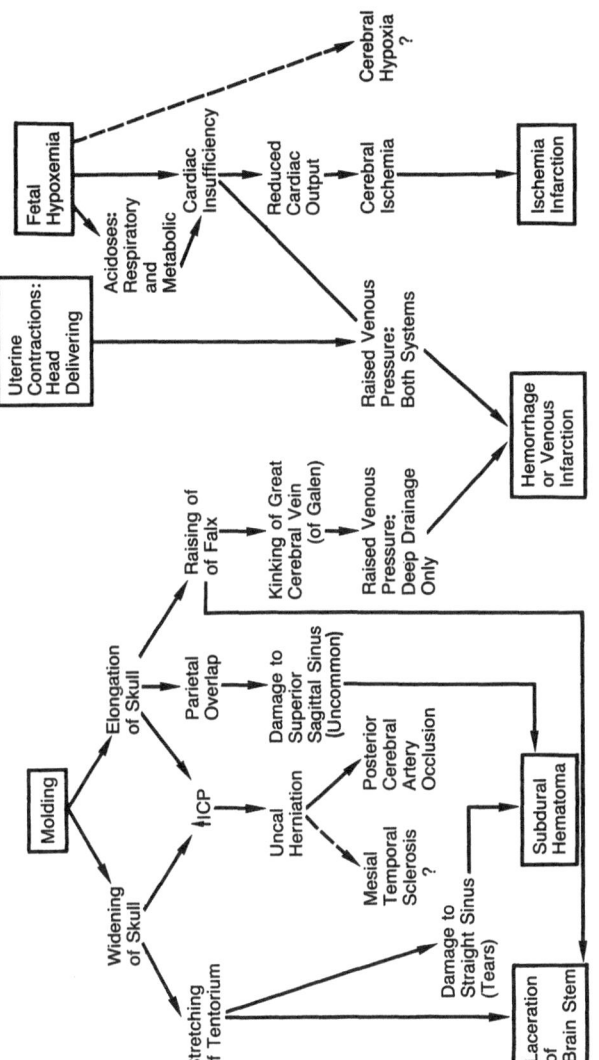

Figure 2.3. Probable pathogenetic mechanisms in birth injury. (Adapted from Reference 29.)

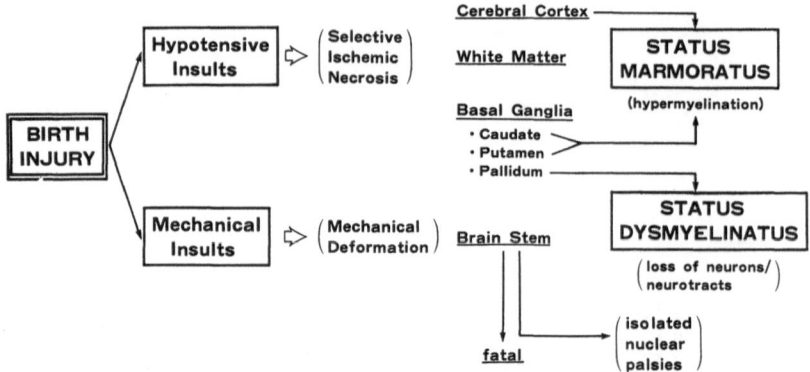

Figure 2.4. Effects of birth injury on neurons and neurotracts. (Derived from Reference 19.)

differ from those of adults in their distribution and pathogenesis. A typical example is birth injury, in which an immature brain with underdeveloped neurons and neural tracts receives injuries in unusual, pathogenetic mechanical modes resulting in a unique pathophysiologic status[19] (Fig. 2.3). The distribution of the lesion and neuronal changes are also characteristic in birth injuries. The injuries are generally divided into two major categories, hypotensive (hypoxic) and mechanical. The former causes selective ischemic necrosis of the brain as widely distributed lesions, if the neural structure is not completely destroyed. In those lesions, "status marmoratus" (hypermyelination) associated with gliosis and neuronal loss is seen, especially in the cerebral cortex, putamen, and caudate nuclei. Mechanical injury, in contrast, causes loss of myelinated fibers ("status dysmyelinatus") especially in the pallidum; this in turn causes neuronal loss and neural tract destruction. Mechanical injury to the brain stem is often fatal; if not, it may represent one cause of isolated nuclear palsies. Figure 2.4 is a summary derived from Lewis' explanation of birth injury.[19]

Development of the Subarachnoid Space and the Arachnoid Membrane

Shortly after closure, the neural tube is surrounded by a dense cell layer called "meninx primitiva." The primitive subarachnoid space develops within this "meninx primitiva" by gradual expansion of the intercellular space and decrease of its cellular component (Fig. 2.5). The subarachnoid space is essentially the opened connective tissue space, formed in late

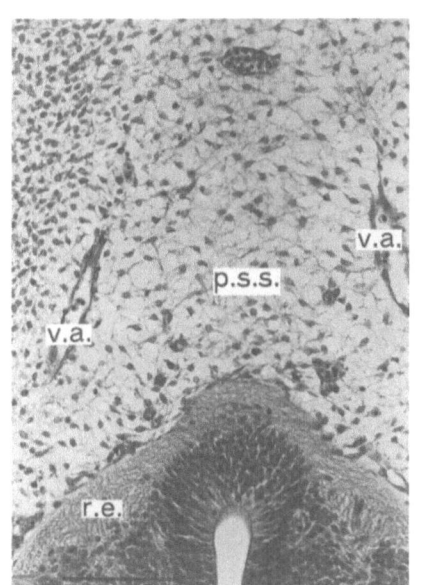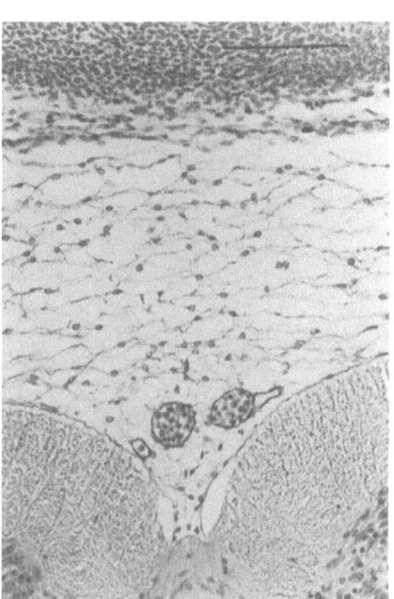

A   B

Figure 2.5. Development of the primitive subarachnoid space. **A.** Primitive sub-arachnoid space in the region ventral to the rhombencephalon of the embryo, Carnegie stage 14. Note the increase of the intracellular space of the meninx primitiva. The primitiva dura mater is not yet formed. **B.** Primitive subarachnoid space in the region ventral to the spinal cord of the embryo, Carnegie stage 21. The intercellular space is much widened. The primitive dura mater is going to be formed.   (pss = primitive subarachnoid space; re = rhombencephalon; va = vertebral artery)

embryonic life. It is different from the true space (i.e., the lumen in the neural tube) in which the lumen is created by closure of the neural plate and is covered by the epithelium.

Increase of the intercellular space (an early sign of the formation of the primitive subarachnoid space) is first observed in the region ventral to the mes- and rhombencephalon at Carnegie stage 14.[21] Further development of the primitive subarachnoid space is summarized in Figure 2.6. Formation of the primitive subarachnoid space seems to spread caudally from the ventral portion of the mes- and rhombencephalon to the spinal cord and cranially to the prosencephalon. It also tends to spread from the ventral to the dorsal portions of the neural tube. At Carnegie stages 18 to 20 some portion of the fourth ventricle roof becomes thin, forming the "area membranacea" superior and inferior of Weed.[28] An increase of the intercellular space is also observed in that area. At Carnegie stages 21 to 23, an increase of the intercellular space becomes evident in the whole

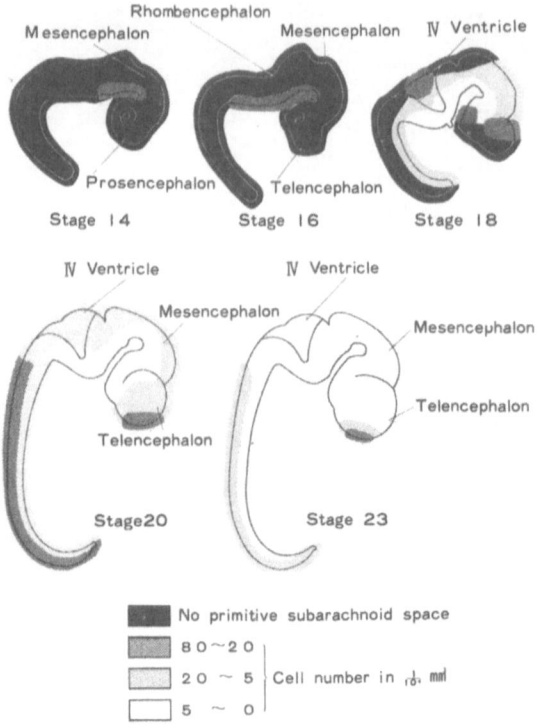

Figure 2.6. Further development of the primitive subarachnoid space.

neural tube.[21,28] At this stage, the developed embryonic subarachnoid space is covered by the primitive dura mater, not the arachnoid membrane, as the arachnoid membrane has not yet appeared. Some authors[25] term this primitive subarachnoid space the embryonic "subdural space" because the arachnoid membrane is not yet developed. This term is somewhat misleading, however, as the space is actually the precursor of the subarachnoid space and should not be confused with the subdural space of an adult.

The main factor contributing to the formation of the subarachnoid space is considered to be the CSF, which flows out from the fourth ventricle into the perineural "meninx primitiva." According to Weed's observation,[28] appearance of the choroid plexus is followed by leakage of CSF through the permeable areas of the rhombic roof ("area membranacea superior" and inferior), and the escaping fluid dissects open the intercellular space of the "meninx primitiva" to form the subarachnoid space. Cohen and Davis[9,10] studied the development of the CSF pathway in chickens, rats, rabbits, and guinea pigs. They supported Weed's observation. This universally accepted interpretation was challenged by the present authors.[21] Our observations, which are not in agreement with Weed's interpretation, are as follows:

1. Cavity formation in the "meninx primitiva" is seen before the appearance of the choroid plexus.
2. The cavity formation is first seen in the region ventral to the rhombencephalon, not in the region around the rhombic roof where CSF supposedly leaks from the ventricle.
3. Development of the primitive subarachnoid space has been observed in the abnormal embryo with dysraphism involving the rhombencephalon and the high cervical cord; in this embryo there was no connection between the ventricular system and the perineural primitive subarachnoid space (Fig. 2.7). This observation indicates that the primitive subarachnoid space can be formed without the escape of CSF from the fourth ventricle.

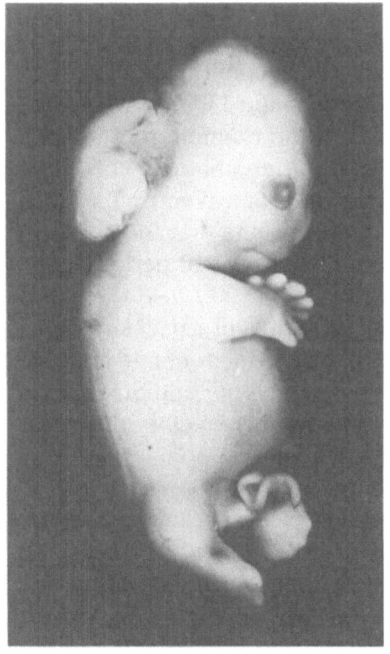
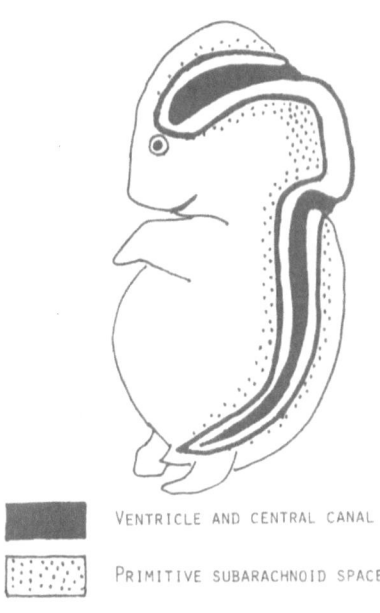

A

■ VENTRICLE AND CENTRAL CANAL

▒ PRIMITIVE SUBARACHNOID SPACE

B

Figure 2.7. An embryo with dysraphism involving the rhombencephalon and the high cervical cord in Carnegie stage 20 (**A**). In this embryo, there is no connection between the ventricular system and the perineural primitive subarachnoid space as shown schematically in **B**. Even in this embryo, the primitive subarachnoid space is well developed.

When Weed, Cohen, and Davis made their observations, CSF was believed to originate from the choroid plexus. However, recent studies have presented substantial evidence for the extrachoroidal formation of CSF.[5,12,20] Bering and Sato[5] reported as much as 50% of CSF may be extrachoroidal in origin. Our observation of human embryos may be interpreted as indicating that extrachoroidal formation of CSF occurs early in embryonic life.

At present, little information is available about when the communication between the ventricle and the newly developed primitive subarachnoid space is established. In 1917, Weed[28] reported that in a pig embryo with a CR length of 14 mm (that is, at approximately Carnegie stage 16 in human embryo development), dye injected into the lateral ventricle leaked out through the rhombic roof into the developing primitive subarachnoid space, and the dye flowed to cover the neural tube in the pig embryo of 18-mm CR length (at about Carnegie stage 18 in a human embryo). This communication is through the thin membrane of the rhombic roof ("area membranacea" inferior). Direct communication through the foramina of Magendie and Luschka is developed later in fetal life. According to Weed's observations,[28] the foramen of Magendie is not yet open in the human fetus of 52-mm CR length. However, Brocklehurst[7] observed it to be open in human embryos of 37 mm, 46 mm, 48 mm, 50 mm, and 54 mm in CR length. Its opening has been confirmed in the fetus of 124-mm CR length by Wilson[29] and of 125-mm and 130-mm CR length by Blake.[6] Significantly, histological studies of the rhombic roof suggest that its opening is due to an active process of differentiation, not to the bursting of the membrane induced by a buildup of intraventricular pressure.[7] From presently available information, it appears that the development of the foramen of Magendie begins in the early fetal period and is practically always evident in human adults.[3]

The development of the other outlets, the foramina of Luschka, seems more inconsistent. The foramina are described as evident in late fetal life (220-mm CR length by Brocklehurst[7] and by Rasmussen[22] and Strong[26] (in fetuses of 195-mm CR lengths). They may not be open even in the adult, however.[7] The size of the fetus when the foramina first opens has never been ascertained.

As stated earlier, the primitive subarachnoid space is well developed by the end of the embryonic stage and is covered only by the dura mater; the arachnoid has not yet appeared. The primitive dura mater is formed by gradual concentration of the cells of the "meninx primitiva" along their peripheral margin, and the intercellular space increases to form the primitive subarachnoid space in more central regions. The dura mater is almost fully developed around the neural tube by the end of the embryonal stage. The arachnoid is the last of the meninges to develop, and its development has not been fully ascertained. The primitive subarachnoid space develops into the subarachnoid space of the adult only after the arachnoid is separated from the dura mater. According to Sensenig,[25] the development of the arachnoid begins in the fetus of about 80-mm CR length and is almost complete when the fetus has reached a 120-mm CR length. However, at this stage the arachnoid seems closely attached to the dura mater, and the subdural space appears not to be present.

The development of the subdural space is significant for the pediatric clinician in conjunction with subdural hematoma, but it has not been well studied. Sensenig[25] observed the "spinal" subdural space in a restricted area in fetuses of 180 and 245 mm in CR lengths. More detailed observations on this space are offered by Lemire (see Table 2.1), but the development of the cranial subdural space remains to be studied.

The source of CSF absorption has been generally attributed to arachnoid granulations.[13,15] However, in embryos, the arachnoid membrane has not emerged, and the arachnoid villi (protruding into the sinus) have not developed. Therefore, CSF absorption must be carried out through a route other than arachnoid granulations, at least until the midfetal period when the arachnoid villi appear. Turner[27] reported that the arachnoid villi were present in a fetus with a CR length of 80 mm. However, the present authors did not find the arachnoid villi even in a fetus of 100-mm CR length in which the saggital sinus was serially sectioned and microscopically studied. Arachnoid granulations are not visible to the naked eye until 3 to 6 months after birth.[8,14,27] Full development of arachnoid granulations occurs only in late childhood to adulthood.[4,13,14] Therefore, the role of arachnoid granulations in CSF absorption should not be considered as important in the fetus and infant as in the adult. Gilles and Davidson[13] and Gutierrez et al.[15] reported cases with congenital agenesis of the

Table 2.1. Ages of fetuses showing separation of arachnoid from dura mater.

CR length (mm)	Level of the spinal cord		
	Cervical	Thoracic	Lumbar
180	Not separated	Not separated	
200	Separating in several places	Separating in several places	Complete separation
225	Separating in several places	Attached at one point	Separating in several places
280	Complete separation	Complete separation	Complete separation
290	Complete separation	Separating in several places	Separating in several places
330	Complete separation	Complete separation	Complete separation

villi causing congenital hydrocephalus. Because the arachnoid villi are so poorly developed in infants, the relationship of hydrocephalus to the absence of the arachnoid villi needs re-evaluation.

References

1. Alexander L: Die Anatomic der Seitentaxhen der vierten Hirnkammer. Z Anat 1931;95:531–707.
2. Bailey P, Cushing H: Tumors of the Glioma Group. Philadelphia, JB Lippincott Co., 1926.
3. Barr ML: Observations on the foramen of Magendic in a series of human brain. Anat Rec 1948;71:281–289.
4. Basmajcian JV: The depression for the arachnoid granulations as a criterion of age. Anat Rec 1952;112:843–846.
5. Bering EA Jr, Sato O: Hydrocephalus: Changes in formation and absorption of cerebrospinal fluid within the cerebral ventricles. J Neurosurg 1963;20:1050–1063.
6. Blake JA: The roof and lateral recesses of the fourth ventricle, considered morphologically and embryologically. J Comp Neural 1900;10:79–108.
7. Brocklehurst G: The development of the human cerebrospinal fluid pathway with particular reference to the roof of the fourth ventricle. J Anat 1969;105:467–475.
8. Clak LG: On the Pacchionian bodies. J Anat 1928;55:40–48.
9. Cohen H, Davis S: The development of the cerebrospinal fluid spaces and choroid plexus in the chick. J Anat 1937;72:23–53.
10. Cohen H, Davis S: The morphology and permeability of the roof of the fourth ventricle in some mammalian embryos. J Anat 1938;72:430–458.
11. Cooper ERA: Arachnoid granulations in man. Acta Anat 1958;34:187–200.
12. Curl FD, Pollay M: Transport of water and electrolytes between brain and ventricular fluid in the rabbit. Esp Neural 1968;20:558–574.
13. Gilles FH, Davidson RI: Communicating hydrocephalus associated with deficient dysplastic parasaggital arachnoid granulations. J Neurosurg 1971;35:421–426.
14. Grassman CB, and Potts DG: Arachnoid granulations, radiology and anatomy. Radiology 1974;113:95–100.
15. Gutierrez Y, Friede RL, Kaliney WJ: Agenesis of arachnoid granulations and its relationship to communicating hydrocephalus. J Neurosurg 1975;43:553–558.
16. His W: Die Neuroblosten und deren Entstehung im embryonalen Mark. Arch F Anat U Phyiol 1889;1889:249–300.
17. Kahle W: Studien über die Matrixphasen und die örtlichen Reifungsunterschiede im embryonalen menschlichen. Gehirn Dtsch Z Nervenheilk 1951;166:273.
18. Lemire RJ, Loeser JD, Leech RW, Alvord EC Jr: Normal and Abnormal Development of the Human Nervous System. New York, Harper & Row, 1975.
19. Lewis AJ: Mechanisms of Neurological Disease. Boston, Little Brown & Co, 1976.

20. Milhorat TH: *Hydrocephalus and the Cerebrospinal Fluid.* Baltimore, The Williams & Wilkins Co, 1972.
21. Osaka K, Handa H, Matsumoto S, Yasuda M: Development of the cerebrospinal fluid pathway in the normal and abnormal human embryos. *Child's brain* 1980;6:26–38.
22. Rasmussen AT: Additional evidence favoring the normal existence of the lateral apertures of the fourth ventricle in man. *Anat Rec* 1926;33:179–182.
23. Rogers L, West CM: The foramen of Magendie *J Anat* 1931;65:457–467.
24. Sauer FC: Mitosis in neural tube. *J Comp Neural* 1935;62:377.
25. Sensenig EC: The early development of the meninges of the spinal cord in human embryos. *Carnegie Inst Contr Embryol* 1951;34:147–157.
26. Strong RM, Green LD, Oliverio JV: The lateral aperature of the fourth ventricle in man *Anat Rec* 1926;32:323 (abstract).
27. Turner L: The structure of arachnoid granulations with observations on their physiological and pathological significance. *Ann R Coll Surg* 1961;29:237–264.
28. Weed LH: The development of the cerebrospinal spaces in the pig and in man. *Carnegie Inst Contr Embryol* 1917;5:1–116.
29. Wilson JT: On the nature and mode of origin of the foramen of Magendie. *J Anat* 1937;71:423–426.

CHAPTER 3

The Cerebrospinal Fluid Pathways: Structure and Development

David G. McLone

Introduction

Ancient anatomists identified and dissected two of the three meningeal coverings of the brain. Breasted[16] found the first known reference to them in *The Edwin Smith Surgical Papyrus,* a manuscript written in 1700 BC and regarded as a copy of a manuscript composed in 3000 BC. Hippocrates knew of thin membranes separating the two cerebral hemispheres, and Aristotle identified an inner membrane with blood vessels and an outer membrane closely applied to bone.[89] Galen[44] recognized a space between the pachy and lepto-meningeal layers and noted that the cranial dura mater consisted of an inner and outer portion.[140] Galen also established the early nomenclature when he restricted the term "meninx" to the coverings of the brain; previously, it had referred to the linings of all body cavities. Stephen of Antioch introduced the terms "dura mater" and "pia mater" in his translation of Galen; "mater," from the Latin, means mother in the sense of "mother of pearl."[89] Ancient anatomists thought that the pia mater supplied nourishment to the brain and protected the brain from the harsh dura mater. Vesalius[127] described the meninges essentially as Galen had but failed to identify two layers in the dura mater. In 1666 Blasius finally identified the third membrane, the arachnoid.[88]

Species variations in the meninges have evoked controversy. The study of the meninges of avian and mammalian species led to two separate conclusions about the number of layers of meninges. One group, including Cohen and Davis,[26,27] Cuvier,[30] Owen,[97] Streeter,[121,122] and Hansen-Pruss,[49] described three layers. A second group, including Sterzi,[118,119] Farrar,[35] Kappers,[63] and Kappers et al.,[64] found only two layers. The confusion probably occurred because the meninges of these animals were studied with gross and light microscopic techniques and with a variety of methods of fixation. All investigators now agree with the concept of three layers—dura mater, arachnoid, and pia mater—in higher mammals.

There are problems, however, in applying a three-layered classification to all animals. For instance, the cranial dura mater has two distinct layers.

Also, in lower mammals the transition from dura to arachnoid is gradual, with no distinct line of demarcation; and both pia and arachnoid appear to be the same cell type, with one cell often participating in both layers. Also, in primates the spinal pia mater must be subdivided further into a pial layer and an epipial layer.

The modern anatomical work most often cited as the basis of our present knowledge is the detailed study by Key and Retzius[66] in the 1800's. They first identified the continuity between the spinal and cerebral SAS.[77] Weed,[129-136] in the early 1900's, added a physiological and developmental study. Millen and Woollam[87-91] and Clark[25] contributed a detailed macro- and microscopic description of the adult human meninges. At present, most anatomists describe the meninges essentially as Woollam and Millen[144] did. The innermost pia is seen as a thin layer of cells enveloping the central nervous tissue. The epipial tissue is seen as a more superficial layer of pial cells and blood vessels (Fig. 3.1). The cerebral pial layer contains collagen, which increases in amount in higher mammals[14,64] (i.e., mouse, rat, monkey, and man); blood vessels ensheathed with pial cells[143,144]; and an occasional macrophage.[93,94] Thin trabeculae, which often contain collagen, cross the SAS to reach the pial network. His[57,58] and Held[55] described spaces associated with SAS which are now considered artifacts of fixation. A second space, the Virchow–Robin spaces, is lined with leptomeninges and communicates with the SAS. They pass for a

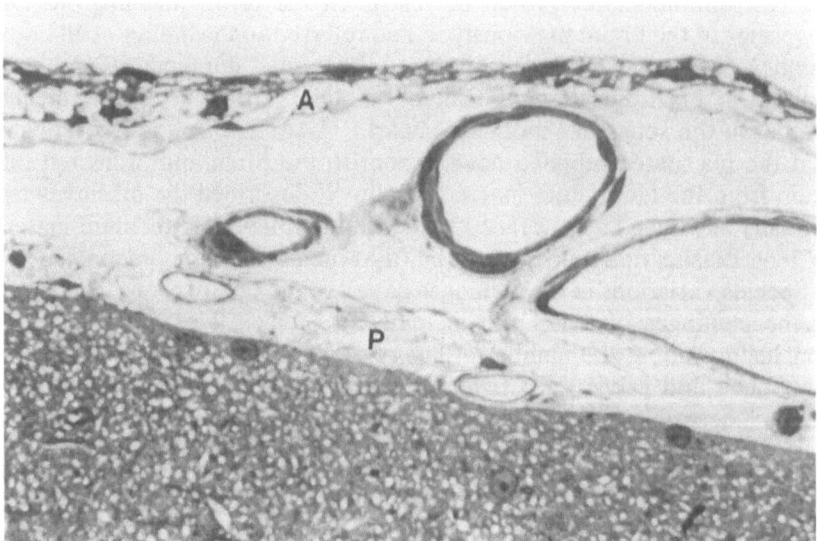

Figure 3.1. A light micrograph of the mature subarachnoid space shows the arachnoid (A), vessels ensheathed by pia-arachnoid processes, and pial surface (P) adjacent to the cerebral cortex.

short distance into the cerebral tissue surrounding the large vessels before ending blindly.[11,114]

The arachnoid adjacent to the dura is well described as overlapping tiers of cells with few organelles and a relatively clear cytoplasm in contrast to the cells of the dura.* The cytoplasm has been described as watery or hydrated. It contains a prominent Golgi complex, small clusters of rough endoplasmic reticulum, scattered ribosomal rosettes, and numerous pinocytotic and coated vesicles.[89] In the human arachnoid, desmosomal junctions are found between the cells; in rodents, zonula adherens[36,68] is more common.[14] The cells of the pia seem essentially the same as those of the arachnoid except for long, thin processes tending to run parallel to the cortical surface. Collagen fibrils, reported to have 550 nm period[92] and elastic fibers, both resting on a basal lamina, are scattered between the pia and limiting glial cells of the central nervous system. Gaps or fenestrae exist in the pial layer, where (CSF) bathes the cerebral cortex.[103]

The cerebral dura mater consists of two portions: an outer periosteal layer forming the periosteum of the inner table of the skull, and an inner fibrous or meningeal portion, which corresponds to the entire dura of the spinal cord. The periosteum consists of a lamination of fibroblasts oriented parallel to the skull,[5] between which are layers of collagen fibers and scattered elastic fibers. The dura immediately adjacent to the inner table of the skull is made up of plump osteoblasts and osteoclasts with particulate calcium coating the adjacent collagen fibers.[92] The inner border of the dura is formed by elongated squamous fibroblasts adjacent to the arachnoid cells. Between the dura mater and the arachnoid a potential space, the "subdural space," exists.[74,99,100] A dense material has been shown to occupy this space.[99] The innervation of the cranial dura is from branches of the trigeminal, upper cervical, and sympathetic fibers from the plexus around the meningeal arteries.

The origin of embryonic meninges has been a subject of debate for many years. Bischoff[10] thought that the neural tube, along with forming gray and white matter, formed the fibrous dura, the serous arachnoid tissue, and the vascular tissue of the pia. Bischoff's view was modified by Remak,[106] who regarded the pia and the arachnoid as neural derivatives and the dura as a derivative of the skeletal layer. Reichert[105] further modified this by stating that the arachnoid consists of two layers, a visceral layer arising with the neural tube pia, and a parietal layer associated with, and of the same skeletal-layer origin as, the dura.

In 1861, Kollman[71] claimed that the meninges developed from a single Wharton's jelly-like layer between the developing skull and neural tube. This claim was disputed by Kolliker[70] and His,[57] who argued that the meninges developed from somites. The mesodermal origin of the dura and

---

* References 1–6, 46, 99, 100, 115, 124, 128, 134.

the arachnoid was postulated in 1876.[56] Soon afterwards it was fairly well established.*

The controversy was reopened in the 1920's by Harvey and his co-workers.[50–52,73,77] Studying regeneration after selective injury to dura- or pia-arachnoid cells, they found that dura mater regenerated without arachnoid adhesions but pia-arachnoid cells regenerated with adhesions with the dura, thereby suggesting a different embryonic origin. To support their deduction, Harvey et al. made transplants of neural tube tissue from amphibian and avian embryos, one having neural crest cells and the other without them. They also made heterotransplants of Nile blue, sulfate-labeled neural crest cells. These investigators found that in the absence of neural crest cells, only the dura developed. Labeled heterotransplanted crest cells were located only in the primitive pia-arachnoid layer. Their conclusion was that the pia-arachnoid is of neural crest origin and the dura derives from mesoderm. Flexner[40] and later Spofford[117] and others concluded that the majority of the meninges were probably of mesodermal origin, with only a small contribution from the neural crest.[115] The mesodermal origin of all three meningeal layers in the spinal cord was sustained by Hochstetter[59] and Ask.[7]

More recent studies have not lessened the confusion. Pease and Schultz[99] found the ultrastructure of leptomeningeal cells over the rat cerebral cortex to be quite different from that of dural cells—in fact unique—and favored a neural crest origin of the leptomeninges. They were supported by the histology and data of Millen and Woollam.[88] Johnston[62] and Weston[139] used radioautographic techniques to study the migration and fate of cranial neural crest cells in chick embryos. They found that these cells migrated over the anterior and ventral surface of the diencephalon and telencephalon. Johnston[62] showed that these areas of the brain are invested with mesenchyme of mixed origin but mostly derived from neural crest. This suggested that the source of the mesenchyme may be irrelevant, as the developing neural tissue probably induces meningeal formation in the surrounding mesenchyme regardless of its source.

Although the specific embryonic origin of each layer of the meninges remains in doubt, their development has been extensively studied.† Redford[104] first pointed out the sequential development of the mesenchyme around the developing nervous system. He showed that the thinning out of the mesenchyme around the developing nervous system is not haphazard but, in fact, organized in a definite pattern that changes with brain development. Cushing[29] showed that these changes proceded from

* References 35, 45, 47, 61, 112, 117–120, 131.
† References 29, 50–52, 55, 56, 68, 69, 104, 113, 123.

the spinal column to the basicranium and then over the convexity of the cerebral hemispheres. The mesenchyme, which is divided into two layers (the outer forming the dura and the inner a "secondary meninx"), formed the arachnoid and pia. In chicks, a perimedullary condensation at about the 11th to 12th day of incubation was found; it was rapidly followed by the development of an SAS.

Sensenig[115] described the development of the spinal meninges and found that vascularization of the neural tube begins in an 8-mm human embryo with the formation of endothelial channels adjacent to it. In the embryo of 8- to 15-mm crown-rump (CR) length, he found primitive meninges were well defined; by 20-mm CR length the ventral dura was evident. The pia remains one cell thick with a vascular plexus of variable thickness on the outer surface. Kilika[68] studied the submicroscopic developmental anatomy of the human meninges and found the embryonic meninges well developed and essentially in their adult configuration by the 65-mm stage.

Weed[131] described two openings in the rhombencephalic roof of the pig. The "area membranacea" superior opens first and then closes. It is followed by an opening in the "area membranacea" inferior, which persists as a foramen of the fourth ventricle. Because the choroid plexus develops at the same embryonic stages,[63] Weed felt that the CSF passed through these foramina, dissecting open the SAS. Keegan,[65] and Cohen and Davis[26,27] found that the sequence of events varied with species. In fact, in some animals the SAS develops prior to the choroid plexus.[20,81] McLone and Bondareff[81] observed the development of the SAS from a pre-existing space, the mesenchymal extracellular space, and sustained that this was independent of the CSF circulation. Osaka and Oi (Chapter 2) sustain that the development of the rhombencephalic foramina is an active process independent of CSF secretion.

After the studies of Weed,[129–136] Keegan,[65] Cohen and Davis,[26,27] and Sensenig[115] concerning the development of the SAS, no detailed sequential investigation of mammalian meninges was undertaken (most notably at the submicroscopic level) until 1975,[2,81] when the ultrastructural transformations resulting in a functional subarachnoid space were studied. Low and coworkers[2,76,80,107] have employed light, electron, and scanning-electron microscopes to study the SAS. Studies by Bondareff et al[12,13,14] of the comparative submicroscopic anatomy of the mature SAS in mice, cats, monkeys, and man showed striking similarities in the ultrastructure and distribution of this space.

The structure of the arachnoid villi and granulations, the final pathway from the subarachnoid space to venous blood,[67] consists of a two-cell layer: one arachnoid and one endothelial cell separated by a basal lamina.[102,116] The endothelium contains many vesicles thought to represent the transmission of CSF to the venous system (Fig. 3.2).

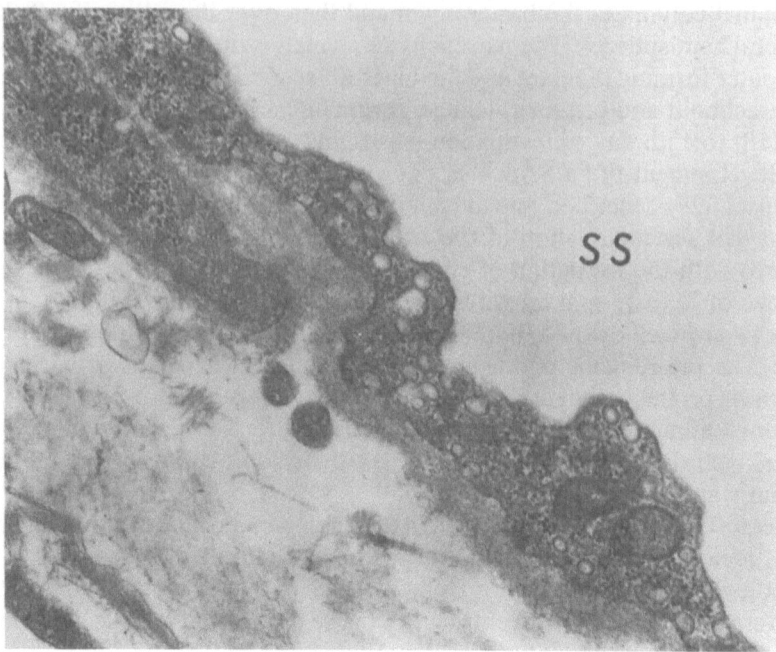

Figure 3.2. An electron micrograph demonstrates the numerous vesicles in the venous endothelium of the sagittal sinus (SS).

Development of the Subarachnoid Space

Following closure of the neural tube, a reticulum of mesenchymal cells is interposed between the ectoderm and the developing nervous system. The extracellular space of this mesenchyme is large (Fig. 3.3) and contains a ground substance conducive to rapid diffusion to and from the neuroepithelium. This pre-existing large space is ultimately transformed into a functional SAS. Growth of the neural mass and its metabolic needs soon exceed the capacity of diffusion alone, and vascular proliferation ensues in the surrounding mesenchyme.

Vessels penetrate the neural surface as vascularization of the nervous system begins. From the outset of vascularization the endothelium (continuous and closed by a tight junction) has most of the characteristics of mature central nervous system (CNS).

As vascularization proceeds, the primitive pia-arachnoid cells above the "vascular tunic" form a compact stratified layer (Fig. 3.4) delineating the outer limit of the subarachnoid space. The cells at the outer margins of this compact layer undergo rapid conversion to connective tissue-type cells. The amount of rough endoplasmic reticulum is markedly increased. From this outer layer the dura mater and skull are formed.

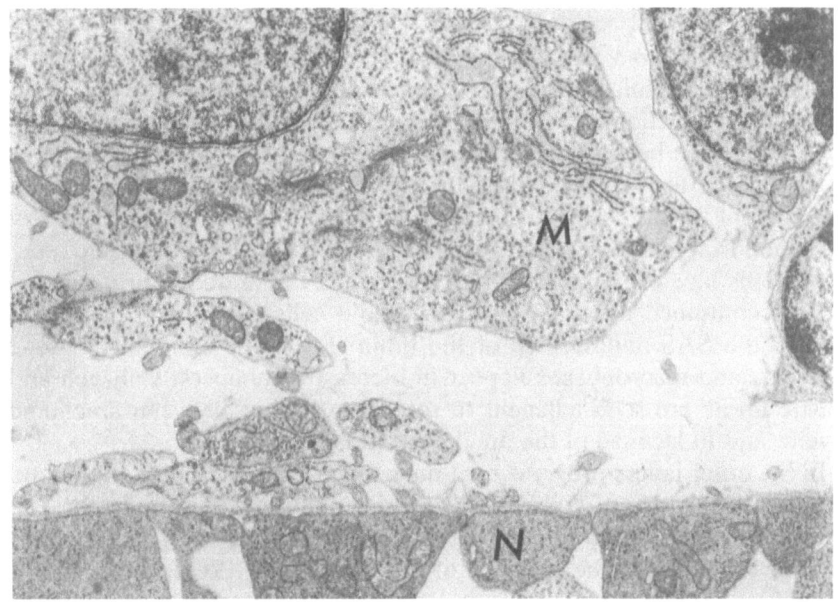

Figure 3.3. An electron micrograph shows the surface of the neural ectoderm (N) adjacent to the large extracellular space of the surrounding mesenchyme (M).

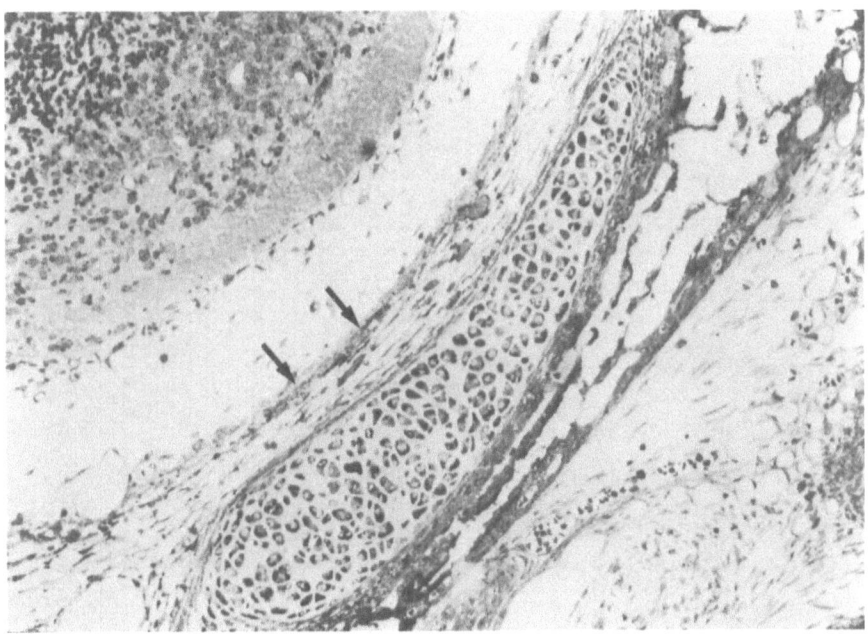

Figure 3.4. A light micrograph of the basal subarachnoid space of a fetal animal. The outer limit of the subarachnoid space has been delineated by arrows. The cartilaginous skull has also begun to form.

Maturation of the pia-arachnoid involves further lateral growth and lamination of cellular processes. Complex interdigitations of processes and cellular junctions wash the circulating CSF off the surrounding tissues. Junctions between pia-arachnoid cells are much more common as one proceeds up the phylogenetic scale. The pia-arachnoid cells' organelle content undergoes little change with maturation. They contain a few mitochondria, ribosomes, and a small amount of rough endoplasmic reticulum. This lace of organelles gives the cells a "hydrated" appearance.

With continued maturation pia-arachnoid cells ensheath the vasculature of the SAS and surface of the brain (Fig. 3.5). Connective tissue elements and macrophages appear in increasing numbers. Collagen and elastic fibrils are seen adjacent to the brain surface between arachnoid layers, and in lacunae in the arachnoid surface.

In the outer layers progress continues toward a mature dura mater and skull. Dense layers of collagen are formed. Fibrils within one layer run parallel, and in each layer the course of the fibrils is at an angle to adjacent layers. This adds to the integrity of this dural layer. Vessels are rare in this layer, but bundles of axons are seen growing between layers of collagen. The outermost cells secrete collagen in what appear to be random bundles that become calcifiable. The deposition of calcium crystals marks the beginning of membranous skull formation.

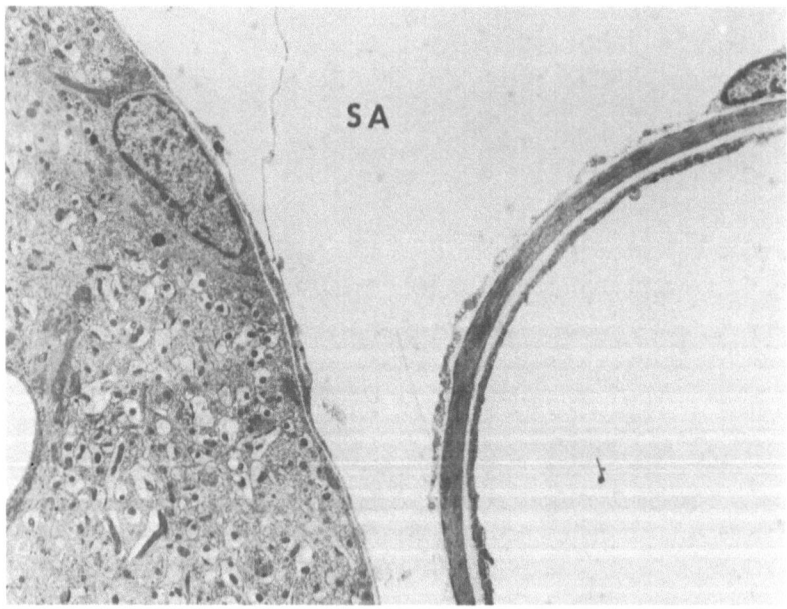

Figure 3.5. An electron micrograph shows the delicate pia-arachnoid processes that envelop the surface of the brain and blood vessels. The subarachnoid space is denoted by SA.

By birth the development of the SAS is near completion. Postnatally the changes are mostly in the size of structures and the amount of connective tissue.

The pia-arachnoid arises from a primary mesenchyme of epiblastic origin, forms junctional complexes, stratifies, and lines a fluid space. All this is typical of epithelium. It arises from the same mesenchyme that forms muscle; can secrete ground substance, collagen, and microfilaments (or their precursors); and has phagocytic capabilities. Yet it appears structurally similar to other subepithelial loose connective tissue. The ground substance of this primary mesenchyme initially appears to be in equilibrium with tissue fluid, presumably of vascular origin, and typical of loose connective tissue. Tissue fluid is replaced by CSF, during the course of normal development, which results in a total restructuring of an extracellular connective tissue compartment and the formation of the subarachnoid space. The macromolecular changes in the extracellular connective tissue compartment which underlie this truly remarkable structural transformation are not known.

Development of the Limiting Glial Membrane

An interface between the subarachnoid CSF and the cortical molecular layer is formed by the cells that postnatally cover the convexity of the vertebrate brain. These cells appear to be functionally unique and comprise a membrane-like structure, the outer-limiting glial membrane described in 1890 by Weigert.[137] They have the general appearance of typical astrocytes with long processes that radiate horizontally over the surface and vertically down into the substance of the brain.* The ultrastructure of these astrocyte-like cells has been described, and differences between them and the astrocytes typically found in cerebral cortical neuropile have been noted.[32,33,61,93,103]

These limiting glial astrocytes appear to derive from glioblasts during early neural tube development.[37] The cytoplasmic processes, which extend to both the marginal and ependymal surfaces, are contiguous laterally and provide a glial envelope for the neural tube.[21,54] Later, during the first few days of postnatal life, the extracellular compartment of the superficial cerebral cortical neuropile increases in volume,[82] resulting in what Haug[54] has described as "loosening." The volume of this enlarged extracellular space then gradually diminishes during the second 2 weeks of postnatal life[15] as the numbers of astrocytic and neuronal cell processes of the neuropile increase and a superficial limiting glial layer is reconstituted. At this time, the glial interface between the SAS and the molecular-layer is established.

---

* References 12, 127, 36–39, 55, 61, 96, 101.

With the outpouching of the telencephalic hemispheres and the concomitant increase in neuroepithelial mass, the metabolic demands of the developing nervous system exceed the ability of the mesenchyme to supply them. As Folkman et al.[41] have shown in central nervous system neoplasms, once a critical cell mass is achieved, vasogenesis must occur or growth ceases. They have isolated a nucleoprotein, the "vasogenic factor," from the developing neoplasm that induces vasogenesis in surrounding tissues. It has also been shown that many of the characteristics of neoplasia result from the derepression of embryonic genetic expression.[43] A similar angiogenic factor has been isolated in fetal mice. It may well be the metabolic needs of the neuropeithelium that initiate the first period of meningeal development, the period of vascularization.

The alterations in organelle content and tissue morphology are consistent with this sequence of events. Neural epithelial cells contain many mitochondria and an abundance of polysomes, which typify cells in active protein synthesis. Immediately adjacent to the basal lamina is a layer of collagen fibrils. As these fibrils are not found elsewhere, they presumably originate from the underlying neuroepithelium. Recent evidence indicates that the superficial glial epithelium of the spinal cord can synthesize collagen and that collagen is essential to many inductive processes.[28] It seems reasonable, then, to suggest that the substrate is present and that a vasogenic factor, perhaps similar to that of Folkman et al.,[41] may be the inducing agent resulting in the development of vessels adjacent to the telencephalon of the mouse beginning at about the tenth day of fetal life.

From the outset, the vascular endothelium of the blood vessels in the central nervous system has intercellular junctions that appear tight, and there are no fenestra in the vascular wall.

The neuroepithelial-vascular interaction first entails the induction of vessels by the neuroepithelium, followed by penetration of the neural tissue by the vascular elements. Because these newly formed vessels are incompletely invested by glia and remain so during most of fetal life, a direct contact results between the neural extracellular space and the vascular endothelium. The former, which might represent a pathway for exchange between primitive neural tissue and the circulatory system prior to establishing a functional glioepithelium and subarachnoid circulation, may also explain the differences between fetal and mature animal's "blood-brain barrier" function.[17-19] This pathway has been shown to be functional in hydrocephalus,[82] which may simply represent utilization of a fetal mechanism under pathological conditions.

During the early postnatal period, the limiting neural epithelial structure begins to change rapidly. Polysomes increase in number; this suggests the onset of another period of rapid protein synthesis, and within the first week of postnatal life, multilaminar membranes can be found within the cytoplasm of these cells. Haug[53,54] first reported these multilaminar membranes in the cytoplasm of postnatal limiting glial epithelial cells of cats. He postulated that they might be utilized in the rapid lateral extension of the limiting glial cells. The plausibility of this is supported by Caley and Maxwell,[23,24] who found that the period of the most rapid growth in cerebral cortical volume and cerebral circumference in rats was from the second to the ninth postnatal days. In that time these multilaminar membranes are continuous within a cell and with the cell's outer membrane. Such studies suggest that these membranes may be stored, as are the cytoplasmic membranes of urinary bladder transitional epithelium. With the rapid increase in cerebral circumference they are drawn over the surface.

Two types of membrane arrays may be seen during the development of glia limitans. One has already been mentioned, the other occurs during early fetal development and is possibly related to glycogen metabolism.[79]

It is possible that the limiting glia acts as a source of energy for the developing neuronal elements and anticipates the rapid cerebral cortical expansion. This possibility is indicated by the accumulation of membranes prior to expansion, coupled with the fact that these glial cells send slender processes deep into the underlying neuropile and subtend a large extracellular space. This decrease with the maturation of neuronal elements, and in turn lends support to Cajal's[21,22] original contention that the limiting epithelium is the lattice upon which the underlying neuronal network forms. However, not all limiting glial epithelial cells participate in this process. Many of the cells retain their fetal appearance and have few polysomes and little rough endoplasmic reticulum, giving them a less dense appearance. Possibly, these cells retain a greater potentiality and are called into play for reparative processes such as gliosis or scar formation in later life.

One of the most prominent organelles of the limiting glia are the large mitochondria. Although many of these are very large, some as much as 2 μm in diameter, most of them are similar in size to the mitochondria of fetal neuroepithelial cells. Their size is accentuated by the fact that mature neuronal mitochondria in the adjacent neuropile are much smaller. Why these large mitochondria persist in large numbers in the limiting glial epithelium is not known.

Gap junctions between cells, typical of adult limiting glia, can occasionally be identified in the early postnatal period but become numerous during the second and third weeks of postnatal life. The presence of gap junctions between limiting glial cells implies continuity between the SAS and the extracellular space of the superficial neuropile. As the glial cells are electrically coupled,[75] a means of communication exists across this layer as well as within it. Processes from these limiting glial cells extend into the underlying molecular layer, where they are spatially associated with neuronal elements, including the synapses. They may participate in electrophysiologic events by affecting the potassium ion concentration of the extracellular fluid in the vicinity of neuronal elements. This enables neurons to fire repetitively without the extracellular accumulation of K+ ions. Possibly the limiting glia modulates superficial cortical events by responding to neuronal activity in the depths and at the cerebral surface. It could also respond to ion fluctuations in circulating CSF.

There are three postnatal periods, each lasting about 7 days. The first is a period of "loosening" when glial perikarya withdraw from the surface and the extracellular space increases; the second, a period of "elongation," is characterized by the spread of glial processes laterally; the third is a period of "maturation."

Changes in the Brain Extracellular Space

In humans and laboratory animals the absence of communication between the ventricular system and the subarachnoid space may result in death from increased intracranial pressure.[9,29,48,138] In spite of continuing production of CSF, the CNS may sometimes adapt,[78] suggesting an alternate or additional pathway for CSF circulation or absorption[8,108,111,142] (other than that between the ventricular system, subarachnoid space, and arachnoid villi), especially during the early phases of hydrocephalus. Another possibility is a diminution in CSF production. The contrary, free communication between the ventricles and the subarachnoid spaces, does not assure adequate CSF circulation and absorption.*

Fixation artifact resulted in low estimates of volume of the brain extracellular space,[95,98] but newer methods reflect changes in this volume.[125,126,141] Changes in volume of the brain extracellular space have been demonstrated in hydrocephalic animals.[72] In addition, the selective accumulation of extracellular fluid in the white matter, expanding the extracellular space, has been demonstrated at the electron microscopic level in the brain edema of congenital hydrocephalus.[83]

Earlier studies indicated that the extracellular space increases in the hydrocephalic mouse,[83] thereby suggesting that it may function as an alternate pathway for CSF circulation and absorption.[86]

Intraventricular pressure elevations typical of hydrocephalus have been reported by some authors to have no effect on halting CSF production but to be inversely related to it by others.[109,110] Although the SAS or ventricular system may not be evident, some CSF absorption continues, and intracranial volumes and pressures compatible with life are temporarily maintained. The effect of increased CSF volume and pressure on normal cellular function, nerve conduction, and so forth is not yet completely understood.

---

* References 31, 60, 84, 85, 129.

References

1. Alksne JF, Lovings ET: Functional ultrastructure of the arachnoid villus. *Archs Neurol* 1972;27:371–377.
2. Allen DJ, Low FN: SEM of subarachnoid space of dogs. *J Comp Neurol* 1975;161:515–539.
3. Anderson DR: Ultrastructure of meningeal sheaths. *Archs Ophthal* 1969;82:659–674.
4. Anderson DR, Hoyt WF: Ultrastructure of intraorbital portion of human and monkey optic nerve. *Archs Ophthal* 1969;82:506–530.
5. Andres KH: Uber die Feinstruktur der Arachnoidea und Dura mater von Mammalia. *Z Zellforsch Mikrosk Anat* 1967;79:272–295.
6. Andres KH: Zlur Feinstruktur der Arachnoidalzotten bei Mammalia. *Z Zellforsch Mikrosk Anat* 1967;82:92–100.
7. Ask O: Studien uber die embryologische Entwicklung des menschlichen Ruckgrats und seines Inhaltes unter normalen Verhaltnissen und bei gewissen Formen von Spina Bifida. *Uppsala Lakfor Forh* 1941;46:243–348.
8. Bering EA Jr, Sato O: Hydrocephalus: changes in formation and absorption of cerebrospinal fluid within the cerebral ventricles. *J Neurosurg* 1963;20:1050–1063.
9. Berry RJ: The inheritance and pathogenesis of hydrocephalus-3 in the mouse. *J Path Bact* 1961;81:157.
10. Bischoff TLW: Entwicklungsgeschichte der Saugethiere und des Menschen. Leipzig, Vieweg, 1842.
11. Bohme G: Die marginale Glia des Cortex cerebri der Ratte. *Z Zellforsch Mikrosk Anat* 1966;70:269–278.
12. Bondareff W, McLone DG, Myers R: The external glial limiting membrane in Macaca: ulatrastructure of a laminated glioepithelium. *Am J Anat* 1973;136:277–296.
13. Bondareff W, McLone DG, and Myers R: Morphogenesis of astroglial scars resulting from perinatal asphyxia. *Anat Rec* 1972;172:273.
14. Bondareff W, McLone DG, Decker SJ: Ultrastructure of glioepithelia in the brains of mice and men. *Anat Rec* 1973;1975:487.
15. Bondareff W, Pysh JJ: Distribution of ECS during postnatal maturation of rat cerebral cortex. *Anat Rec* 1968;1960:773–780.
16. Breasted JH: The Edwin Smith Surgical Papyrus, Chicago, The University of Chicago Press, 1930, vol. 1 and 2.
17. Brightman, MW, Reese TS: Junctions between intimately opposed cell membranes in the vertebrate brain. *J Cell Biol* 1969;40:648.
18. Brightman MW: The distribution within the brain of ferritin injected into cerebrospinal fluid compartments: I. Ependymal destruction. *J Cell Biol* 1965;26:99–123.
19. Brightman MW: The intracerebral movement of proteins injected into blood and cerebrospinal fluid of mice. *Prog Brain Res* 1968;29:19–41.
20. Brocklenhurst G: The development of human cerebrospinal fluid pathway with particular reference to the roof of the fourth ventricle. *J Anat* 1969;105:467–475.
21. Cajal RS: Studien uber die Sehrinde der Katze. *J Psychol* 1923;29:161–181.

22. Cajal RS: Studies on Vertebrate Neurogenesis. Springfield, Charles C Thomas Publishers, 1960, p 325.
23. Caley DW, Maxwell DS: Light and electron microscopic study of the developing rat cerebral cortex: Abstract. *Anat Rec* 1966;154:325–326.
24. Caley DW, Maxwell DS: Development of the blood vessels and extracellular spaces during postnatal maturation of rat cerebral cortex. *J Comp Neur* 1970;138:31–48.
25. Clark LG: On the pacchionian bodies. *J Anat* 1928;55:40–48.
26. Cohen H, Davis S: The development of the cerebrospinal fluid spaces and choroid plexus in the chick. *J Anat* 1937;72:23–43.
27. Cohen H, Davis S: The morphology and permeability of the roof of the fourth ventricle in some mammalian embryos. *J Anat* 1938;27:430–458.
28. Cohen A, Hay ED: Secretion of collagen by embryonic neuroepithelium at the time of spinal cord somite interaction. *Dev Biol* 1971;26:578–605.
29. Cushing H: Studies on the cerebro-spinal fluid. *R Med Res* 1914;31:1.
30. Cuvier GL: Leçons d'anatomie comparée Paris, Crochard, 1809.
31. Dandy WE: Where is cerebrospinal fluid absorbed? *J Am Med Assn* 1929;92:2012–2014.
32. Farquhar MG: Neuroglial structure and relationships as seen with the electron microscope. *Anat Rec* 1955;121:291.
33. Farquhar MG, Hartmann JF: Neuroglial structure and relationships as revealed by electron microscopy. *J Neuropath Exp Neurol* 1957;16:18.
34. Farquhar MG, Palade G: Junctional complexes in various epithelia. *J Cell Biol* 1963;17:375–412.
35. Farrar CB: The embryonic pia. *Am J Insan* 1907;63:295–299.
36. Fleischhauer K: Fluoroeszenzmikroskopische Untersuchungen an der faserglia. *Z Zellforsch Mikrosk Anat* 1960;51:467–469.
37. Fleischhauer K: Uber die postnatale Entwicklung der subependymalen und marginalen Gliafaserschichten im Gehirn der Katze. *Z Zellforsch Mikrosk Anat* 1966;75:96–109.
38. Fleischhauer K, Hillebrand UH: Uber die Vermehrung der Gliazellen bei der Markscheidenbildung. *Z Zellforsch Mikrosk Anat* 1966;69:61–68.
39. Fleischhauer K: Regionale Unterschiede im Bau der marginalen Glia. *Anat Anz* 1964;113:Erg.-Heft, 191–193.
40. Flexner LB: The development of the meninges in Amphibia: A study of normal and experimental animals. *Contr Embryol* 1929;20:31–49.
41. Folkman J, Merte E, Abernathy LC, Williams G: Isolation of a tumor factor responsible for angiogenesis. *J Exp Med* 133:275 (1971).
42. Frederickson RG, Haller FR: The subarachnoid space interpreted as a special portion of the connective tissue space. *Proc NY Acad Sci* 1971;24:142–159.
43. Frenster JH, Herstein PR: Gene derepression. *New Engl J Med* 1973;288:124–129.
44. Galen ADC: On anatomical procedures; Singer C (trans). London, Cumerlege, 1956, pp 129–200.
45. Gelderen C van: Uber die Entwicklung der Hirnhaute bei Teleostiern. *Anat Anz* 1925;60:48–57.
46. Gomez DG, Potts DG: The surface characteristics of arachnoid granulations. *Archs Neurol* 1974;31:88–93.

47. Gronberg G: Die Ontogenese eines niedern Saugergehirns nach Untersuch-ungen and *Erinaceus europaeus. Zool. Jb: Abt 2, Anat. Ontol. Tiere* 1902;15:261–384.

48. Gruneberg H: Congenital hydrocephalus in the mouse, a case of spurious pleiotropism. *J Genetics* 1943;45:1.

49. Hansen-Pruss OC: Meninges of birds, with a consideration of the sinus rhomboidalis. *J Comp Neurol* 1923;36:193–217.

50. Harvey SC, Burr HS: An experimental study of the origin of the meninges. *Proc Soc Exp Biol Med* 1924;22:52–53.

51. Harvey SC, Compenhout E van: Development of the meninges in the chick. *Proc Soc Exp Biol Med* 1931;28:974–976.

52. Harvey SC: Development of the meninges: Further experiments. *Archs Neurol Psychiat* 1933;29:683–690.

53. Haug H: Die Membrana limitans glia superficialis der Shrinde der Katze. *Z Zellforsch Mikrosk Anat* 1970;155:79–87.

54. Haug H: Die postnatale Entwicklung der Gliadeckschicht der Shrinde der Katze. *Z Zellforsch Mikrosk Anat* 1972;123:544–565.

55. Held H: Uber die Neuroglia marginalis der mensch: lichen Grosshirnrinde. *Mschr Psychiat Neurol* 1909;26:360.

56. Hensen V: Beobachtungen uber die Befruchtung und Entwicklung des Kaninchens und Meerschweinchens. *Z Anat Entw Gesch* 1876;1:213–273, 353:423.

57. His W: Uber ein perivasculares Canalsystem in den nervosen Centra-lorganen und uber die Beziehungen zum Lymlphsystem. *Z wiss Zool* 1865;15:127.

58. His W: Die Haute und Hohlen des Korpers (Wiederabdruck eines akademis-chen Programmes vom Jahre 1865). *Arch Anat Physiol Anat Abt* 1903:368–404.

59. Hochstetter F: Uber die Entwicklung und Differenzierung der Hullen des Ruckenmarkes beim Menschen. *Morph Jb* 1934;74:1–104.

60. Hochwald GM, Wallenstein M: Exchange of albumin between blood, cere-brospinal fluid and brain in the cat. *Am J Physiol* 1967;212:1199–1204.

61. Janzen RW: Topographische Besonderheiten im Bau der Glia marginalis des Menschen. *Z Zellforsch Mikrosk Anat* 1967;80:570–584.

62. Johnston MC: Radioautographic study of the migration and fate of cranial neural crest cells in the chick embryo. *Anat Rec* 1966;156:143–156.

63. Kappers JA: Structural and functional changes in the telencephalic choroid plexus during ontogenesis. In Wolstenholme JT, O'Connor S, *The Cerebro-spinal Fluid.* Boston, Little Brown & Co, 1958, pp 3–31.

64. Kappers A, Huber GC, Crosby EC: The comparative anatomy of the ner-vous system of vertebrates including man. New York, Hafner Printers, 1960, vol 1.

65. Keegan JJ: A comparative study of the roof of the fourth ventricle. *Anat Rec* 1917;11:379.

66. Key A, Retzius G: Studien in der Anatomie des Nervensystems und des bindegewebes. Stockholm, Samson and Wallin, 1875–76.

67. Klatzo I, Miquwl J, Ferris PJ, Prokop JD, Smith DE: Observations on the passage of fluorescein labelled serum proteins (FLSP) from cerebrospinal fluid. *J Neuropathol Exptl Neurol* 1964;23:18–35.

68. Klika E: The ultrastructure of meninges in vertebrates. *Acta Univ Carol Medica* 1967;13:53–71.
69. Klika E: L'ultrastructure des meninges en l'ontongénese de l'homme. *Z. Mikrosk Anat Forsch* 79:209–222 (1968).
70. Kolliker A von: Grundriss der Entwicklungsgeschichte des Menschen und der hoheren Thiere. Leipzig, Engelmann, 1880.
71. Kollmann J: Die Entwicklung der Adergeflechte: Ein Beitrag zur Entwicklungsgeschichte des Gehirns. Leipzig, Engelmann, 1861.
72. Lawson R, Raimondi AJ: Hydrocephalus-3, a murine mutant: Alterations in fine structure of choroid plexus and ependyma. *Surg Neur* 1973;1:115–128.
73. Lear M, Harvey SC: The regeneration of the meninges. *Ann Surg* 1924;80:536–544.
74. Leary T, Edwards EA: The subdural space and its linings. *Archs Neurol Psychiat* 1933;29:691–701.
75. Loewenstein WR: Communication through cell junctions: Implications in growth control and differentiation. *Dev Biol* 1968 (suppl 2):151–183.
76. Low FN: Microfibrils: fine filamentous components of the tissue space. *Anat Rec* 1962;141:131–137.
77. Locke CE, Naffziger HC: The cerebral subarachnoid system. *Archs Neurol Psychiat* 1924;12:411.
78. Lorenzo AV, Page LK, Watters GV: Relationship between cerebrospinal fluid formation, absorption and pressure in human hydrocephalus. *Brain* 1970;93:679–692.
79. Luck DJ: Glycogen synthesis from uridine diphosphate glucose. *J Biophys Biochem Cytol* 1961;10:195–209
80. McCabe JS, Low, FN: The subarachnoid angle: An area of transition in peripheral nerve. *Anat Rec* 1969;164:15–34.
81. McLone DG, Bondareff W: Developmental morphology of the subarachnoid space and continuous structures in the mouse. *Am J Anat* 1975;1421:2173–293.
82. McLone DG, Bondareff W, Raimondi AJ: Hydrocephalus-3, a murine mutant: II. Changes in the brain's extracellular space. *Surg Neurol* 1973;1:233–242.
83. McLone DG, Bondareff W, Raimondi AJ: Brain edema in the hydrocephalic hy-3 mouse: Submicroscopic morphology. *J Neuropathol Exptl Neurol* 1971;39:627–637.
84. McLone DG, Bailey O, Bondareff W, Raimondi AJ: Neonatal communicating hydrocephalus in the hy-3 mouse. Houston, American Association of Neurological Surgeons, April 1971.
85. Milhorat TH, Clark RG, Hammock MK, McGrath PP: Structural, ultrastructural, and permeability changes in the ependyma and surrounding brain favoring equilibration in progressive hydrocephalus. *Arch Neurol* 1970;22:397–407.
86. Milhorat TH, Hammock MK: Isotope ventriculography. *Arch Neurol* 1971;25:1–8.
87. Millen JW: Some aspects of the anatomy of the pia mater and the choroid plexus. *Scient Basis Med Ann Rev* 1963:125–136.
88. Millen, JW, Woollam DHM: On the nature of the pia mater. *Brain* 1961;84:514–520.

89. Millen JW, Woollam DHM: The Anatomy of the Cerebrospinal Fluid. London, Oxford University Press, 1962.
90. Millen JW, Woollam DHM: The reticular perivascular tissue of the central nervous system. *J Neurol Psychiat* 1954;17:286.
91. Millen JW, Woollam DHM: Observations on the nature of the pia mater. *Brain* 1961;84:514.
92. Morse DE, Low FN: The fine structure of the pia mater of the rat. *Am J Anat* 1972;133:349–367.
93. Nelson B, Blinzinger K, Hager H: Electron microscopic observations on subarachnoid and perivascular spaces of the Syrian halmster brain. *Neurology* 1961;11:285–295.
94. Nelson E: An electron-microscopic study of bacterial meningitis: I. Experimental alterations in the leptomeninges and subarachnoid space. *Archs Neurol* 1962;6:390–403.
95. Nevis AH, Collins GH: Electrical impedance and volume changes in brain during preparation for electron microscopy. *Brain Res* 1967;5:57–85.
96. Niessing K: Uber systemartige Zusammenhange der Neuroglia im Grosshirn und uber ihre funktionelle Bedeutung. *Morph Jb* 1936;78:537–584.
97. Owen R: Comparative anatomy and physiology of vertebrates, London, Longmans' Green, 1868, vol 3.
98. Palay SL, McGee-Russel SM, Gordon A Jr, Grillo MA: Fixation of neural tissues for electron microscopy by perfusion with solution of osmium tetroxide. *J Cell Biol* 1962;12:385–397.
99. Pease DC, Schultz RL: Electron microscopy of rat cranial meninges. *Am J Anat* 1958;102:301–321.
100. Penfield WG: The cranial subdural space (a method of study). *Anat Rec* 1924;28:173–175.
101. Petrovieky P: Uber die Glia marginalis und oberflachlichte Nervenzellen im Hirnstamm der Katze. *Z Anat Entw Gesch* 1968;127:221–231.
102. Potts DG, Reilly KF, Deonarine V: Morphology of the arachnoid villi and granulations. *Radiology* 1972;105:333–341.
103. Ramsey HJ: Fine structure of the surface of the cerebral cortex of human brain. *J Cell Biol* 1965;16:323–333.
104. Redford LL: Unpublished work referred to by Cushing (17).
105. Reichert KB: Der Bau des menschlichen Gehirns durch Abbildungen mit erlauterndem Texte dargestellt. Leipzig, Engelmann, 1859–61.
106. Remak R: Untersuchungen uber die Entwicklung der Wirbeltiere. Berlin, Reimer, 1850–1855.
107. Rybroek JU, Low FN: Intercellular junctions in the developing arachnoid membrane in the chick. *J Comp Neurol* 1982;204:32–43.
108. Sahar A, Hochwald GM, Ransohoff J: Alternate pathway for cerebrospinal fluid absorption in animals with experimental obstructive hydrocephalus. *Exp Neurol* 1969;25:200–206.
109. Sahar A, Hochwald GM, Ransohoff J: Experimental hydrocephalus: Cerebrospinal fluid formation and ventricular size as a function of intraventricular pressure. *J Neurol Sci* 1970;11:81–91.
110. Sahar A, Hochwald GM, Ransohoff J: Cerebrospinal fluid turnover in experimental hydrocephalic dogs. *Neurology* 1971;21:218–224.
111. Sahar A, Hochwald GM, Sadik AR, Ransohoff J: Cerebrospinal fluid absorp-

tion in animals with experimental obstructive hydrocephalus. *Arch Neurol* 1959;21:638–644.

112. Salvi G: L'istogenesi e la struttura delle meningi. *Memorie Soc Tosc Sci Nat* 1898;161:187–228.

113. Sayad WY, Harvey SC: The regeneration of the meninges. *Ann Surg* 1923;77:129–141.

114. Schaltlenbrand G, Bailey P: Die perivaskulare Piagliamembran des Gehirns. *J Psychol Neurol* (Leipzig) 1928;35:199.

115. Sensenig EC: The early development of the meninges of the spinal cord in human embryos. *Contr Embryol* 1951;34:147–157.

116. Shabo AL, Maxwell DS: The morphology of the arachnoid villi: A light and electron microscopic study in the monkey. *J Neurosurg* 1968;29:451–463.

117. Spofford WR: Observations on the posterior part of the neural plate in Amblystoma. *J Exp Zool* 1945;99:35–52.

118. Sterzi G: Richerche intorno all' anatomia comparata ed all' ontogenesi delle meningi e considerazioni sulla filogenesi. *Atti I° Veneto Sci* 1901 (part 2);60:1101–1372.

119. Sterzi G: Recherches sur l'anatomie comparée et sur l'ontogenèse des meninges. *Archs Ital Biol* 1902;37:257–260.

120. Strasser H: Uber die Hullen des Gehirns und des Ruckenmarks: Ihre Functionen und ihre Entwicklung. *C R Ass Anat* 1901 (suppl):175–184.

121. Streeter GL: Developmental horizons in human embryos: Description of age group XV, XVI, XVII, and XVIII, being the third issue of a survey of the Carnegie collection. *Contr Embryol* 1948;321:133–230.

122. Streeter GL: Developmental horizons in human embryos: Description of age group XIX, XX, XXI, XXII, and XXIII being the fifth issue of a survey of the Carnegie collection. *Contr Embryol* 1951;34:165–196.

123. Tiedemann F: Anatomie und Bildungsgeschichte des Gehirns im Fotus des Menschen nebst einer vergleichenden Darstellung des Hirnbaues in den Thieren. Nuremberg, 1816.

124. Turner L: The structure of arachnoid granulations with observations on their physiological and pathological significance. Ann R Coll Surg 1961;29:237–264.

125. Van Harreveld A, Crowell J, Malhotra SK: A study of extracellular space in central nervous tissue by freeze-substitution. *J Cell Biol* 1965;25:117–137.

126. Van Harreveld A, Malhotra SK: Extracellular space in the cerebral cortex of the mouse. *J Anat* 1967;101:197–207.

127. Vesalius A: De humani corporis fabrica libri spetem. Basel, 1543.

128. Waggener JD, Beggs J: The membranous coverings of the neural tissues: an electron microscopy study. *J Neuropath Exp Neurol* 1967;26:412–426.

129. Weed LH: Studies on cerebrospinal fluid: II. The theories of drainage of cerebrospinal fluid with an analysis of the methods of investigation. *J Med Res* 1914;31:21–50.

130. Weed LH: Studies on cerebrospinal fluid: III. The pathways of escape from the subarachnoid spaces with particular reference to the arachnoid villi. *J Med Res* 1914;31:51–93.

131. Weed LH: The development of the cerebrospinal spaces in pig and in man. *Contr Embryol* 1917;5:3.

132. Weed LH: The experimental production of an internal hydrocephalus. *Contr Embryol* 1920;9:425.
133. Weed LH: The cerebrospinal fluid. *Physiol Rev* 1922;2:171.
134. Weed LH: The absorption of cerebrospinal fluid into the venous system. *Am J Anat* 1923;31:191.
135. Weed LH: in Penfield W, *Cytology and Cellular Pathology of the Nervous System*. New York, Hoeber, 1932, vol 2.
136. Weed LH: Meninges and cerebrospinal fluid. *J Anat* 1938;72:181–215.
137. Weigert C: Bemerkungen uber das Neurogliagerust des menschlichen Centrainervensystems. *Anat Anz* 1890;5:543–551.
138. Weller RO, Wisniewski H: Experimental hydrocephalus in rabbits. *Brain* 1969;82:818–828.
139. Weston JA: The migration and differentiation of neural crest cells. *Adv Morphogen* 1970;8:41–114.
140. Wiberg J: The anatomy of the brain in the works of Galen and 'Ali' Abbas: A comparative historical-anatomical study. *Janus* 1914;19:17–84.
141. Wiebel ER, Kistler GS, Scherle WF: Practical stereological methods for morphometric cytology. *J Cell Biol* 1966;39:23–38.
142. Wislocki GB, Putnam TJ: Absorption from the ventricles in experimentally produced internal hydrocephalus. *Am J Anat* 1921;29:313–320.
143. Wolff J: Beitrage zur Ultrastruktur der Kapillaren in der normalen Grosshirnrinde. *Z Zellforsch Mikrosk Anat* 1963;60:409–431.
144. Woollam DHM, Millen JW: The perivascular spaces of the mammalian central nervous system and their relation to the perineuronal and subarachnoid spaces. *J Anat* 1955;89:193.

CHAPTER 4

The Postnatal Development of the Brain and Its Coverings

Warwick J. Peacock

Introduction

Until recently, it was thought that the important stages in the development of the brain occurred before birth and that postnatal growth merely represented an increase in size, not complexity. This concept has been shown to be incorrect. It is now known that the rapid expansion of the brain after birth reflects ongoing maturational processes that increase connections among neurons and facilitate neuronal function.[1,2] Many of these refinements continue until well into adulthood and may be utilized in the brain's response to injury.[12,13,14]

The postnatal growth of the brain is not merely an expansion of volume but is an increase in structural complexity. Maturity reflects a tremendous extension of interneuronal connections allowing the vastly variable behavior of adult humans to emerge. Neurons appear at about 10 to 18 postmenstrual weeks, and neuroglia from 15 postmenstrual weeks to 2 postnatal years. Cortical maturity can be assessed by studying the extent of dendritic growth, dendritic-spine formation, and the degree of myelination. These factors correlate well with functional maturity. Nerve cell body regeneration is not possible, but nerve processes proliferate in response to injury and establish functional or nonfunctional new connections. Functional connections may reduce neurological deficit or, if inappropriately situated, may lead to increasing disability such as spasticity.

The evolutionary success of humans is due to their intellectual capacity, which reflects the remarkable complexity of their brain. It is said that the human brain contains about (1×10^{12}) neurons and that each cortical neuron receives up to 30,000 presynaptic terminals.[3] A prolonged time period is required to achieve this enormous structural complexity, and the human brain must reach a certain minimum size to provide sufficient space for the vast number of nerve processes and their connections. The size to which the brain can grow during intrauterine life is limited by the dimensions of the birth canal, although birth itself is not a significant milestone in the continuing process of neuronal maturation. By the time

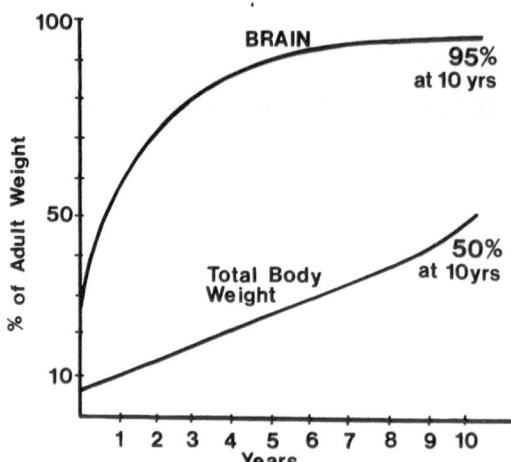

Figure 4.1. Precocious growth of the brain compared to that of the whole body.

of birth the coverings of the brain have achieved a subtle compromise between rigidity and mobility, thus allowing molding of the head to occur in its course through the birth canal.

The growth of the skull vault is secondary to the increase in brain volume and occurs as a result of the laying down of bone in distracted sutures and by endocranial absorption and pericranial accretion. The shape of the vault is molded in part by the interactions of the surrounding functional matrices but essentially by the gentle and insistent expansive force of the brain.

The rapid development of the brain compared with that of most other organs indicates that from early fetal life its weight is nearer that of the adult than any other organ except perhaps the eye (Fig. 4.1). At birth the brain has reached 25% of the adult weight; at 6 months, about 50%; at 2 years, 75%; and at 5 years, 90% of its final weight. At 10 years the figure is 95%. This contrasts with the weight of the whole body, which at birth is 5% of young adult weight and at 10 years only about 50%.[4]

Developmental Dynamics of Brain Growth

The dynamic processes involved in the development of the brain begin within ten days of conception, and some are still active well into adult-hood. Division into ante- and postnatal stages is thus somewhat arbitrary as far as the growth of the brain is concerned. Many processes, such as myelination[2] and dendrite maturation,[1] start during fetal life and continue postnatally for many years (Fig. 4.2). The timing of birth itself in relation-ship to the development of the fetus is variable; viability is possible at least as early as 28 gestational weeks. The important processes involved

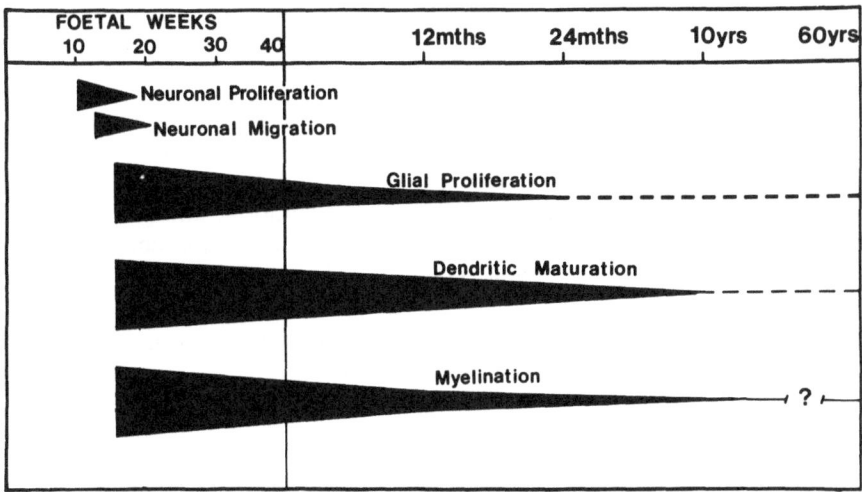

Figure 4.2. Timetable of the important processes involved in brain development.

in the growth and maturation of the brain are cell division and migration, followed by dendrite production with synapse formation, and finally myelination.

Cell Division and Migration

The neuroepithelial cells lining the neural tube divide repeatedly and give rise to two types of cells, neuroblasts and glioblasts. After the cells have passed through a number of multiplication cycles, they migrate outward to form a second cellular region composed of young neurons and glial cells. Neurons and neuroglia develop at different times and at different rates. Most of the neurons of the cerebral cortex are produced during the period from 10 to 18 post-menstrual weeks,[3] and once formed they lose the ability to divide again (Fig. 4.2). Glial cells are formed from about 15 post-menstrual weeks and continue to be produced postnatally for 2 years, probably retaining the ability to divide throughout life.[1] The timing of these major periods of multiplication is fixed; if, for any reason, cell division is suppressed during critical periods, the neurodevelopmental timetable does not permit a compensatory "catch-up" period later. Neuronal or glial cell populations will thus be forever depleted.[5]

Oligodendrocytes, the glial cells responsible for the myelination of neuronal processes, multiply immediately prior to the onset of myelination.[2] Microglial cells, the potential phagocytes within the brain, are of mesenchymal origin and reach the brain as soon as the cerebral circulation has been established. Microglia respond to infection or ischaemia by expanding to take on their phagocytic role, and the resident cells are joined by invading monocytes that play the same role.[6]

The migration of neurons and glial cells occurs in waves in a precisely ordered sequence. The large cells migrate first, forming the deeper layers of the cortex; the smaller neurons migrate later, contributing to the superficial layers and probably acting as interneurons. Cells of a similar type tend to aggregate and adopt a preferential orientation. In the cerebral cortex the majority of the large pyramidal neurons are consistently aligned, with their prominent apical dendrites directed toward the surface and their axons directed toward the underlying white matter. Once the neurons and glial cells have reached their destination, maturational processes contribute to the increase in brain size.

Cell Differentiation and Dendrite Formation

One of the most striking features in the development of neurons is the progressive elaboration of their outgrowths, a phenomenon that continues postnatally for years. The degree of process formation can be used as a measure of cortical maturity.[7] Most neurons in the mammalian brain are multipolar, with several tapering dendrites functioning as receptor sites and a single axon as the cell's effector process. The young outgrowths bear distinctive structures at their growing ends, called growth cones, which are endowed with amoeboid properties enabling them to explore their immediate environment and to push aside obstacles until they reach their destination. Axons are able to find their way to their specific synaptic sites even though they extend for considerable distances within the brain and give off one or more branches before finally reaching their predetermined destination. Although the evidence is largely indirect, it is possible that the growth cone has encoded within it the necessary molecular features that enable it to detect appropriate substrates along which to grow and to identify correct targets, responding to structural or chemical cues along its way. The growth cones at the end of the axonal branches establish contact with target cell bodies or their dendrites, thereby forming synapses.[8]

In the brain, as in other organs, the number of cells produced exceeds the number that survive.[9] Not only are more nerve cells generated than survive, but also more dendrites and synapses develop than can be maintained. To remove the excess cells, a period of carefully programmed cell death occurs at the time the nerves are forming synaptic connections with target structures. The limiting factor determining the final number of cells and dendrites seems to be the number of functional contacts or synapses that can be established and maintained. If a limb is experimentally removed from a developing fetus, the magnitude of naturally occurring cell death in the areas within the central nervous system that would normally innervate that limb is increased enormously. In contrast, the amount of cell death can be reduced by grafting a supernumerary limb onto the side of a chick embryo. Thus, competition apparently exists, and only neurons and processes with functional connections survive.[9]

One criterion used for assessing cortical maturity before and after birth is the amount of dendrite development and the degree of dendritic specialization.[1,7] Dendrites and especially the dendritic spines along their length are the major targets for the exploring axonal growth cones in the establishment of synapses. Development of synapses provides the functional basis of the brain, and the onset of function correlates well with what is seen histologically. Purpura[1] examined histologically the degree of dendritic development in the brains of stillborn fetuses and of older normal children who died at various ages. He found that the apical dendrites at 14 weeks of fetal life are well developed, but basilar dendrites are barely detectable on pyramidal cells. Basilar dendrites make their appearance at about 18 weeks and elongate rapidly through to term (Fig. 4.3).

The shape and length of the dendritic spines is also a good index of cortical maturation.[1] Before term the dendrites are covered by long, thin spines, whereas in the 6-month-old infant the number of long, thin spines is significantly reduced, and the number of stubby and mushroom-shaped spines increases steadily until about 7 years of age (Fig. 4.4). The nature of the dendritic spines is also helpful in assessing the functional integrity of the cerebral cortex. Long, thin dendritic spines indicate immaturity, and stubby, mushroom-type spines show an advanced degree of maturation. Dendritic spine differentiation commences at about midgestation and continues throughout early childhood.

A structure–function relationship exists between the visual cortex of the preterm infant and the visual evoked potential (VEP). Purpura[10] found the VEP of very young preterm infants to be immature and poorly organized. In infants of 34 weeks' gestation the dendritic development was

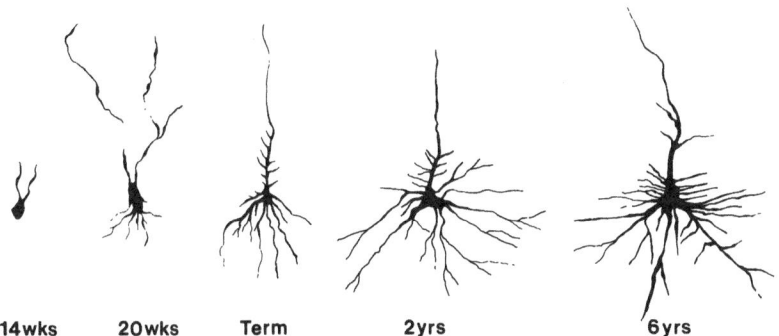

14 wks   20 wks   Term   2 yrs   6 yrs

Figure 4.3. Apical dendrites appear at 14 postmenstrual weeks and basal dendrites at 20 postmenstrual weeks. Secondary branches have appeared by term, and new dendrites develop up to about 6 years of age. (Adapted from Reference 1.)

A   B   C

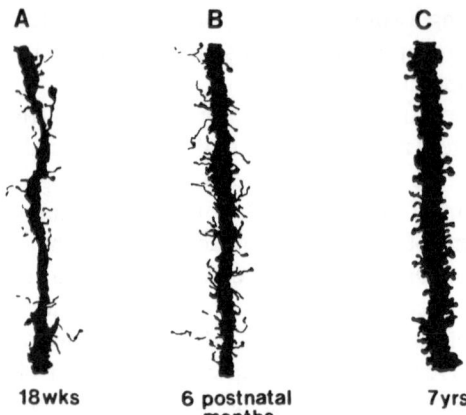

18 wks   6 postnatal   7 yrs
          months

Figure 4.4. Long, thin dendritic spines appear at about 18 post-menstrual weeks. Stubby and mushroom spines can be seen at 6 postnatal months and are well developed at 7 years of age. (Adapted from Reference 1.)

prominent, and dendritic spines were extensively produced. At this stage the VEP was better organized and more mature.

Illness affecting the brain in the perinatal and early postnatal periods leads to abnormalities in dendritic growth.[10] Huttenlocher[11] examined the brain in mentally defective patients and found that the cortex also showed reduced dendritic branching and a sparsity of spines on the apical and basal dendrites; this would, of course, be associated with a decreased number of synaptic sites. Defective dendritic development may be an important anatomical substrate for severe mental deficiency.

As cortical maturation progresses the density of nerve cell bodies decreases because the cell bodies enlarge. With the growth of axons and dendrites the distance between cells increases.

Myelination

Another very important factor in the assessment of the regional maturation of the brain is the degree of myelinaton of fibers within that area. The onset of function in a neuron probably correlates well with its acquisition of a myelin sheath. Yakovlev[2] showed that myelination is preceded by a proliferation of oligodendrocytes and that fiber systems begin to myelinate at different stages during fetal life or after birth. He noted that the timing of myelination of a fiber system correlates well with the onset of its function. He examined over 200 brains varying in age from the fourth month of fetal life to one postnatal year and then looked at a large collection of brains available from the third and later decades of life. His findings (Fig. 4.5) were that the first structures to myelinate were the spinal and cranial nerve roots, beginning with the spinal motor roots at the end of the fourth fetal month; these completed their cycle by term. One of the earliest intrinsic systems to myelinate is the vestibulo-acoustic system,

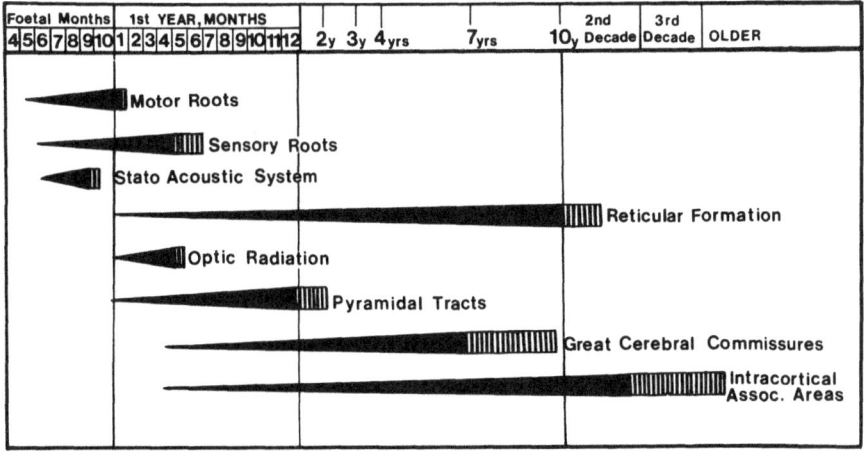

Figure 4.5. Myelogenetic cycles within the nervous system. (Adapted from Reference 2.)

probably because the maternal environment is a noisy one for the fetus and gravitational forces make demands for postural adjustment in utero. The optic nerves and tracts and the lateral geniculate nuclei begin to myelinate late in the ninth fetal month, but this cycle is rapidly completed in the first few months after birth.

Myelination of the pyramidal tracts commences during the eighth month of fetal life and is completed only after about 2 years of postnatal life. The reticular formation shows very little myelination up to term and then myelinates very slowly, continuing well into adult life. The reticular formation is known to be involved in such functions as concentration and attention span, which become well developed only in adolescence. The corticopontine tracts are the last of the long, descending transcapsular projections to begin myelinating and have the longest cycle, starting during the second postnatal month and continuing into the second postnatal year. The fibers that connect corticopontine fibers with the cerebellar cortex lie in the middle cerebellar peduncle and also myelinate late. Their cycle runs from one postnatal month through to the fourth postnatal year. These tracts are associated with coordination of fine motor function, which develops slowly in the young child. The long association and commissural fiber systems of the cerebral hemispheres begin myelinating during the fourth postnatal month and continue until the end of the first decade. Structures involved with the highest intellectual functions, the short intracortical connections of the association areas in the frontal, parietal, and temporal lobes, begin to myelinate in the third postnatal month and may continue even into the sixth decade.

Fibers carrying impulses to specific cortical areas myelinate at the same time as those carrying impulses away from the same area to the periphery. Maturation, therefore, occurs in arcs or functional units rather than simply in geographical regions. The first cortical area to show maturation is the primary motor cortex in the precentral gyrus followed by the primary sensory cortex in the postcentral gyrus. The motor and sensory areas representing the arms and upper trunk mature before those for the legs; this correlates well with the sequence of motor development in the young infant.

Regeneration and Plasticity

How do nerve cells respond to injury? New neurons cannot replace lost ones, but each cell can proliferate new processes to replace those that have been damaged. Within the central nervous system a vivid demonstration of regeneration has been provided by the experimental work of Goldman-Rakic and her colleagues.[12] Tritiated amino acids were injected into the frontal association cortex of monkeys on one side (Fig. 4.6) and were found to be transported through fibers of the corpus callosum to the

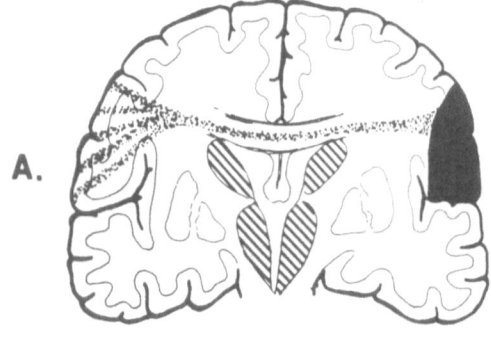

A.

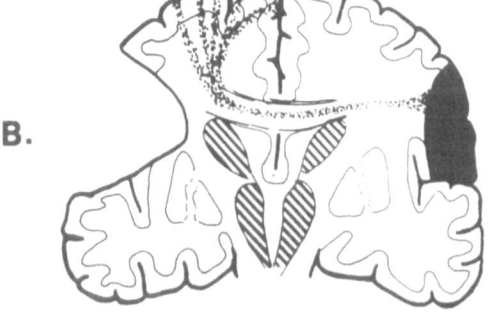

B.

Figure 4.6. Experiment to show nerve process regeneration. **A.** Tritiated amino acids injected into the right frontal cortex are transported to the contralateral cortex. **B.** Part of frontal lobe has been excised on the left; regenerating axons grow to new sites in the left hemisphere. (Adapted from Reference 12.)

same cortical region of the opposite side. The experiment was repeated in animals in which part of the contralateral frontal lobe had been ablated. The callosal fibres regenerated, but when they reached the opposite side and found the normal targets were absent, they swerved and terminated in a neighboring region of the cortex.

Liu and Chambers[13] transected one pyramidal tract in the spinal cord of cats and several years later examined the axonal terminations of dorsal root fibers in both sides of the cord. They found that the field of terminations was larger on the side of the tract lesion, which suggested that the dorsal root fibers had given off collateral sprouts that took over the vacated synaptic sites. This phenomenon probably accounts for the increasing spasticity that occurs following damage to descending motor tracts in stroke, paraplegia, and cerebral palsy.

Raisman[14] studied the effect of dividing one or the other of the two main tracts that connect with the septal nucleus of the adult rat (Fig. 4.7). The septal nucleus receives two well-defined inputs, one from the hippocampus and the other from the median forebrain bundle, each making characteristic synaptic connections onto the septal nucleus. When the hippocampal input is cut, there is an increase in the number of synaptic contacts from the median forebrain bundle. In contrast, when the median forebrain bundle is cut, the synaptic sites on the cell bodies are taken over by the hippocampal terminals.

The foregoing experiments illustrate that when one input is transected, another input expands its terminal field onto the vacated synaptic sites on the cell bodies or dendrites. The compensatory sprouting suggests that a cell is programmed to receive a certain number of synaptic connections and reacts to injury by attempting to restore its appropriate number of synapses. These experiments carry the hope that we may not only reveal more of the normally occurring plastic capabilities of nerve cells but eventually may use them to compensate for the effects of injuries to the human brain.

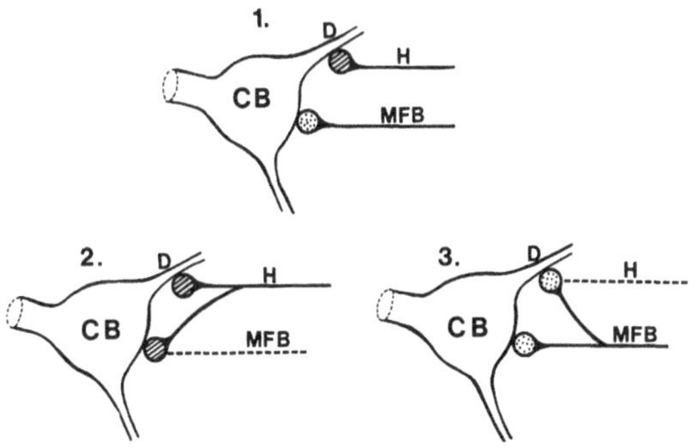

Figure 4.7. Regeneration of connections to cells of septal nucleus: CB (cell body), D (dendritic), H (hippocampal fibres) MFB (medial forebrain bundle fibres). 1. Normal state; 2. MFB divided and H occupies vacated synaptic sites; 3. MFB occupies vacated H synaptic sites. (Adapted from Reference 14.)

Postnatal Development of the Coverings of the Brain

The cranium supports and protects the underlying brain. These two functions must be combined with the capacity for rapid expansion resulting from brain growth and the malleability required during birth. The cranium is divided into two parts: the vault or calvaria and the base. The vault develops by ossification in membrane, a type of ossification that allows for rapid expansion by molding and distraction of sutures. The base develops in cartilage and therefore has a slower growth rate. Although there are many theories concerning the dynamics of skull growth, most workers in this field believe that the skull grows secondarily to the functional structures that it supports or protects.[15] The skull supports and protects a number of functional matrices, all of which influence its growth; these include the brain, the eyeball and its associated oculomotor structures, the respiratory passages, and the upper part of the digestive system. The interrelating forces and demands of these functional units produce the shape and size of the bony skeleton of the skull.

The exact mechanisms by which deforming mechanical forces produce structural bony change are obscure but appear to be mediated through piezoelectric currents.[16] Bone, being highly crystalline as a result of its collagen and apatite content, behaves as a crystal by generating a minute electrical current when it is mechanically deformed, thereby producing polar electric fields.[17] Bioelectric effects may be generated in several ways, and electrical potential differences are a feature of all cell membranes. It is conceivable that osteoblasts and osteoclasts, and the matrices within which they operate, react to electrical potential by building up bone in negatively charged fields and, conversely, by resorbing bone in positively charged fields. The ultimate shape of a bone and its internal architecture is probably a reflection of its genetically determined form as well as the mechanical demands to which it is subject. Throughout life, bone shape is constantly remodelled because of changes in functional requirements. Because of the precocious growth of the brain, the vault at birth is large in proportion to other parts of the body, and the facial skeleton is relatively small because of the rudimentary condition of the mandible and maxillae, noneruption of the teeth, and the small size of the sinuses and nasal cavities. In the newborn the bones of the vault are smooth and unilaminar and lack diploë, and the glabellar, supraciliary, and mastoid processes have not as yet developed. Because of the absent mastoid processes, the stylomastoid foramen lies on the lateral aspect of the skull, exposing the facial nerve.

The Calvaria

The frontal, parietal, squamous temporal, and squamous occipital bones arise from primary ossification centers that appear at about 6 weeks of

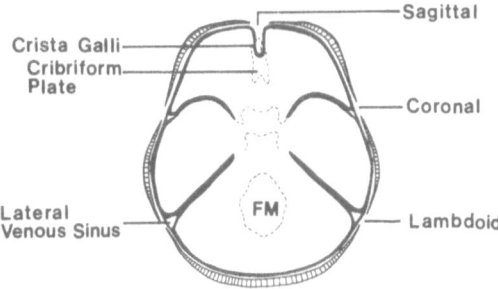

Figure 4.8. Skull base showing the five points of attachment of dural bands.

intrauterine life. Bone grows in a radiating fashion until the sites of the sutures are reached. These sites are predetermined and rise from five points at which the dura is attached to the base of the skull (Fig. 4.8): at the crista galli, the lateral tips of the lesser wings of the sphenoid bone, and at the posterior angles of the two petrous bones.[15] Well-oriented fiber tracts in the dura run upward from these five points towards the calvaria and underlie the future sites of the major sutures. The fiber tracts transmit mechanical forces reciprocally between base and vault and direct the forces resulting from the growth of the brain in specific directions. Without such dural tracts the neurocranium would tend to assume a perfectly spherical shape. Osteogenesis is inhibited at the suture sites by an as-yet unknown mechanism that determines the location of sutures between adjacent bones. The metopic-sagittal suture system runs upward from the crista galli in the median plane; the coronal sutures extend upward parallel to the fiber tracts connected to the tips of the lesser wings of the sphenoid bone; and the lambdoid sutures overlie the fiber tracts attached to the base of the skull at the posterior angles of the petrous bones. Two midline fontanels and two pairs of laterally placed fontanels are formed at the angles of the two parietal bones. As the brain increases in volume the skull bones are displaced outward and away from each other, thereby calling into play two adaptive processes. First, the curve of each bone must be flattened to accommodate the arc of a circle with a greater diameter by absorption of bone on the periphery of the inner surface and by laying down of bone on the periphery of the outer surface (Fig. 4.9). Second, the gap created at the sutures is passively filled in by bony growth at the bone edges.

Skull Base

Early in fetal life the entire skull base is formed in cartilage, and ossification centers develop in the basiocciput and pre- and postsphenoid cartilages and in the mesethmoid. At birth the pre- and postsphenoid cartilages

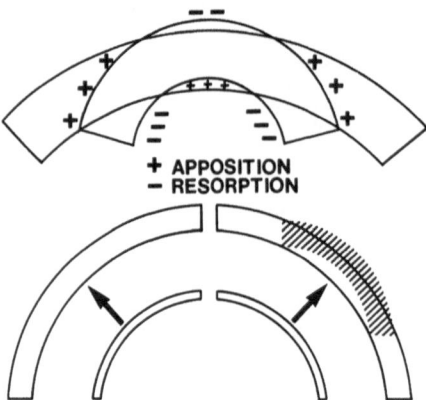

+ APPOSITION
− RESORPTION

Figure 4.9. Diagram to show mecha-
nisms of skull growth and moulding.
(Adapted from David DJ, Poswillo
D, Simpson D (eds): *The Cranio-
synostoses.* New York, Springer-
Verlag New York Inc, 1982.

have united to form the body of the sphenoid, which remains separated
from the basiocciput by the spheno-occipital synchondrosis. Subsequent
growth changes in the cranial base result from remodelling of the bony
surfaces and endochondral ossification at the synchondroses. Although
growth at the spheno-occipital synchondrosis continues until early adulthood, it occurs mainly in the first 3 to 4 years of life, the period characterized by rapid brain growth; it is therefore probably passive.[18]

Combined Calvarial and Basal Growth

Antero-posterior growth of the cranial vault occurs at the coronal and
lambdoid sutures and in the base at the sphenooccipital synchondrosis,
sphenoethmoidal, and frontosphenoidal sutures. Growth in width takes
place in the vault at the sagittal suture and in the base at the sutures
bordering the greater wing of the sphenoid, the occipitomastoid suture,
and the cartilaginous petrooccipital joints. Increase in height is due to
growth at the frontozygomatic, sphenoparietal, and squamosal sutures.
The posterior fontanel closes 2 months after birth. The anterolateral fontanel closes next, at 3 months, and the posterolateral fontanel closes by
the end of the first year. Aisenson[19] examined 1677 children serially over
the first few years of life. He found that the anterior fontanel closed
between 4 and 26 months, with 90% of all cases closing between 7 and 19
months. By the end of the first year 41.6% were closed.

By the second year of life the bones of the vault are interlocked at the
sutures, and further growth occurs by accretion and absorption on their
superficial and deep surfaces, respectively. The cranial vault, unilaminar
at birth, develops two tables and intervening diploë by about the fourth
year.[20] The appearance of muscular markings on the outer table is related
to the development of the muscles of mastication and the posterior muscles of the neck. The mastoid process forms a visible bulge on the surface
in the second year and is invaded by air cells during the sixth year.

The three paranasal sinuses that develop adjacent to the cranial vault—the frontal, ethmoid, and sphenoid sinuses—are rudimentary or absent at birth. Their primary expansion occurs with the eruption of the first deciduous molars. The two frontal sinuses are usually fairly well formed between the seventh and eighth years, but reach their full size only after puberty. They vary in size in different individuals but are larger in males, where they give the profile of the forehead an obliquity that contrasts with the vertical or convex outline seen in children and females. The enlargement of the frontal sinuses is associated with the appearance of the supraciliary arches, which are produced to resist the mechanical stresses generated by the masticatory apparatus. The ethmoid sinuses in the floor of the anterior fossa and in the medial walls of the orbit are small but of clinical importance at birth. They grow rapidly between the sixth and eighth years and again after puberty. The two sphenoid sinuses in the body of the sphenoid bone vary in size and shape. They are rarely symmetrical because of the displacement of the septum. Their main development takes place after puberty since they are only rudiments at birth.

References

1. Purpura DP: Dendritic differentiation in human cerebral cortex: Normal and aberrent developmental patterns, in Kreuteberg GW (ed): *Advances in Neurology*. New York, Raven Press Publishers, 1975, vol 12.
2. Yakovlev PI, Lecours AP: The myelogenetic cycle of regional maturation of the brain, in Minkowski A (ed): *Regional Development of the Brain in Early Life*. Oxford, Blackwell, 1967, pp 3–70.
3. Tanner JM: *Growth and Development of the Brain in Foetus into Man*. London, Open Books, 1978, pp 103–116.
4. Cheek DB: *Fetal and Postnatal Cellular Growth*. New York: John Wiley & Sons Inc, 1975.
5. Davison AN, Dobbing J: The developing brain, in Davison AN, Dobbing J (eds): *Applied Neurochemistry*. Oxford, Blackwell, 1968, pp 253–286.
6. Imamoto K, Leblond CP: Presence of labelled monocytes, macrophages and microglia in a stab wound of the brain following an injection of bone marrow cells labelled with ^{3}H-uridine into rats. J Comp Neurol 1977;174:225–80.
7. Conel JL: *The Postnatal Development of the Human Cerebral Cortex*. Cambridge: Harvard University Press, 1939–1959, vol 1–4.
8. James DW: Growth cones and synaptic connections in tissue culture, in Bellairs R, Gray EG (eds): *Essays on the Nervous System*. Oxford, Clarendon Press, 1974.
9. Hamburger V: Cell death in the development of the lateral motor column of the chick embryo. *J comp Neurol* 1975;160:535–546.
10. Purpura DP: Structure-dysfunction relationships in the visual cortex of preterm infants, in Brazier MAB, Coceani F (eds): Brain Dysfunction in Infantile Febrile Convulsions. New York, Raven Press Publishers, 1976.
11. Huttenlocher PR: Dendritic development in neocortex of children with mental defect and infantile spasms. *Neurology* 1974;24:203–210.
12. Goldman-Rakic PS: Development and plasticity of primate frontal association

cortex, in Schmitt FO (ed): *The Organization of the Cerebral Cortex.* Cambridge, The MIT Press, 1981, pp 69–97.

13. Liu CN, Chambers WW: Intraspinal sprouting of dorsal root axons. *Arch Neurol* 1958;79:46–61.
14. Raisman G: Neuronal plasticity in the septal nuclei of the adult rat. *Brain Res* 1969;14:25–48.
15. Moss ML: Functional Anatomy of Cranial Synostosis. *Child's Brain* 1975;1:22–33.
16. Sperber GH: Characteristics of Bone Development and Growth, in Sperber GH (ed): *Craniofacial Embryology.* Littleton: Wright, 1981.
17. Friedenberg ZB, Harlow MC, Heppenstall RB et al.: The cellular origin of bioelectric potentials in bone. *Calc Tiss Res* 1973;13:53.
18. Melsen B: Time and mode of closure of the spheno-occipital synchondrosis determined in human autopsy material. *Acta Anat* 1972;83:112.
19. Aisenson RM: Closing of the anterior fontanelle. *Pediatrics* 1950;6:223–225.
20. Williams PL, Warwick R: Cranial characteristics at different ages, in Williams PL, Warwick R (eds): *Gray's Anatomy,* ed 36. New York, Churchill Livingstone, 1980, pp 344–350.

CHAPTER 5

Normal Developmental Milestones, the Significance of Delayed Milestones, and Neurodevelopmental Evaluation of Infants and Young Children

Marianne Larsen

Introduction

The clinical neurological assessment of a newborn should begin with a history: parental and obstetric, as well as a detailed history of the infant's intrapartum and neonatal course. Important factors in the obstetric history, which should include complete information regarding the pregnancy, are the age of the mother and her medical background, prior pregnancies, and familial neurological disorders. Important factors in the history of the neonatal course are feeding, sucking, and crying patterns. Questions should be asked about seizures, cyanotic spells, apneic spells, infection, jaundice, and muscle tone.

Examinations

An examination of the newborn should include a general (pediatric) and a neurological examination; some of the general pediatric findings may be significant with respect to the neurological examination. The initial physical examination of the newborn is done in the delivery room. At that time the examiner should be able to detect significant anomalies, birth injuries, and cardiorespiratory disorders that may compromise successful adaptation to extrauterine life. A simple examination may suffice to document neurological integrity in the newborn and may be adequate when signs of disease are obvious or definite; however, when the findings are marginal or only suggestive of abnormality, a second examination may yield more reliable information regarding the nature of the problem.

Apgar Scoring

Immediate and repeated Apgar scoring provides a rapid and dependable measurement of the infant's physiological status. The Apgar system is based on a simple assignment of 0, 1, or 2 points for vital functions such as color, respiratory effort, heart rate, and (for the central nervous system)

Table 5.1. Interpretation of the Apgar scores.

Features evaluated	Apgar score		
	0 points	1 point	2 points
Heart rate	None	< 100	> 200
Respiratory effort	Apnea	Irregular, shallow, or gasping respirations	Vigorous and crying
Color	Pale, blue	Pale or blue extremities	Pink
Muscle tone	Absent	Weak, passive tone	Active movements
Reflex irritability	Absent	Grimace	Active avoidance

oxygenation, as well as tone and reflex irritability. The components of the Apgar score correlate well with the infant's ease of transition from fetal to newborn life; hence, routine scoring at 1 and 5 minutes after delivery has become the practice. The 1-minute score correlates closely with the pH of the umbilical cord's arterial blood, whereas the 5-minute score most closely correlates with the neurological outcome. A 5-minute Apgar score of less than 6 indicates asphyxia; a score below 3 is a strong indication of severe asphyxia (see Table 5.1). In interpreting the Apgar score one should note that low scores encountered in infants with low birth weight (less than 1500 g) or of less than 32 weeks' gestational age may be present in the absence of asphyxia.

Ontogenesis of the Central Nervous System

To assess accurately neurological findings, the examiner must consider the ontogenesis of the central nervous system, which can be divided into four stages. The initial stage of embryogenesis and induction occurs during the first 30 days of development. During this period, the neural tube is formed. Interference with ontogenesis during this period results in such dysraphic or facial forebrain anomalies as anencephaly, meningomyelocele and the holoprosencephaly.[8] The second ontogenetic stage begins at the end of the first month. It is one of neuronal proliferation and outward migration from the area surrounding the neural tube. By the 25th week of gestation, the cerebral cortex reaches its full neuronal complement, neuronal proliferation ceases, and electrical activity becomes measurable. Insult to morphogenesis during this period gives rise to various disorders of cellular proliferation and migration such as microcephaly, schizencephaly, and polymicrogyria. The third stage starts at the beginning of the last trimester of gestation and includes a rapid multiplication of glial cells accompanied by an arborization of the neural processes, the formation of synapses, and the ultimate alignment and orientation of the cortical neurons. A number of insults, including perinatal ones, may affect this developmental stage. The fourth and last stage, myelination, occurs over a long time span. It commences during the second trimester, is maximal during the first year of postnatal life, and may continue into the third decade.

The brain of the term newborn infant weighs between 325 and 435 g and accounts for approximately 10% of total body weight at birth. All primary and secondary fissures and sulci are present, but tertiary sulci are only partially developed. The four major lobes are clearly distinguishable, and on microscopic examination, the cerebral cortex of the term newborn infant exhibits lamination similar to that of the adult brain. Nissl bodies are not yet present in cortical neurons, except in certain Betz cells in the motor cortex. The cerebellum in the newborn contains the prominent external granular cell layer, which gradually disappears during the first postnatal year.

At birth, all cranial nerves except the optic nerve are myelinated, as are the spinal roots, the olivary and cerebellar connections, and the tracts of the spinal cord posterior columns. Myelination of the corticospinal tract, the cortical cerebellar fibers, and optic nerves begins just prior to birth. The rapid brain growth that occurs during the first postnatal year is largely the result of continued myelination and arborization of dendritic processes; these establish the neuronal connections necessary for the complex behavioral characteristic of the older infant and child.

Neurological Examination of the Premature Infant

In the past the term "premature infant" included all babies weighing less than 2500 g at birth. However, in evaluating a small, low-birth-weight newborn one must recognize that the infant of low birth weight may be small either because of retarded intrauterine growth (i.e., a small-for-date infant) or because of shortened gestation (i.e., a premature infant). An infant who has a relatively low birth weight in relation to length of gestation (a small-for-date infant) does not manifest the same neurological patterns of growth as does the infant whose weight is appropriate for his or her gestational age (a premature infant). Infants of diabetic mothers may be born considerably before term and yet weigh more than 2500 g; such infants should be considered premature for purposes of neurological evaluation.

The physician examining the newborn baby should, therefore, make a reasonable estimation of gestational age to assess fully the significance of the observations. Certain external physical characteristics are useful in making this estimation. These include the amount of breast tissue, the ear cartilage, the degree of development of external genitalia, and skin color and texture (see Table 5.2). Another bit of objective information useful in differentiating between premature infants and small-for-date infants is

Table 5.2. External characteristics useful for estimation of gestational age.

External characteristics	Gestational age			
	28 weeks	32 weeks	36 weeks	40 weeks
Ear cartilage	Pinna soft, remains folded	Pinna slightly harder but remains folded	Pinna harder, springs back	Pinna firm, stands erect from head
Breast tissue	None	None	1–2 mm nodule	6–7 mm nodule
External genitalia: male	Testes undescended, smooth scrotum	Testes in inguinal canal, few scrotal rugae	Testes high in scrotum, more scrotal rugae	Testes descended, pendulous scrotum covered with rugae
External genitalia: female	Prominent clitoris, small, widely separated labia	Prominent clitoris, larger separated labia	Clitoris less prominent, labia majora cover labia minora	Clitoris covered by labia majora
Plantar surface	Smooth	1–2 anterior creases	2–3 anterior creases	Creases cover sole

Source: Volpe JJ: *Neurology of the Newborn.* Philadelphia, WB Saunders Co, 1981. Modified from Usher R: *Ped Clin N Am* 1966;13:835.

nerve conduction velocity. The mean conduction velocity of the ulnar nerve of a term infant is about 30 meters per second; this velocity is progressively slower with shorter gestational age.[6,29]

An accurate estimation of gestational age requires that the infant be in an alert, quiet, restful state—awake if possible, preferably 30 to 60 minutes before feeding, as significant diminution in awareness and muscle tone occurs immediately after feeding, and the infant may be irritable before a scheduled meal. In a premature infant, the various phases of sleep, stupor, and wakefulness alternate rapidly and tend to fuse. The 28 week premature infant often needs to be aroused by repetitive stimulation.[12] It has been suggested that preterm infants of 25 to 30 weeks' gestation are more readily awakened than had been previously thought, but that they do not tend to stay awake as long as do full term infants.[7] Others[9] have emphasized that a considerable degree of waking alertness exists in infants of 31 weeks' gestation.

By term, alertness clearly becomes more acute and a lower threshold is required for arousal. At this time the infant remains alert for longer periods without requiring tactile and auditory stimulation to react. Various EEG recordings in premature infants suggest that 80% to 85% of their time is spent sleeping compared to 60% for the term baby. At 28 weeks the infant demonstrates eye closure when confronted by a bright light; by 32 weeks light stimulation induces persistent lid closure. Pupillary light reflex appears as early as 29 weeks, but is consistently present at 32 weeks. At 36 weeks the infant is able to turn the head toward the light source. With funduscopy the newborn's optic disk has a greyish-white appearance (pseudo optic atrophy). Retinal hemorrhages are reported to occur in 50% of newborns, and the macular light reflex is normally absent. Eye movement can be judged by the doll's head maneuver. This response is first present at 28 to 32 weeks of gestation and can usually be elicited in the full-term infant. Ocular-vestibular responses can best be elicited by spinning the infant while it is held in an upright position, facing the examiner. With this maneuver the infant usually opens the eyes, thereby enabling extraocular movements to be noted. At 28 weeks the infant blinks or startles to loud noises.

The cry of the smallest premature infant is generally not responsive to stimuli; by 36 to 37 weeks the cry has become more frequent, continuous, vigorous, and lasting. It is easily provoked by noxious stimuli.

Neurological maturity can be evaluated with the use of Table 5.3[23], which presents five reflex responses, including pupillary reaction, traction response, glabellar tap, neck righting, and head turning to diffuse light. In the neurologic examination of the premature infant, an evaluation of muscle tone is of major importance.[1,27] It is particularly helpful in differentiating between small-for-date and premature infants. The premature infant of 26 to 28 weeks' gestation is flaccid and, in vertical suspension, it hangs limply without extending the extremities, spine, or head. The gradual

Table 5.3. Reflexes of value in assessing gestational age.

Reflex	Stimulus	Positive response	Gestation (in weeks) if reflex is:	
			Absent	Present
Pupil reaction	Light	Pupil contraction	<31	29 or more
Traction	Pull up by wrists from supine	Flexion of neck or arms	<36	33 or more
Glabellar tap	Tap on glabella	Blink	<34	32 or more
Neck righting	Rotation of head	Trunk follows	<37	34 or more
Head turning	Diffuse light from one side	Head turning to light	Doubtful	32 or more

Note: Twenty-nine weeks means 203 days after the first day of the last menstrual period. If there is a conflict between two results, the reflex placed higher in the table is more likely to give the true gestational age.
Source: Robinson RJ: *Arch Dis Child* 1966;41:437.

development of the hypertonic flexed posture that is characteristic of the full-term infant progresses in a caudocephalic direction, so that by 34 weeks a supine infant assumes the frog-leg position with the legs flexed at the hips and knee; the upper extremities are still hypotonic and extended. In general, measurement of the various body angles offers some objective evidence for the degree of tone. The popliteal angle measured by maximal extension of the leg at the knee with the hip fully flexed decreases from 180 degrees at 28 weeks to less than 90 degrees at term. Similarly, the adductor angle of the hip and dorsiflexion angle of the foot diminish to an angle approaching zero degrees at term. The so-called Scarf sign, obtained by drawing the arm medially across the chest towards the opposite shoulder, allows the elbow to reach the opposite shoulder in the smallest premature infant; in the full-term infant, however, the elbow barely approaches the midline. Additional evidence of muscle tone may be observed in various righting and posture reactions. When placed upright, the 28-week premature infant will not support his or her weight, the 34-week infant does so briefly several weeks later and then generally has a good supporting response. In the premature infant, profound muscle hypotonia allows the legs to be flexed passively toward the head (heel-to-ear maneuver), but the range of this maneuver is lessened in the older infant because of increased muscle tone. At 30 weeks the head exhibits a considerable amount of head lag. By 38 weeks the head follows the trunk, is maintained briefly, and then falls forward when the infant is pulled from a supine to a sitting position during the traction maneuver.

Primarily during the waking state but during sleep as well, the small premature infant exhibits a repetitive stretching movement of extremities; these movements tend to generalize to involve the head and trunk. Tremulousless and even clonic movements are prominent, but become increasingly rare after 32 weeks' gestation. The reflexes in the premature infant are weak, but become brisk and fully developed at 34 weeks. The

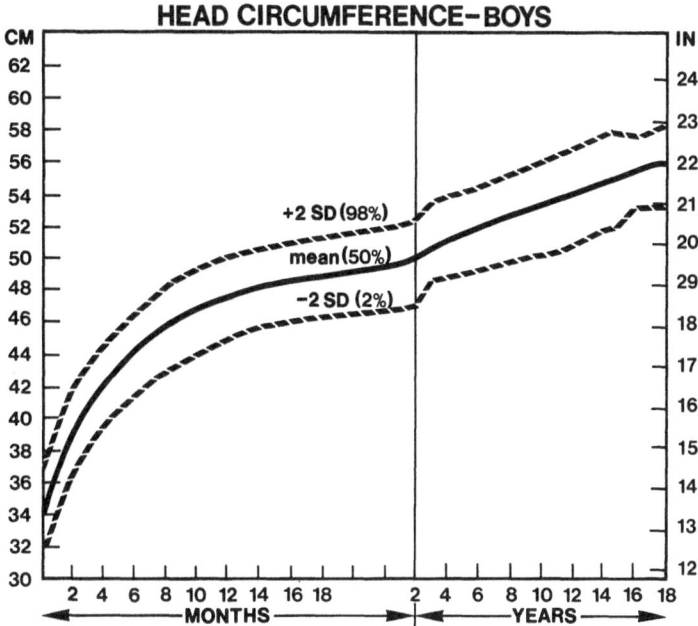

Figure 5.1. Head circumference (boys). (*Source:* Nellhaus G: Composite international and interracial graphs. *Pediatrics* 1968;41:106.)

grasp reflex is barely present at the fingers at 28 weeks, but by 36 weeks is strong. The Moro reflex is partially present at 24 weeks and is well developed by 28 weeks, although it fatigues easily. At 38 weeks the entire range of responses characteristic of the term infant may be observed (see Fig. 5.1).

Overall, the most valuable diagnostic tool remains the serial evaluation of the neurological status of the infant. From the neurological standpoint, it is noteworthy that when the short-gestation infant has reached the postnatal equivalent of term, the examination reveals findings that are quite different from those for a term infant.[11] The premature infant persists in toe-walking, not attaining the heel-toe progression of the term child. The reduced tone of the premature infant is maintained to some extent so that incomplete dorsiflexion of the foot and larger popliteal angle may persist.

Neurological Examination of the Term Infant

As with the premature infant, the initial portion of the examination of a term infant should include a general physical examination. Congenital abnormalities of the cranial vault, face, limbs, trunk, genitalia, spine, and skin are easily noticeable by the experienced and careful examiner. Special attention must be directed to midline defects of the spine, face, and palate. Alteration of skin pigmentation in the form of hyper- or hypopigmentation should be noted. Congenital vascular abnormalities, such as seen in infants with Sturge-Kalischer-Weber syndrome, should be noted. The shape of the head (dolicocephalic, brachycephalic, etc.) should be reported; molding of the head may obscure significant alterations in head shape that will not become apparent until some days later. The most common alteration of the head is caput succedaneum, which is an intrapartum edema of the scalp, not subperiosteal in that it crosses suture lines. Cephalohematomas represent subperiosteal bleeding and do not cross suture lines. Cephalohematomas are most commonly located in the parietal areas and, at times, may be bilateral. They are occasionally associated with an underlying fracture, but rarely with anemia and hyperbilirubinemia.[12]

Head size should be measured at the largest occipital-frontal circumference and plotted on the appropriate head circumference sheet (see Figs. 5.1 and 5.2). Length and weight charts should also be plotted. Usually there is a greater correlation between head circumference and length than between head circumference and weight. The 50th-percentile head circumference of the newborn male is 35 cm with an expected rate of growth

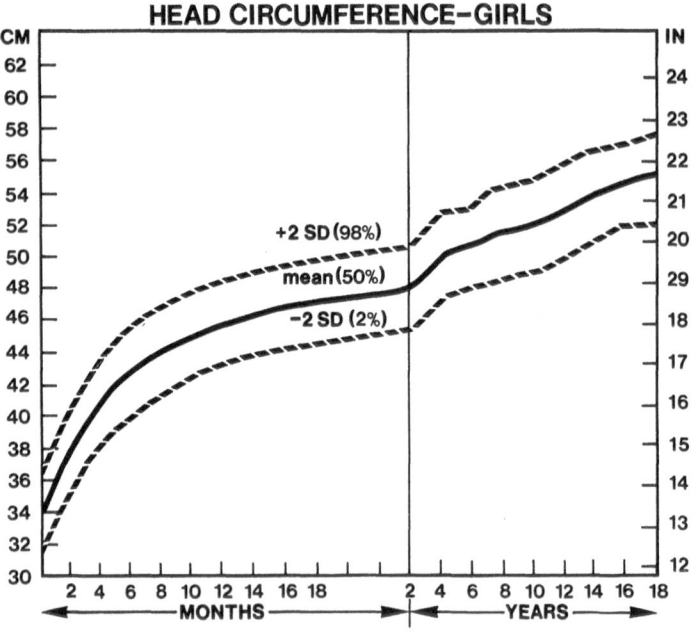

Figure 5.2. Head circumference (girls). (*Source:* Nellhaus G: Composite international and interracial graphs. *Pediatrics* 1968;41:106.)

of 2 cm per month for the first 3 months, 1 cm per month for the next 3 months, and 0.5 cm per month from the 6th through the 12th months.

The fontanel should be assessed for size, flatness, fullness, or tenseness. Examining for fullness of the fontanel is best done with the infant held quiet and in a sitting position. The examiner should palpate the sutures; absent suture separations are as significant as excessive spreading of the lines. Since molding may alter these parameters, a better estimate can be obtained after the first few days of life. Large fontanels and split sutures are usually a normal variant but can be associated with increased intracranial pressure (see Table 5.4). Small fontanels and overriding sutures are generally of little significance, but may be associated with conditions (such as microcephaly, in which volumetric delay in brain growth fails to stimulate growth of the skull. Cranial synostosis, either total or partial, should be considered and excluded by appropriate examination and tests. If a bruit is audible, persistent, and focal, an arteriovenous malformation should be considered, but very unlikely.

The infant's state of alertness should be noted, as it indicates mental status; this is accomplished partly by observing the infant and partly by direct physical examination. The newborn baby's cry should be vigorous and easily elicited. Abnormalities such as high-pitched, hoarse, cat-like (deletion of chromosome 5), or an unsustained or inability to cry, are indicators of probable neurological abnormalities. Muscle tone is evaluated by passive movements of various parts of the body, ideally with the infant awake and not crying. When muscle tone is being evaluated, it is important to have the child's head in a neutral position, since the tone may be altered by tonic neck reflexes.

The term infant assumes a flexed posture of both upper and lower extremities with a certain degree of resistance at the elbows and knees. Muscle tone should be symmetric. Reduced muscle tone with hypotonia

Table 5.4. Disorders in which large fontanel for age may be one feature.[22]

Types of disorders	
Skeletal disorders	Chromosomal abnormalities
Achondroplasia	Down's syndrome
Aminopterin-induced syndrome	13 Trisomy syndrome
Apert's syndrome	18 Trisomy syndrome
Cleidocranial dysostosis	Other conditions
Hypophosphatasia	Athyrotic hypothyroidism
Kenny's syndrome	Hallerman-Streiff syndrome
Osteogenesis imperfecta	Malnutrition
Pyknodysostosis	Progeria
Vitamin D deficiency rickets	Rubella syndrome
	Russell-Silver syndrome

Source: Popick G, Smith : Fontanels, range of normal size. *J Ped* 1972;80:749.

Table 5.5. Developmental reflexes.

Reflex	Appearance age	Disappearance age
Adductor spread of knee jerk	Birth	7 to 8 months
Moro	Birth	5 to 6 months
Palmar grasp	Birth	6 months
Plantar grasp	Birth	9 to 10 months
Rooting	Birth	3 months
Asymmetric tonic neck	Birth	5 to 6 months
Truncal incurvation	Birth	1 to 2 months
Parachute	8 to 9 months	Persists
Landau	10 months	24 months

and frog-leg position is abnormal but has no localizing value. Flaccidity is most often encountered in the comatose infant (but can also result from traumatic injury to the upper portions of the spinal cord), disease of the anterior horn cells, or abnormality of the neuromuscular juncture.

Neonatal reflexes are specific reflexes characteristic of certain periods of infancy (see Table 5.5). They are generally attributed to mechanisms at the brain stem level which may be provoked by appropriate stimuli because of the relative lack of cerebral inhibition.[18] Abnormalities of these reflexes are an asymmetrical response, absence of an expected response, and persistence of a reflex that should have disappeared. When testing the reflexes, the presence of symmetry as an indicator of normalcy is critical. Normal deep tendon reflexes are always symmetric. The knee jerk is often brisk in newborn, and generally is associated with adductor spread. Unsustained ankle clonus may normally be present. The plantar response may be either flexor or extensor. When eliciting plantar responses the examiner should take care that this maneuver does not interfere with the plantar grasp. It is important that the infant be awake and supine with the head in midline, legs extended either spontaneously or by the examiner, and the foot perpendicular to the leg. The stimulus is applied to the lateral plantar surface of the foot, beginning at the heel and moving toward the fifth toe. The movement of the great toe determines the response. If it dorsiflexes, the response is extensor; if the first movement is plantar flexion, the response is flexor. In 93% of normal infants, the response is dorsiflexion. The most important factor in the evaluation of the toe reflex is symmetry.[10]

Muscle tone of the trunk, the shoulder, and the pelvic girdle may be assessed by holding the child horizontal and in vertical suspension. Hypotonicity may become evident with the child in the inverted U posture, in horizontal suspension. Lack of shoulder girdle fixation is present if the child slides through the examiner's hands in vertical suspension (shoulder slip) or is unable to maintain an erect standing posture with the feet placed on the examining table.

The *Moro* (startle) reflex is the best known and can be elicited in a number of ways: most easily with the infant supine, allowing the lifted head to fall about 30° below the level of the trunk.[21] This maneuver results in adduction and extension of the arms, opening of the hands, and then adduction of the arms. This response diminishes steadily, disappearing by 4 months of age (later in prematurely born infants). Marked or persistent asymmetry of the response occurs with brachial plexus injuries, fractured clavicle, or hemiparesis. The palmar grasp response, present at birth, is symmetric and normally disappears by 2 to 4 months of age. The *asymmetric tonic neck response (ATN)* is elicited by rotation of the head around the vertically held body, and consists of extension of the extremity to which the face has been rotated and flexion of the contralateral upper extremity (fencing-soldier position). It may be elicited during the newborn period, peaks at 2 to 6 weeks, and disappears at 5 to 6 months of age, though extensive studies of the ATN employing electromyographic techniques have indicated that such a reflex may persist into later childhood and adult life in normal individuals.[21] The ATN, however, should never be sustained by enforcement. A normal infant should always be able to break the imposed reflex by struggling. The reflex may be unilaterally or bilaterally abnormal. The abnormality implies cerebral dysfunction that is usually greatest in the cerebral hemisphere opposite the direction to which the face is turned. This reflex is particularly useful in determining the presence of cerebral dysfunction in the hypotonic child in whom the site of the disease producing hypotonicity is unclear. The presence of a strong ATN also tends to mitigate against satisfactory sitting or standing balance. The *symmetric tonic neck* (Landau) reflex is elicited by holding the infant prone, in horizontal suspension. The examiner first flexes, and then extends the infant's head. With flexion of the head, the infant flexes the legs; with extension of the head it extends the legs. This reflex appears at 3 months and disappears by 24 months.[4] *Plantar grasp* reflexes are assessed by placing an object in the palm of the infant's hand, thusly eliciting flexion of the fingers in grasping of the object. Again, symmetry is the normal response. The involuntary grasp disappears at approximately 3 months, at which time it is replaced by voluntary, purposeful symmetric grasping, initially with a raking hand grasp and by 9 months with a clearly developed thumb-forefinger pincer grasp. The *placing* reflex is elicited by holding the infant in an upright position and bringing the dorsi of the infant's feet against the under edge of the table top. Upon contact the infant will briskly flex the legs at the hip and knees to terminate contact with the table. The *traction* response is elicited with the infant in a supine position. The examiner grasps the infant's hands and gently pulls him to a sitting position. With this maneuver, one notices head control; normally, the head lags as the infant assumes the sitting position and falls forward when the infant is upright.

By 3 to 4 months the infant should hold the head and trunk in a straight line, indicating good head control; also at about that time, the child should actively participate in sitting. A *parachute* response may be obtained in the infant at or beyond 9 months by holding the infant in horizontal suspension and then suddenly thrusting him in a head-first direction toward the floor or table top. The arms should immediately extend and adduct slightly. Again, symmetry should be present; asymmetry of the response is seen in infants with unilateral upper limb weakness or spasticity. Total lack of response is seen in severe quadriplegia.

The sensory examination of the term newborn begins with touch over the limbs. The infant's perception of touch is manifested by withdrawal or turning of the face and eyes toward the stimulated area. Pinpricks cause similar withdrawal or associated crying. The cranial nerves in the newborn can be examined by watching the infant. Facial asymmetry, either peripheral or central, can clearly be observed when the infant is crying. Care should be made not to mistake congenital hypoplasia of the depressor anguli oris muscle for facial nerve palsy. The depressor anguli oris muscle defect consists of a localized facial weakness in which the lower lip on one side fails to be depressed on crying, thereby causing asymmetry. Association of this defect with other anomalies has been reported, most commonly congenital heart defect.[3] Urinary anomalies have also been reported.[19]

The pupils of the newborn should be evaluated for light reaction. Extraocular movements can best be observed through the doll's eye maneuver or ocular vestibular response. Hearing can be assessed by ringing a bell or making a loud click in either ear. The movement of the tongue and masseter muscles can best be examined by watching the infant sucking; the rooting and tongue retrusion responses should also be noted. Finally, tongue fasciculation should be sought; this is best done when the infant is quiet.

Neurological Examination of the Infant and Young Child

Although the nervous system of the infant and young child functions according to the same principles as that of the older child and adult, the morphologic and physiologic immaturity of the infant's nervous system produces variations in the norms of clinical examination. Familiarity with the infant's development and the development of reflexes plays a major role in the examination (see Table 5.6). The evaluation should be of the mental status and motor development. Mental status is determined by evaluating visual and auditory alertness and awareness, social awareness, development of sounds and language, and the ability to understand and take directions. An 18-month-old child is able to identify body parts and use at least five or six single words. A 24-month-old child is expected to speak phrases and sentences. Attention should be paid to both receptive and expressive speech. A child normally sits in the tripod position at 7 to 8

Table 5.6. Child development from 2 months through 2 years.*

2 months
Keeps hands predominantly fisted
Lifts head up for several seconds while prone
Startles to loud noise
Follows with eyes and head over 90-degree arc
Smiles responsively
Begins to vocalize single-vowel sounds

3 month
Occasionally holds hands fisted
Lifts head up above body plane and holds position
Holds an object briefly when placed in hand
Turns head toward object, fixes and follows fully in all directions with eyes
Smiles and vocalizes when talked to
Watches own hands, stares at faces
Laughs

4 months
Holds head steady while in sitting position
Reaches for an object, grasps it, brings it to mouth
Turns head in direction of sound
Smiles spontaneously

5 to 6 months
Lifts head while supine
Rolls from prone to supine
Lifts head and chest up in prone position
Exhibits no head lag
Transfers object from hand to hand
Babbles
Sits with support
Localizes direction of sound

7 to 8 months
Sits in tripod fashion without support
Stands briefly with support
Bangs object on table
Reaches out for people
Mouths all objects
Says "da-da," "ba-ba"

9 to 10 months
Sits well without support, pulls self to sit
Stands holding on
Waves "bye-bye"
Drinks from cup with assistance

11 to 12 months
Walks with assistance
Uses pincer grasp
Uses two to four words with meaning
Creeps well
Assists in dressing
Understands a few simple commands

13 to 15 months
Walks by self—falls easily
Says several words, uses jargon
Scribbles with crayon
Points to things wanted

18 months
Climbs stairs with assistance, climbs up on chair
Throws ball
Builds two- to four-block tower
Feeds self
Takes off clothes
Points to two to three body parts
Uses many intelligible words

24 months
Runs, walks up and down stairs alone (both feet per step)
Speaks in two- to three-word sentences
Turns single pages of book
Builds four- to six-block tower
Kicks ball
Uses pronouns "you," "me," "I"

* Represents the age at which the average child acquires the skill.
Source: Data from Gesell A, Amatruda CS: *Developmental Diagnosis.* New York, Paul C. Hoeber, 1956; Illingworth RS: *The Development of the Infant and Young Child,* ed. 5. Baltimore, Williams & Wilkins Co, 1972.

months, crawls and pulls to a stand at 9 to 11 months, and begins to walk independently at 11 to 14 months. An 18-month-old infant climbs stairs with assistance and at 24 months walks up and down stairs alone. Hand preference is not present in the infant; therefore, if present it indicates focality, as does reflex asymmetry.

Normally the mental status of the infant and young child is at the same level as motor development and chronological age. The examiner has to make a judgment as to the significance of any degree of difference and should be able to localize abnormalities. The neurological examination should be a pleasurable experience for both the examiner and the child. The examiner should be flexible and should reserve the funduscopy, testing of the gag reflex, and painful stimuli to the very last.

References

1. Amiel-Tison C: Neurological evaluation of the maturity of the newborn infant. *Arch Dis Child* 1968;43:89.
2. Apgar V: A proposal for a new method of evaluation of the newborn infant. *Anesth Analg* 1953;32:260.
3. Cayler CG; Cardiofacial syndrome. *Arch Dis Child* 1969;44:69.
4. Cupps C, Plescia MG, Houser C. The Landau reaction: A clinical and electromyographic analysis. *Dev Med Child Neurol* 1976;18:41.
5. DeKaban A: *Neurology of Early Childhood.* Baltimore, Williams & Wilkins Co, 1970, pp. 50.
6. Dubowitz V, Whittaker, Brown BH, Robinson A: Nerve conduction velocity: An index of neurological maturity of the newborn infant. *Dev Med Child Neurol* 1968;10:741.
7. Fenichel GM: Neurological assessment of the 25–30 Week premature infant. *Ann Neur* 1978;4:92.
8. Friede RL: Developmental Neuropathology. New York, Springer-Verlag New York Inc, 1975.
9. Hack M, Mostow A, Miranda SB: Development of attention in preterm infants. *Pediatrics* 1976;58:669.
10. Hogan, Milligan: The plantar reflex of the newborn. *N Engl J Med* 1971;285:502.
11. Illingworth RS: *The Development of the Infant and Young Child,* ed. 5. Baltimore, Williams & Wilkins Co, 1972.
12. Kozinn, PJ, Ritz ND, Moss AH, Kaufman A: Massive hemorrhage in scalps of newborn infants. *Am J Dis Child* 1964;108:413.
13. MacDonald HM et al.: Neonatal asphyxia. *J Ped* 1980;96:898.
14. Nelson KB, Ellenberg JH: Children who outgrew cerebral palsy. *Pediatrics* 1982;69:529.
15. Nelson KB, Ellenberg JH: Neonatal signs as predictors of cerebral palsy. *Pediatrics* 1979;64:225.
16. Nelson KB, Eng GC: Congenital hypoplasia of the depressor anguli Oris muscle, differentiation from congenital facial palsy. *J Ped* 1972;81:16.
17. Menkes J: Neurologic evaluation of the newborn infant, in Schaffer's *Diseases of the Newborn,* ed 5. Philadelphia, WB Saunders Co, 1984.

18. Paine RS, Oppe TE: Neurologic examination of children. *Clin Dev Med* 1966;20:1.
19. Pape KE, Pickering D: Asymmetric crying facies, and index of other congenital anomalies. *J Ped* 1972;81:21.
20. Parmelee AH: A critical evaluation of the Moro reflex. *Pediatrics* 1964;33:773.
21. Parr C, Routh DK, Byrd, McMillan: A developmental study of the asymmetrical tonic neck reflex. *Dev Med Child Neurol* 1974;16:329.
22. Popick G, Smith: Fontanels, range of normal size. *J Ped* 1972:80:749.
23. Robinson R: Assessment of gestational age by neurological examination. *Arch Dis Child* 1966;41:437.
24. Robinson R: Cerebral functions in the newborn. *Dev Med Child Neurol* 1966;8:561.
25. Paine RS: Neurologic examination of infants and children. *Ped Clinics N Am* 1960;7:41.
26. Saint-Anne Dargassies S: Neurodevelopmental symptoms during the first year of life. *Dev Med Child Neurol* 1972;14:235.
27. Saint-Anne Dargassies S: La Maturation neurologique du prémature. *Etud Neonatal* 1955;4:71.
28. *Schaffer's Diseases of the Newborn*, ed 5. Philadelphia, WB Saunders Co, 1984.
29. Schulte, FJ, Michaelis R, Linke I, Nolte R: Motor nerve conduction velocity in term, preterm, and small-for-dates newborn infants *Ped* 1968;42:17.
30. Tooley WH, Phibbs RH, Schlueter MA: *Intra-uterine Asphyxia and the Developing Fetal Brain*. Chicago, Year Book Medical Publishers, Inc, 1977, pp 251–261.
31. Zelson D, Lee SJ, Pearl M: The incidence of skull fractures underlying cephalhematomas in newborn infants. *J Ped* 1974;85:371.

CHAPTER 6

Effects on Head Form of Intrauterine Compression and Passage Through the Birth Canal

Niels Sörensen

Introduction

During birth the infant's head is exposed to contractions of the uterine muscles and to intra-abdominal pressure. These mechanical influences are the cause of transitory physiological or enduring pathological changes on the skull. The exact effect of the uterus on the skull in utero is not fully understood. Studies on head molding during labor have been based mainly on x-rays.[4] Moloy concluded from x-rays taken as early as 1 hour after birth that the infant's head was usually not deformed during normal labor. He also observed, however, a dislocation of the parietal bones resulting from pelvic narrowness. Borell and Fernström[2,3] examined radiologically the deformation of heads in 27 newborn children during normal and pathological births, observing that skull deformaties differ according to the size of the pelvic opening. Therefore, the developmental dynamics of skull form at birth are a result of the relative volumes of the fetus' skull and the parturient's pelvis, relative to the birth presentation.

Occipito-Anterior Vertex Presentation

The infant's head changes its shape during the course of (a normal) birth, although the extent of the deformation varies. The parietal bones are pressed out from between the frontal and occipital bones. This causes the formation of a step between the coronal and lamdoid sutures. The parietal bones are symmetrically displaced so that no difference in level occurs within the region of the sagittal suture, no sheering force exerted upon the sagittal sinus or bridging cortical veins. Observations of overlapping skull bones have not been made in surviving infants. The trapezoidal form (broader superomedially than inferolaterally) of the parietal bones permits the frontal and occipital bones to approach one another as the parietal bones are displaced, so that they are not pressed underneath the parietal bones. The occipitofrontal diameter may thus be reduced 1 cm, facilitating passage through the birth canal.

Other deformations of the skull are clinically not as distinct as these. They are also difficult to observe radiologically. As the parietal bone is displaced toward the vertex, the *sutura lateralis* is enlarged. This may cause a difference in level between the bones that border this suture, with the parietal bones sliding beneath the temporal bones. The degree of deformation changes with the position of the head within the birth canal. It can be shown that the parietal bones are already displaced while the head is in the pelvic inlet. The greatest displacement of both parietal bones occurs in the upper part of the birth canal, however. As the head passes through the bony pelvis into soft tissue, the deformation decreases or disappears. Deformation recurs when the skull passes through the vulva and the muscular portion of the *introitus vaginae* compresses it.

Deflexion Presentation

The infant's head is characteristically deformed during brow or face presentation. The parietal bones are pressed inward relative to the frontal and occipital bones, opposite to what occurs in normal presentation. The brow presentation presents a smaller mentoparietal diameter to the bony and muscular pelvic outlets, thus facilitating passage and diminishing skull deformation. Likely, deformations are not caused by contact of the infant's head with the bony pelvis during its passage through the birth canal since significant deformities have been observed even in those instances when a distinct gap between the bony pelvis and the skull bones was observed.[6] In fact, displacement of the skull bones is especially prominent when the parturient has a hypertonic uterus and may be absent during weak uterine contractions. During contractions in the explusion period the external mechanical pressure on the skull bones and brain is greater than the pressure of growth, thereby causing deformation (configuration) that is reversed after birth (reconfiguration). In extrauterine life the pressures exerted by the brain determine skull form provided that no pathological brain or bone injuries are present. Configuration is more pronounced the longer the birth process and the more the neonatal skull differs from the usual spherical form. Thus, infants with dolichocephaly suffer especially severe configuration. In such cases the changes in sutures and fontanels are more distinct.

After normal birth, deformations are soon reversed. Reconfiguration may be demonstrated neuroradiologically within 4 days of an uncomplicated birth. Evidently, during this period, reconfiguration depends on an undamaged brain whose form is determined by turgor and growth and which transmits its shape to the skull through the dura capsule.[8] The sutures appear to widen as a result of mild postpartum cerebral edema, which disappears rapidly. Should deformation occur abruptly and be severe, intracranial bleeding may result from tearing of the falx cerebri and the tentorium cerebelli. Narrowness of the pelvis is not a *sine quo non* for this to occur.[5]

It has been suggested that during breech delivery, occipital osteodiastasis—an overriding of the squamous and lateral portions of the developing occipital bone—is caused by pressure from the *symphysis pubica* against the suboccipital region; however, this may also occur during forcible engagement of the head.[9]

Various nonlife-threatening pathologic changes may occur at the basicranium during passage through the birth canal. Injury to the basicranium may distort synchondroses; thus weakened during birth, the basicranium might progressively deform during neonatal life until fusion of the elements constituting the base of the skull occurs. In later life this may be detectable as basilar impression, atlantooccipital assimilation, or indentation of the occiput behind the foramen magnum, sometimes called nuchal impression.[1] Secondary suture fusion may be the result of birth trauma across the neonatal skull sutures.

As stated earlier, the above-mentioned studies on head molding during labor were based mainly on x-ray investigations. Increasing sophistication of ultrasonic techniques and computed axial tomography should provide more precise data on the physiologic and pathologic changes of the infant's head during the birth process.

References

1. Battersby R, Williams B: Birth Injury: A possible contributory factor in the aetiology of primary basilar impression. *J Neurol Neurosurg Psych* 1982;45:879–883.
2. Borell V, Fernström I: Die Umformung des kindlichen Kopfes bei engem Becken. *Geburtsh U Frauenheilk* 1958;18:1245–1256.
3. Borell V, Fernström I: Die Umformung des kindlichen Kopfes während normaler Entbindung in regelrechter Hinterhauptlage. *Geburtsh U Frauenheilk* 1958;18:1156–1166.
4. Henderson SG, Sherman LS: The roentgen anatomy of the skull in the newborn infant. *Radiology* 1946;46:107–118.
5. Holland E: Cranial stress in the foetus during labour and on the effects of excessive stress on the intracranial contents with an analysis of eighty-one cases of tentorium cerebelli and subdural cerebral haemorrhage. *J Obstet Gynec Brit Emp* 1922;29:549–571.
6. Lindgren L: The lower parts of the uterus during the first stage of labour in occipito-anterior vertex presentation. *Acta obstet gynec scand* 1955;2:7–79 (suppl).
7. Moloy HC: Studies on head molding during labor. *Amer J Obstet Gynec* 1942;44:762–782.
8. Müller D: *Die subakuten Massenverschiebungen des Gehirns unter der Geburt*. Leipzig, VEB Georg Thieme 1973.
9. Wigglesworth JS, Husemeyer RP: Intracranial birth trauma in vaginal breech delivery: The continued importance of injury to the occipital bone. *Br J Obstet Gyn* 1977;84:684–691.

CHAPTER 7

Traumatic Birth Injuries

Karl H. Hovind

Introduction

Birth trauma has been defined[55] as any condition that adversely affects the fetus during labor or delivery. Here, however, only the mechanical factors affecting the fetus during labor and delivery will be addressed. Although the obstetrician must cope with primary birth injuries, the actual problems of birth injuries should be considered the combined concern of both the obstetrician and the pediatrician. Infants who have sustained serious injury may experience permanent sequelae that, in turn, may be of concern to the pediatric neurologist, physiotherapist, psychologist, orthopedist, pediatric surgeon and neurosurgeon. The possibility of birth injury must be considered in the case of an obscure death of an infant during or shortly after delivery; medico-legal problems may then arise and need resolution.

In general, the physiopathology and dynamics of birth injuries have been sparingly discussed in the literature.[49] Various authors have focussed mainly on the concrete injury, its clinical aspects, and its sequelae. Perinatal craniocerebral injuries may be divided into two main groups:

1. Injuries that, because of their etiology and posttraumatic course, do not differ from those which may occur at any time during postnatal life (such as skin injuries, extracranial hemorrhages, fractures, neural damage). These injuries may be so moderate that complete recovery ensues, or so severe as to give rise to fatal complications.
2. Injuries that may occur after birth as well, but that give rise to structural or functional disturbances meriting special attention when occurring during birth (such as intracranial hemorrhages, plexus and nerve lesions, medullary injuries, hypoxia).

Historical Review

It was not until the beginning of the 19th century that attention was drawn to the fact that there might be a connection between head injuries occurring during delivery and pathological conditions of infancy. In ancient

Greek medicine, Hippocrates (460–377 B.C.) distinguished between epilepsy and infantile convulsions. Cerebral palsy was recognized long before it attracted the interest of the medical profession. Shakespeare (1564–1616) indicates the pathogenesis as well as the clinical aspects of cerebral palsy in his portrayal of King Richard III.[40] (It is a fact that this king was born prematurely in a foot presentation and that difficulties were involved in resuscitating the infant.)

Little (1819–1894), in 1843,[40] proposed that cerebral diplegia in children must be considered in relation to birth.[18] He considered prematurity and asphyxia as predisposing factors. Gowers (1888) fully supported Little's concept of cerebral palsy.[22] He reported a number of cases with the following etiology: first-born delivery, asphyxia, complicated (breech) delivery. Roberts (1925),[56] in his studies of the CSF, pointed out that the incidence of intracranial hemorrhage was directly proportional to the number of pathological labors; these were highest among premature infants. Salomonsen (1928)[58] emphasized that even a normal delivery represents a trauma to the infant: "The traumatic effects of labor upon the brain give rise to demonstrable lesions in such a large proportion of cases that it attains the character of a physical law." Ehrenfest (1931), in his extensive monograph,[14] found nystagmus in 35% of "normally" born infants and retinal hemorrhages in 12%. He considered these findings indicative of "physiological birth injuries."

Incidence of Perinatal Trauma

It is often impossible to distinguish between disorders caused by cardiovascular ischemic-hypoxic factors and those caused by perinatal trauma. (Ischemic-hypoxic lesions are beyond the scope of this chapter and will be discussed only briefly.) Consequently, it is difficult to estimate the frequency of actual traumatic injuries to the nervous system. One may conclude that in such injuries a combination of causes occur simultaneously.

A drastic reduction in traumatic lesions of the central and peripheral nervous system has occurred in industrialized countries during recent decades. This reduction is mainly due to improvements in diagnosis and management of complicated pregnancies. Another factor is the increased tendency of women to give birth to children in specialized clinics with access to modern obstetrical equipment. Still another contribution to the safety of the unborn child is the introduction of real-time ultrasound scanners for continuous recording of the condition of the fetus. As a result, Caesarean sections have become increasingly common.

Trauma nonetheless continues to be the predominant cause of about 2% of all neonatal mortality. Gresham[23] indicates that for every death due to birth trauma, at least 20 babies suffer a major birth injury.

Types of Perinatal Trauma

There are seven types of perinatal trauma, each with various subtypes. These are:

1. extracranial hemorrhage;
2. cranial fractures;
3. intracranial hemorrhage;
4. cerebral contusion;
5. cerebellar contusion;
6. medullary injury;
7. peripheral nerve injury.

These traumas are discussed in detail below.

Extracranial Hemorrhage (Fig. 7.1)

Caput Succedaneum

This type of edematous swelling of the skin, dense and loose connective tissue, and Galea is very common following vaginal delivery. It is caused by compression exerted mainly by the cervix. The edema is soft and superficial, does not involve the peristeum. No treatment is necessary, as the edema resolves in a few days.

Subgaleal Hemorrhage (Fig. 7.2)

This lesion is much less common than the caput succedaneum. The hemorrhage is beneath the aponeurosis (Galea), peripheral to the periosteum. Coagulapathies may be present, so emergency coagulation and bleeding studies should be performed. The lesion frequently enlarges after birth and presents itself as a fluctuant, firm mass. The blood is liquid, and

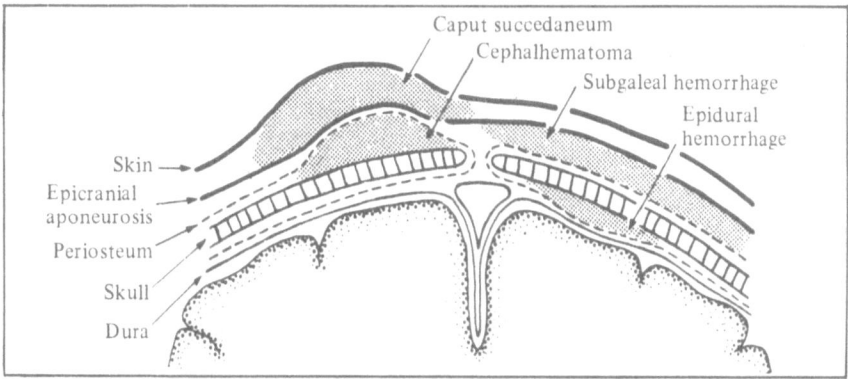

Figure 7.1. Various locations where traumatic hemorrhages occur in the newborn.

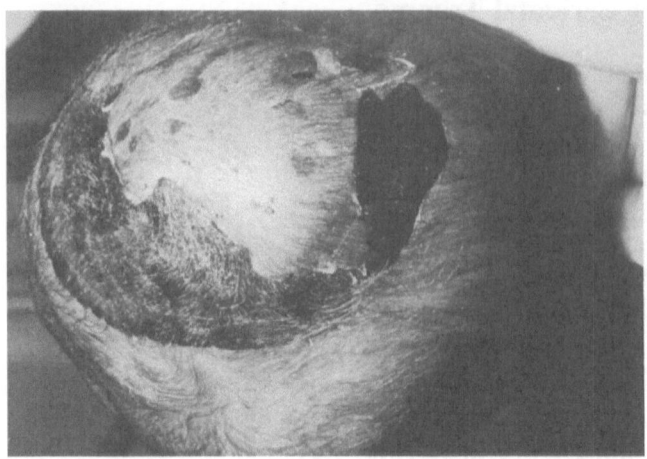

Figure 7.2. Skin lesion in a full-term infant delivered by vacuum extractor.

aspiration is frequently necessary. The procedure is easily performed under local anesthesia after the area has been shaved. Aspiration must be done with all necessary surgical asepsis. Following aspiration a compressive dressing is applied. Blood transfusion may be necessary since the subgaleal space is large. Repeated aspirations may occasionally be necessary.

Cephalohematoma

Incidence

Cephalohematoma is confined to the space between the outer table of the skull and the periosteum, and is located between the cranial sutures. It is present in from 1% to 2% of "normal" deliveries. Years ago, when midforcep deliveries were common, the incidence of cephalohematoma was higher. Midforceps are rarely used in modern obstetrical practice; thus, the incidence of cephalohematoma is decreasing.

Pathology

The hemorrhage in cephalohematoma is subperiosteal, which explains why the hematoma is confined by the sutures. Most hematomas are unilateral and located over the parietal bone. From 10% to 25% of the cases are caused by an underlying skull fracture.

Pathogenesis

Both skull fracture and stripping of the periosteum from the underlying skull result from the crushing and sheering forces that uterine compression and squeezing of the skull within the pelvic outlet cause.

Clinical Features

The lesion presents as a tense, firm mass after birth, frequently enlarging during the first few days. Along the margin of the lesion, the elevated periostium can be palpated by the finger as a ridge with a recessed center, a configuration that is often mistaken for a depressed skull fracture. From a neurosurgical point of view, cephalohematoma is rarely of clinical importance unless an intracranial complicating lesion is present. Infected cephalohematomas and mengigitis are extremely rare. Usually, cephalohematomas resolve in a few weeks. Calcifications may occur, but they gradually disappear over several months.

Management

In most cases no treatment is necessary. In rare cases aspiration is indicated. This procedure is performed in the same way as with subgaleal hematomas.

Skull Fractures

There are three different types of skull fractures: (1) linear, (2) depressed, and (3) occipital osteodiastasis.

Linear Fractures

Incidence

Linear fractures are most commonly located in the parietal bones. The identification of this type of fracture depends on the frequency of x-ray examination.[27] Even with a picture of good quality, a linear fracture may not be detected in about 20% of the cases examined. Consequently, it is very difficult to determine precisely the incidence. Gresham mentions a rate of about 10%.[23]

Pathology and Pathogenesis

Associated lesions may be cephalohematoma, epidural hematoma, subdural hematoma, dural tears, and cerebral contusion. Except for cephalohematomas, the other lesions are rare. Linear fractures are all of traumatic origin.

Management

Linear fractures are of no clinical importance and no therapy is indicated except if any of the above-mentioned associated lesions are present.

Depressed Fractures

These fractures are commonly referred to as "ping-pong ball" lesions. They may be compared to a "green-stick" fracture of the long bones, as there is no loss of continuity. Actually, the depressed fracture is not a real fracture but an inward buckling of the unusually soft bone. Little has been written about the incidence of depressed fractures among a random group of deliveries, although one per thousand seems to be a reasonable figure.

The parietal bone is the most common site for this lesion, followed by the frontal bone. Associated lesions are extremely rare. This "ping-pong ball" fracture is caused by a compressing force on the skull, such as forceps, the thumb, or the pressure of the head against pelvic structures during delivery.

Management

Little is known about spontaneous elevation or the natural course of this fracture. Recently, there have been reports of elevation by vacuum extractor,[65] breast pump,[59] and digital pressure.[41] The use of a vacuum extractor is not without danger and is not recommended. When neurosurgical expertise is available and digital compression or breast pumping has been unsuccessful, operative elevation should be undertaken.[46] This is easily done under local anesthesia after a small area over the nearest suture line has been shaved. An incision of 1 cm in the skin down to the bone exposes the suture. A sharp periostal elevator is then gently introduced under the bone. The tip of the elevator is moved toward the center of the fracture; the impression is then easily elevated, but the surgeon must take care not to use the edge of the skull as a fulcrum lest he extend the depression.

Occipital Osteodiastasis

This lesion consists of a separation of the squamous and basal portions of the occipital bone. It may result in tentorial laceration, posterior fossa epidural hematoma,[64] cerebellar contusion, or medullary compression. Prior to the use of the CT scan, this lesion was detected only postmortem.

Intracranial Hemorrhages

Epidural Hemorrhage

This hemorrhage occurs between the dura and the periosteum on the inner side of the bone. The lesion is rare in neonates.[63] According to autopsy reports only about 2% of neonatal intracranial hemorrhages are epidural hematoma. The source of bleeding is one of the branches from the middle meningeal artery, a major venous sinus, or the diploe secondary to skull fracture. Linear skull fracture is usually present. If an infant, after experiencing a difficult labor or delivery, is eventually delivered by forceps or vacuum extractor and presents signs of increased intracranial pressure (bulging fontanels or separation of the sutures), an epidural he-

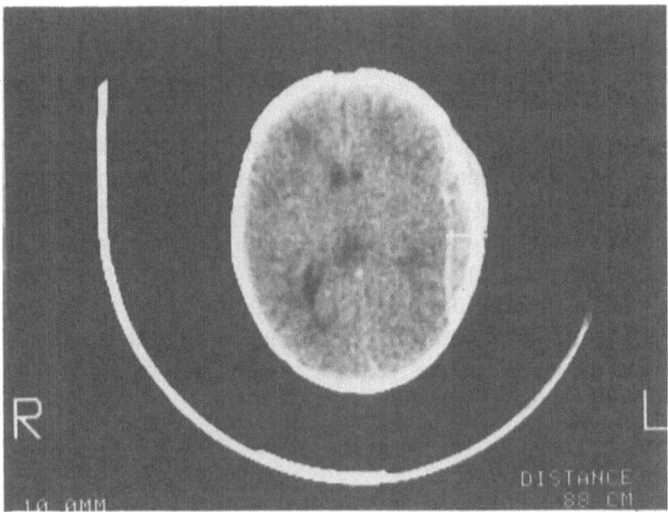

Figure 7.3. Acute subdural hematoma on the left side, 10 days following delivery by vacuum extraction.

matoma should be suspected. An emergency CT scan should be performed, followed by operation as soon as the diagnosis has been established.

Subdural Hemorrhage (Fig. 7.3)

Because therapeutic intervention may be necessary, it is important to diagnose subdural hemorrhage.[50] This type of hemorrhage is almost exclusively caused by rupture of the veins: the transverse sinus, the straight sinus, vein of Galen, occipital sinus, inferior sagittal sinus, or superficial cerebral veins. Cerebral contusion is a frequent finding along with subdural hemorrhage. Infratentorial hemorrhage is predominantly caused by tentorial laceration or occipital osteodiastasis. The clot may very rapidly result in lethal compression of the brain stem.

Pathogenesis

Subdural hemorrhage in the newborn is always a traumatic lesion. The percentages of full-term babies and premature infants with subdural hemorrhage are now approximately similar. The hemorrhage may occur when there is cephalopelvic disproportion, in premature infants whose skulls are particularly compliant, and in primiparous and older multiparous women whose labor is unusually long or precipitous. Additional causes are brow or face presentations, breech deliveries, rotational maneuvers, or forcep/vacuum extractions. Fortunately, improved obstetrical practise has reduced the incidence of subdural hemorrhage; it is now an uncommon lesion.

Clinical Diagnosis

The symptoms and signs depend upon the location and extent of the hemorrhage. Irritability may be the only symptom of a minor hemorrhage. Nuchal rigidity and opisthotonus, followed by bradycardia, pupil dilatation, respiratory failure, and finally cardiac arrest, may follow a massive infratentorial hemorrhage.

CT scan and real-time sonography are definite means of diagnosing the extent and severity of subdural hemorrhage. Subdural taps may be performed when these modes of investigation are not available. Skull x-rays rarely give additional information.

Prognosis

The prognosis is exclusively dependent upon the location and extent of the hemorrhage. With smaller posterior fossa hematomas, early diagnosis followed by craniotomy and evacuation of the clot has improved the outcome. The prognosis with convexity subdural hemorrhage is relatively good. All infants who have survived must be closely observed in the following months, preferably with CT or ultrasonography in order to detect hydrocephalus.

Subarachnoid Hemorrhage

Primary subarachnoid hemorrhage refers to blood in the subarachnoid space, which is not an extension from a subdural, intracerebral, or intraventricular hemorrhage, nor from vascular anomalies. Such hemorrhage is very common in premature infants.[56,57,62] There is a close correlation between bloody CSF in the newborn and retinal hemorrhage. Thus, extensive retinal hemorrhage generally indicates severe subarachoid hemorrhage. According to Volpe,[69] the frequency of periventricular and intraventricular hemorrhage is much higher than that of the primary subarachnoid hemorrhage. In infants weighing less than 2000 g, Volpe's findings were 63% versus 29%, respectively.

The source of bleeding in primary subarachnoid hemorrhage is presumably venous—that is, bridging veins within the subarachnoid space or small vessels in the meningeal plexus. Complications from primary subarachnoid hemorrhage in the newborn are difficult to identify, except for hydrocephalus. Adhesions around the cisterna magna and the IV ventricle may result in an obstruction to CSF circulation. Adhesions over the cerebral convexities may also impair CSF absorption or flow.

Late sequelae from primary subarachnoid hemorrhage are extremely difficult to prove. There is, however, some indication that children who sustain such hemorrhages have a higher incidence of pathological EEG,

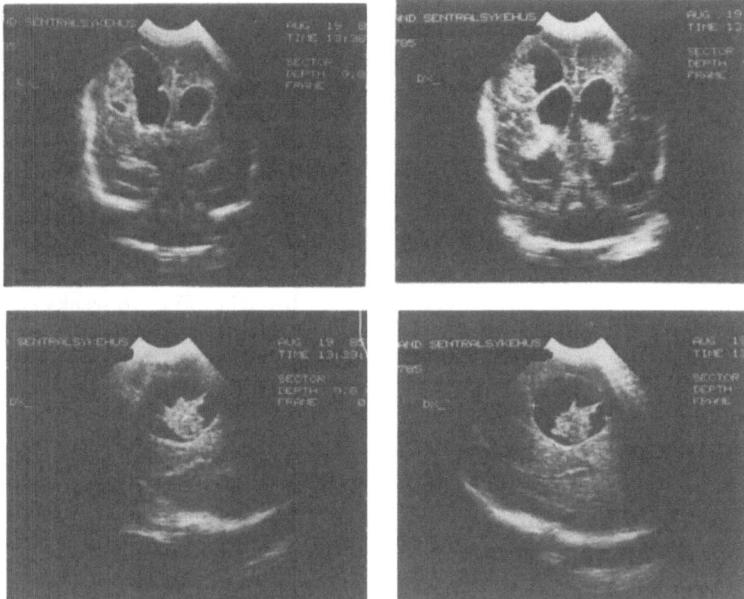

Figure 7.4. Trans-fontanel serial ultrasonic scans, 3 weeks post-partum. Birth weight 1830 g, 10 weeks premature. A porencephalic cavity with a clot is visualized, communicating with the right lateral ventricle. The lateral ventricles are enlarged. Blood may be seen along the floor of the ventricles.

lower school performances, and higher incidence of minimal brain dysfunction. From an intellectual point of view, it is difficult to accept that even a small subarachnoid hemorrhage is of no importance for the growing brain, particularly for immature or premature infants. No extensive reports have been published in this field so far, however.

Intraventricular Hemorrhage (Figs. 7.4 and 7.5)

Subependymal and intraventricular hemorrhages are caused mainly by hypoxic/ischemic factors.[4,10,31] Before the introduction of CT and sonar scans, information about the extent and incidence of intracranial hemorrhage was obtainable only through postmortem examination.[32] With modern real-time ultrasonography, information concerning cerebral blood flow has been greatly improved.[72] These sonar investigations are noninvasive and without side effects.[25,31]

Disturbances of autoregulation in asphyxic premature infants is of importance in understanding the pathogenesis of intraventricular hemorrhage. The anatomical factors in the pathogenesis of subependymal/intraventricular hemorrhage now seem more clear. The localization of the

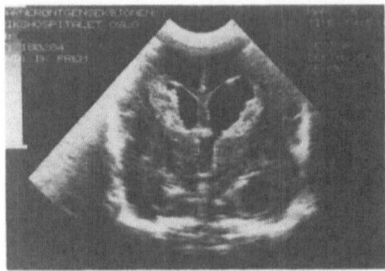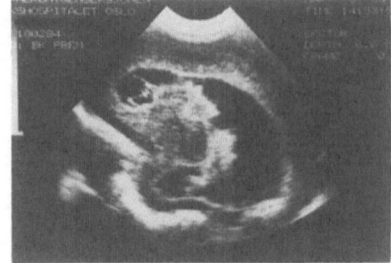

Figure 7.5. Transfontanel serial sonar scans. Birthweight 875 g, 16 weeks premature. Coronal and sagittal scans. Extensive subependymal hemorrhage penetrates the ventricles. The lateral ventricles are enlarged.

hemorrhage is dependent upon the brain's degree of development. During the first 24 to 32 weeks of gestation, the function of the basal ganglia, midbrain, and brain stem has developed. There are many newly formed vessels in this part of the brain. The capillaries and veins here are very fragile, so that the hemorrhage occurs within this subependymal germinal matrix network. In infants of less than 28 weeks' gestation the hemorrhage usually starts below the head of the caudate nucleus and the thalamus. After 32 weeks, subependymal/intraventricular hemorrhages are relatively rare.[62] Hemorrhage in cortical and white matter increases with the length of gestation.

The disturbance of hemodynamics in the cerebral vessels is of utmost importance in the pathogenesis of ventricular hemorrhage in premature infants.[19] Normally, the cerebral blood flow is essentially independent of arterial pressure.[26,29] This vascular autoregulation is disturbed in premature infants, however.[43,47] A sudden increase in arterial blood pressure may lead to a rupture of the fragile capillaries in the germinal matrix. Especially important is perinatal asphyxia, which can lead to hypoxia, hypercapnia, and acidosis. Depressed autoregulation will finally produce cerebral vascular dilation. Increased cerebral perfusion leads to rupture of the vessels.[4,61] In contrast, decreased venous return may induce an increase of the central venous pressure. This in turn increases cerebral perfusion pressure, thereby causing venous stasis, followed by rupture of vessels.

All of those factors which may disturb cerebral perfusion can induce intracerebral hemorrhage in the premature infant: soft cranial bones, traumatic delivery, asphyxia, hypertension, hypotonia, apnea, patent ductus arteriosus, hypoxia, hypercapnia, fast expansion of volume, respiratory disturbance, rupture of pulmonary alveoli, or careless transport and handling of the baby. About 50% of infants with a gestational age of 30 weeks or less have intracerebral hemorrhage.[12] The incidence decreases after 30 weeks of gestation. The reason for this is possibly the maturing of the vascular system and better autoregulation. Hemorrhaging takes place in about 80% of infants within 72 hours following delivery. Later hemorrhages are generally rare.

A frequent complication following hemorrhage is posthemorrhagic hydrocephalus.[35,36,42,48,71] Sonographical investigations[25] have shown the following (Fig. 7.6):

1. transitory hydrocephalus;
2. persistant but not progressive hydrocephalus;
3. persistant, fast, and progressive hydrocephalus;
4. cerebral atrophy.

Sonography has further shown that the hydrocephalic process starts about 2 weeks after the hemorrhage. It is important to realize that the process starts about 2 weeks before a pathological increase of the head circumference can be measured. Sonographically, posthemorrhagic hydrocephalus can be visualized while the head circumference still follows the normal curve.

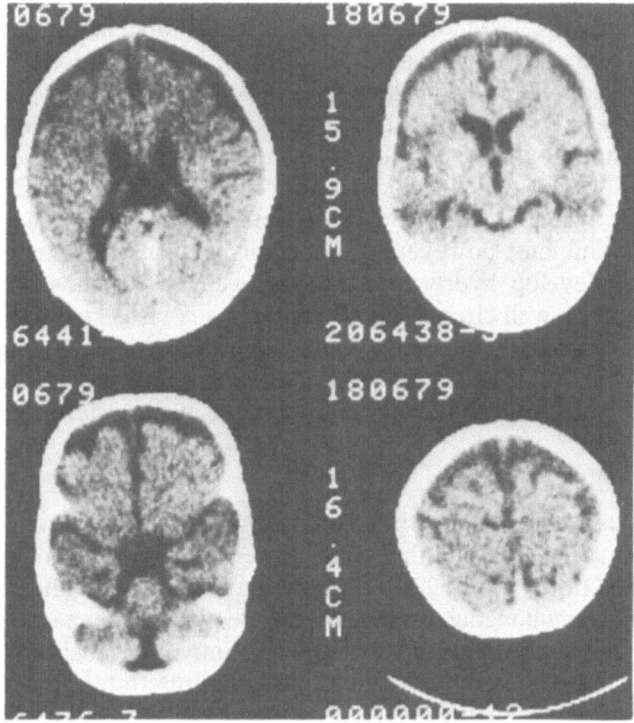

Figure 7.6. Three-month-old infant with an enlarging head. Collection of fluid in the subarachnoid space and cisterns. Previously such a picture was diagnosed as "subdural effusion." The pathology is due to defective resorption of the CSF.

A typical lesion found in the immature brain is caused by hypoxia/ ischemia in the periventricular areas.[52,53,54] Hypoperfusion starts this process. Secondarily, hemorrhagic infarctions are formed, which later may be transformed into cysts and porencephalic cavities. Such lesions close to the ventricles affect the pyramidal tracts in the internal capsule, resulting in a spastic diplegia.

Intracerebellar Hemorrhage

This lesion is a relatively common postmortem finding in premature babies. Recent reports indicate an increasing frequency of such findings in modern neonatal intensive care units. The reason for this seems to be the active attitude toward treatment of low birthweight premature infants. The neuropathology and pathogenesis is very similar to those for cerebral hemorrhage and there seems to be a strong correlation between intraventricular hemorrhage and cerebellar hemorrhage. As pointed out by Donal et al., this indicates that there is a secondary extension of blood through the aqueduct into the IV ventricle, with secondary dissection into the cerebellum.

Clinically, there is a strong association between respiratory distress and perinatal asphyxia. The most consistent signs are rapid deterioration with bradycardia, apnea, hemorrhagic CSF, and falling hematocrit.

The suspicion of cerebellar hemorrhage is essential for proper diagnosis. A premature infant with brain stem dysfunction and bloody CSF should promptly be referred for a CT scan. The possibility of cerebellar herniation always exists when spinal taps are performed. If a CT scan is immediately available, the spinal tap is better deferred. The prognosis is usually very dubious, however. Some infants who survive intracerebellar hemorrhage develop hydrocephalus. Management depends on the CT scan finding. If a well circumscribed hematoma is visualized on the scan, an emergency suboccipital craniotomy with evacuation of the clot should be performed. Conditions that argue against operation are associated cerebral lesions, serious pulmonary disorders, or other systemic disorders.

Cerebral Contusion

This lesion consists of hemorrhage and necrosis of the cortex and subcortical white matter. Tears in the white matter may extend into the cortex and the walls of the ventricles. Subdural and subarachnoid hemorrhages are frequent simultaneous findings. Prior to the CT scan and ultrasonography, cerebral contusion was only a tentative diagnosis based upon history and clinical symptoms and signs: seizures (often focal), monoparesis, hemiparesis, irritability, and a bulging fontanel. All children with such symptoms should be referred for a CT scan.

The incidence rate for cerebral contusion is unknown; presumably, it is a relatively rare lesion. There is no specific therapy for this perinatal trauma.

Cerebellar Contusion

This lesion is often found with occipital osteodiastasis. The pathogenesis and pathology are very similar to those of cerebral contusions.

Treatment with serial lumbar punctures in order to stop posthemorrhagic ventricular dilation has been recommended. The beneficial effect is the acceleration of CSF absorption by removal of protein and blood, in addition to the reduction of CSF pressure. It is still unclear whether this procedure is really effective, however; controlled studies have to be performed. In addition to serial lumbar taps, drugs that decrease CSF production (e.g., furosemide, acetazolamide, digitoxin, glycerol, and isosorbide) may be used.

Compressive head wrapping to arrest progressive hydrocephalus has been recommended in young infants, particularly when associated with myelomeningocele and Chiari II malformation.[15] Because the premature infant in particular has a very compliant skull, cranial distortion may lead to severe hemodynamic alterations. The possibility of provoking an extension of hemorrhage or lesions is significant; consequently, this treatment is not recommended.

Medullary Injury

Most cases of spinal cord injury are due to excessive lateral or longitudinal traction, or torsion of the spine during delivery.[7,8,17,20,23,39] A few cases of medullary lesions sustained in utero have been reported. Such occurrences are, however, quite rare.

Incidence

The real rate of incidence of medullary injury is difficult to determine, as the spinal cord is rarely examined at autopsy. Towbin[67] states that about 10% of neonatal deaths are caused by spinal cord injuries. In an old report Pierson found intraspinal hemorrhages in 46% of infants examined postmortem following breech delivery. Breech delivery is associated with about 75% of recognized neonatal spinal injuries.[1,5,6,7] The sites of the lesions with breech delivery are the lower cervical and upper thoracic regions. With extreme forcep rotation the lesion occurs in the upper- to midcervical region; it occurs principally with cephalic deliveries.

Pathogenesis

The bony spinal column in the newborn is entirely cartilaginous and very elastic. The muscles are rather hypotonic; in addition, tonus may be depressed by anesthesia or drugs. The spinal cord is anchored above by the medulla and the roots of the brachial plexus, and below by the cauda equina. The cord is the least elastic structure and will rupture at the site of the anchoring—that is, in the lower cervical and upper thoracic regions. Acute lesions are epidural and intramedullary hemorrhages and sometimes laceration of the dura. Vertebral fractures and dislocations are rare. Repeated x-ray investigation may eventually disclose calcifications indicating a previous fracture, subluxation, or dislocation.

Chronic lesions are fibrotic adhesions or focal necrotic areas in the cord with cystic cavities. The latter eventually lead to ischemic infraction of the caudal cord segments.

Clinical Features

There are three clinical syndromes: (1) stillbirth or rapid neonatal death, (2) severe respiratory failure, and (3) varying neonatal neurological deficits. In a lower cervical lesion the neurological deficits are apparent in the first hours after delivery. There is paraplegia of the lower extremities and varying involvement of the upper extremities. The sensory level is at C-7 or T-2. Respiration is diaphragmatic with paradoxial respiratory movements, the abdomen is often bulging with distended urinary bladder, the anal sphincter is atonic. Horner's syndrome is occasionally present.

Therapy

From a surgical point of view, little is to be expected in treating this traumatic injury. Occasionally, a metrizamide myelogram is indicated. If an extradural expansion is diagnosed, laminectomy might be beneficial. A few infants with spinal cord transection at birth recover astonishingly well. By and large, however, conservatism seems justified, and treatment is expected to be mainly supportive. In order to establish the level of the lesion, somatosensory evoked potentials may be helpful in proving complete motor and sensory paralysis.

Prevention is most important. The majority of neonatal spinal cord lesions are associated with breech deliveries.[66] Patients permitted to deliver vaginally must be selected extremely carefully. As soon as a breech position is diagnosed and a turning of the fetus is unsuccessful, a Caesarian section must be seriously considered. It is fair to say that breech deliveries have no place in modern obstetrics.

Prognosis

Three clinical groups with different outcomes as a result of medullary injury can be distinguished:

1. stillbirths or infants who die rapidly because of high cervical or brainstem lesion;
2. infants who die within the first year of life mostly because of respiratory complications;
3. infants who survive; these children can be rehabilitated and will be able to live independently. The relative number in this group has increased during the last few decades.

Peripheral Nerve Injuries

Brachial Plexus

The brachial plexus consists of cervical roots 5–8 (C5–8) and the thoracic root 1 (T-1). Lesions of these roots cause varying degrees of weakness in the innervated muscles. Incidence is in the range of 5 to 10 per 10,000 live births; hence this lesion is at least 10 times more common than lesions of the spinal cord.

Pathology

In 1872 Duchenne[13] ascribed medullary injury to manipulation at delivery. Almost simultaneously, Erb[3] described the lesion in adults. The most frequently traumatized roots of the plexus are the C5–C6; the exit of these roots in the supraclavicular region is called Erb's point.

In 1885 Madame Déjérine-Klumpke[13] was the first to associate pupillary changes on the affected side with the lesion of the C8 and T1 nerve root. In less severe lesions there is hemorrhage and edema of the nerves because of tears of the nerve sheath. In more severe cases a complete avulsion of the root from the cord is present.

Pathogenesis

Injury to the brachial plexus results from overstretching of the nerves, usually because of extreme lateral traction. In breech delivery this may occur when the head is delivered; in cephalic deliveries, when the shoulder is luxated free. The most vulnerable part of the plexus are the upper roots. Brachial plexus lesions are found mainly in large infants with fetal depression and with abnormal labor and delivery. Involvement of the proximal upper limb, Erb's palsy, counts for about 90% of brachial plexus lesions.

Total brachial plexus injury is usually termed Klumpke's palsy. This extensive lesion will cause a Horner syndrome—that is, ptosis and miosis—because the sympathetic branches coming from T-1 are affected. Another manifestation of sympathetic affection is that the pigment formation in the iris is disturbed; thus, the eye will remain blue for months or years.

Neurological Features

Muscle function, tendon reflexes, and sensory disturbances are affected according to the severity of the lesion. Usually, motor deficits are more striking than sensory deficits. A more detailed description of the neurological deficits of proximal brachial palsy, total brachial plexus palsy, and reflex abnormalities can be found in Volpe's extensive monography.[68]

Prognosis

The prognosis obviously depends on the severity of the lesion. According to Gordon et al.,[21] 88% of infants studied were normal when examined at 4 months, 92% were normal at 12 months, and 93% were normal at 4 years. Specht[60] is even more optimistic: In his review of more than 19,000 live births, all 11 cases recovered completely. Wickstrom[70] stressed that it is difficult, if not impossible, to estimate the prognosis with any degree of accuracy except for the known poor return of function in those patients with Horner's syndrome or loss of thoracoscapular muscle power, and most of those patients exhibited marked sensory changes. Eng[13] found the electromyogram to be extremely useful in topographically delineating the extent and severity of the injury. It provides a baseline for later prognostication.

Management

Prevention is the best treatment. Caeserean section is recommended in the presence of abnormal presentations, especially when the fetus is large. Conservative use of maternal drugs to avoid fetal depression is also important. Therapy of the affected child should be directed toward prevention of development of contractures.

Facial Nerve Injury

Facial paralysis refers to weakness of the facial muscles and indicates injury to the facial nerve—that is, involvement of the muscles of the upper as well as lower face.

Incidence

Injury to the facial nerve is the most common manifestation of birth trauma.[45] According to Hepner,[28] the incidence rate was 6.4% when the child was examined on the second day of life. There was no difference in incidence for children delivered manually versus by forceps.

Pathology

In view of the favorable prognosis it is likely that edema or hemorrhage into the nerve sheath are present. The site of the lesion is at the exit of the nerve from the stylomastoid foramen, where the nerve divides into its two major branches: the temporofacial and the cervicofacial nerves.

Pathogenesis

Hepner's work presents strong evidence that intrauterine pressure of the sacral promonotorium on the facial nerve is the cause of the injury. In each of his 56 cases of facial paralysis, there was a direct correlation between the affected side of the face and the position of the head in utero.

Cases associated with midforcep or high-forcep extraction are characterized by marked facial weakness, in contrast to natural delivery and outlet
or low-forcep extractions where facial weakness is usually mild. In Rubin's study[57] all but two of 21 facial nerve injuries were associated with
delivery by forceps.

Clinical Syndrome

About 75% of cases of facial nerve injury are the left side. This, perhaps,
reflects the most common obstetrical position: occiput left transverse or
anterior. When the infant is resting, the palpebral fissure is wide and the
nasolabial fold is flattened. The child is unable to wrinkle the brow and
close the eye firmly.

Prognosis

The prognosis is usually excellent. Most children recover within a few
weeks. A sequela may be contracture and synkinesis, which is unusual.

Treatment

It is important to protect the cornea to prevent injury. Eyedrops during
the day and ointment at night are routine. Taping of the involved eye in
this age group involves the danger of corneal ulceration if the tape slides.

Median Nerve Injury

Injury to the median nerve occurs mainly at two sites: the wrist and the
cubital fossa. At those places the radial and brachial arteries pass close to
the nerve. The two arteries are frequently used for sampling arterial
blood, particularly in the premature infant. The nerve could easily be
pierced by a needle aimed at the brachial or radial artery[51] pulsation.
Another and more likely explanation, however, is related to the extrava-
sation of blood, following the puncture of the artery,[34] into a relatively
enclosed space, thereby causing compression of the median nerve or its
blood supply. Puncture of the brachial and radial arteries should definitely
be avoided, particularly in very small infants.

Radial Nerve Injury

The radial nerve may be injured in association with fracture of the hu-
merus, which may occur with overzealous forceps extractions.[16,38] Clinically, the extensors of the fingers, wrist, and thumb are affected. Therapy
is directed toward preventing the development of contractures.

Laryngeal Nerve Injury

Injury to the laryngeal nerve may occur when the head is in an abnormal
position in the uterus, such as slightly flexed and rotated laterally.[9] This

causes the thyroid cartilage to compress the superior branch of the laryngeal nerve against the hyoid bone above, which in turn results in difficulties of swallowing or vocal cord closure and resulting dyspnea. If lateral flexion of the neck is severe, the phrenic nerve may be injured, and paresis of the diaphragm may occur.[2] The treatment is symptomatic, and recovery usually occurs within a year.

Conclusions

The frequency of birth injuries has steadily diminished in the industrialized world during the last decades. There are several reasons for this. Most deliveries today take place in highly specialized clinics where midwives, gynecologists, anesthetists, laboratory personnel, and pediatricians are available, 24 hours a day. Continuous surveillance of the mother and fetus during the delivery is mandatory. If any life-threatening complication to the child should occur, a Caesarean section is performed within minutes. As a consequence of this an increasing number of children are delivered by Caesarean section today.

The frequency of birth injuries is much higher with breech deliveries. A Caesarean section should be performed if a breech position is diagnosed shortly before the expected delivery. Delivery by vacuum extractor became popular following Malmström's work and publications from 1952,[11,24,44] particularly in northern Europe. From a teleological point of

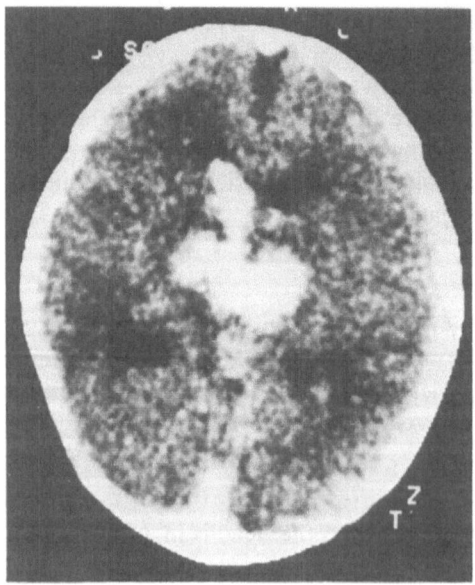

Figure 7.7. Severe intracerebral hemorrhage in a full-term infant delivered by vacuum-extractor.

Figure 7.8. The same child as seen in Figure 7.7, at an age of 4 m. Severe hydrocephalus is present.

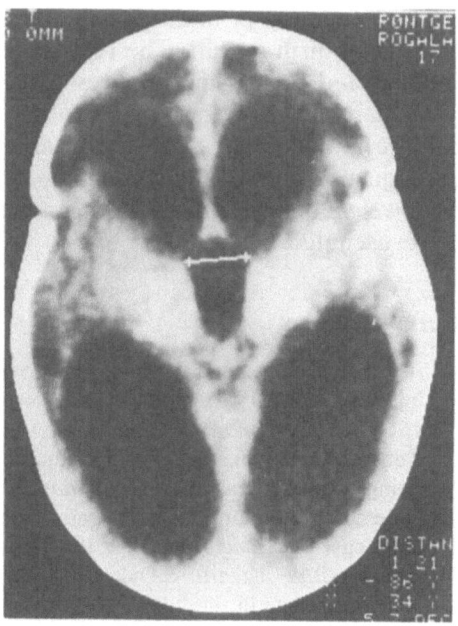

view, it is difficult to accept that the application of such a strong sucking and dragging force to the child's head will leave the underlying brain unharmed. Unfortunately, no extensive investigation has been published to prove this statement. However, it is the author's opinion that the vacuum extractor should be abandoned in modern obstetrics (Figs. 7.7, 7.8).

During the last 10 years an increasing number of units, specializing in the care of premature babies, and examination of all pregnant women with ultrasound in the 20th, 30th, and 38th week of gestation have been established.[37] These units demand extremely qualified personnel, day and night, as severely ill newborn premature infants usually need ventilator assistance. One must, however, remember that there is strong evidence for respiratory therapy being a significant factor in the etiology of intracerebral hemorrhage.[30] Autoregulation of the cerebral blood flow also plays a significant role in the causation of perinatal brain damage. Perinatal asphyxia is followed by hypoxia, acidosis, hypercarbia,[33] and disruption of the blood brain barrier. These factors may be responsible for the loss of autoregulation, thus the CBF becomes pressure passive. An asphyxic child often develops arterial hypotension followed by decreased CBF. Ischemia of the brain is, therefore, further aggravated and necrosis of cerebral tissue results. If arterial hypertension occurs, the increased pressure is transmitted directly to the fragile capillaries, which may rupture and cause an intracerebral hemorrhage.

The frequency of brain damage increases almost proportionally with decreasing birth weight. The real-time ultrasound scanners have shown detailed and depressing pictures of severe intracerebral hemorrhages, particularly in the very low birth weight premature infant. Such brain damage is invariably followed by extensive neurological deficits. As a consequence of this, it is the opinion of this author that any infant with a birth weight below 1000 g, who is not breathing spontaneously, should not be resuscitated.

References

1. Abroms JF, Bresnan MJ, Zuckerman SE, Fisher EG, Strand R: Cervical cord injuries secondary to hyperextension of the head in breech presentation. *Obst et Gyn* 1973;41:369.
2. Adams FH, Gyepes MT: Diaphragmatic paralysis in the newborn infant simulating cyanotic heart disease. *Pediatr* 1971;78:119–121.
3. Adler JB, Patterson RL: Erb's palsy: long term results of treatment in eighty-eight cases. *J Bone Joint Surg* 1967;49A:1052–1064.
4. Ahmann PA, Lazzara A, Dykes FD, Brann AW, Schwartz JF: Intraventricular hemorrhage in the high-risk preterm infant: incidence and outcome. *Ann Neurol* 1980;7:118–124.
5. Allen JP, Meyers GG, Condon VR: Laceration of the spinal cord related to breech delivery. JAMA 1969;208:1019–1022.
6. Bhagwanani SG, Price HV, Lawrence KM, Ginz B: Risks and prevention of cervical cord injury in the management of breech presentations with hyperextension of the fetal head. *Am J Obst and Gyn* 1973;115:1159.
7. Bucher HU, Boltshauser E, Friedrich J, Isler W: Birth injury to the spinal cord. *Helv Pediatr Acta* 1979;34:517–527.
8. Byers RK: Spinal-cord injuries during birth. *Dev Med Child Neurol* 1975;17:103–110.
9. Chapple CC: A duosyndrome of the laryngeal nerve. *Am J Dis Child* 1955;91:56.
10. Cole VA, Durbin GM, Olaffson A, Reynolds EOR, Rivers RPA, Smith JF: Pathogenesis of intraventricular hemorrhage in newborn infants. *Arch Dis Child* 1974;49:722–728.
11. De Villiers JN, Bernman JJ: Vacuum extraction. *SAJ Obst and Gyn* 1963;574–582.
12. Deonna T, Payot M, Probst A, Prod'hom LS: Neonatal intracranial hemorrhage in premature infants. *Pediatr* 1975;56:1056–1064.
13. Eng GD: Brachial plexus palsy in newborn infants. *Pediatr* 1971;48:18–28.
14. Ehrenfest H: Birth injuries of the child. *Obst and Gyn Monogr* 1931;6.
15. Epstein F, Hochwald GM, Ransohoff J: Neonatal hydrocephalus treated by compressive head wrapping. Lancet 1973;1:634.
16. Feldman GF: Radial nerve palsies in the newborn. *Arch Dis Child* 1957;26:469–471.
17. Ford FR: Breech delivery and its possible relation to injury of the spinal cord with special reference to infantile paraplegia. *Arch Neurol and Psychiat* 1925;14:742.

18. Freud S: Die Infantile Cerebrallähmung. *Specielle Pathologie und Therapie* 1897; Band IX, Wien.
19. Friis-Hansen B: Perinatal brain injury and cerebral blood flow in newborn infants. *Acta Pediatr Scand* 1985;74:323–331.
20. Gerlach J, Jensen HP, Koos W, Krause H: *Pädiatrische Neurochirurgie.* Stuttgart, Thieme Verlag, 1967.
21. Gordon M, Rich H, Deutschberger J, Green M: The immediate and long-term outcome of obstetric birth trauma. Brachial plexus paralysis. *Am J Obst and Gyn* 1973;117:51–56.
22. Gowers WR: Clinical lecture on birth palsies. *Lancet* 1888;709–758.
23. Gresham EL: Birth trauma. *Pediatr Clin North Am* 1975;22:317–328.
24. Guardine AN, O'Brien FB: Preliminary experiences with Malmstrøm's vacuum extractor. *Am J Obst and Gyn* 1962;83:300–306.
25. Haller U, Wille L: *Diagnostik Intrakranieller Blutungen beim Neugeborenen.* Berlin, Springer-Verlag, 1983.
26. Harcke HT, Naeye RL, Storch A, Blanc WA: Perinatal cerebral intraventricular hemorrhage. *Pediatr* 1972;80:37–42.
27. Harwood-Nash DC, Hendrick EB, Hudson AR: The significance of skull fractures in children. *Radiol* 1971;101:151–155.
28. Hepner WR: Some observations on facila paresis in the newborn infant. *Pediatr* 1951;8:494–497.
29. Hill A, Volpe JJ: Seizures, hypoxic-ischemic brain injury and intraventricular hemorrhage in the newborn. *Ann Neurol* 1981;10:109–121.
30. Hope PL, Rhorburn RJ, Stewart AL: Timing and antecedents of periventricular hemorrhage in very preterm infants, in: Second Special Ross Laboratories Conference on Perinatal Intracranial Hemorrhage. Columbus, Ohio: Ross Laboratories:78–101, 1982.
31. Hovind KH, Galicich JH, Matson DD: Normal and pathological intracranial anatomy revealed by two-dimensional echoencephalography. *Neurology* 1967;17:253–262.
32. Jean F: Certain causes of neonatal death, intraventricular hemorrhage. *Biol Neonat* 1958;15.
33. Kenny JD, Garcia-Prats JA, Hillard JL, Corbet AJS, Rudolph AJ: Hypercarbia at birth: A possible role in the pathogenesis of intraventricular hemorrhage. *Pediatr* 1978;62:465–467.
34. Koenigsberger MR, Moessinger AC: Iatrogenic carpal tunnel syndrome in the newborn infant. *Pediatr* 1977;91:443–445.
35. Korobkin R: The relationship between head circumference and the development of communicating hydrocephalus in infants following intraventricular hemorrhage. *Pediatr* 1975;56:74–77.
36. Krishnamoorthy KS, Shannon DC, Delong GR, Todres ID, Davis KR: Neurologic sequelae in the survivors of neonatal intraventricular hemorrhage. *Pediatr* 1979;64:233–237.
37. Levene MI, Williams JL, Fawer CL: *Ultrasound of the Infant Brain.* London, Spastics International Medical Publications, 1985.
38. Ligthwood R: Radial nerve palsy associated with localized subcutaneous fat necrosis in the newborn. *Arch Dis Child* 1951;26:436–437.
39. Lindberg V, Hagberg B, Olsson Y, Sourander P: Injury of the spinal cord at birth. *Acta Pedia Scand* 1975;64:546–550.

40. Little WJ: Course of lectures on the deformities of the human frame. *Lancet* 1843:319.
41. Loeser JD, Kilburn HL, Lolley T: Management of depressed skull fracture in the newborn.
42. Lorber J, Bhat US: Posthemorrhagic hydrocephalus. *Arch Dis Child* 1974;49:751–762.
43. Lou H, Lassen N, Friis-Hansen B: Impaired autoregulation of cerebral blood flow in the distressed newborn infant. *Pediatr* 1979;94:118–121.
44. Malmstrøm T: Vacuumextract. *Acta Obst Gyn Scand* 1954;33: suppl 4.
45. Manning JJ, Adour KK: Facial paralysis in children. *Pediatr* 1972;49:102–109.
46. Matson DD: *Neurosurgery of Infancy and Childhood*. Springfield, Thomas, 1969.
47. McDonald MM, Koops BL, Johnson ML: Timing and etiology of intracranial hemorrhage in the newborn. Second Special Laboratories Conference on Perinatal Intracranial Hemorrhage. Columbus, Ohio, Ross Laboratories: 221–232, 1982.
48. Ment LR, Duncan CC, Scott DT, Ehrenkranz RA: Posthemorrhagic hydrocephalus. Low incidence in very low birth weight neonates with intraventricular hemorrhage. *J Neurosurg* 1984;60:343–347.
49. Mørstad O: Birth injuries. A follow up examination. *Acta Obst and Gyn Scand* 1953;33.
50. Natelson SE, Sayers MP: The fate of children sustaining severe head trauma during birth. *Pediatr* 1973;51:169–174.
51. Pape KE, Armstrong DL, Fitzhardinge PM: Peripheral median nerve damage secondary to brachial arterial blood gas sampling. *Pediatr* 1978;93:852–856.
52. Pape KE, Wigglesworth JS: Hemorrhage, Ischemia and the Perinatal Brain: Clinics in Developmental Medicine NOS 69/70. London, Spastics International Medical Publications, 1979.
53. Papile LA, Burstein J, Burstein R, Koffler H: Incidence and evolution of subependymal and intraventricular hemorrhage: A study of infants with birth weights less than 1500 gm. *Pediatr* 1978;92:529–534.
54. Papile LA, Burstein J, Burstein R: Posthemorrhagic dyrocephalus in low-birth weight infants: treatment by serial lumbar punctures. *Pediatr* 1980;97:273–277.
55. Potter EL: Pathology of the Fetus and Infant, 2nd ed. Chicago, Year Book Medical Publishers, Inc., 1961.
56. Roberts MH: Spinal fluid in newborn with special reference to intracranial hemorrhage. JAMA 1925;85:500.
57. Rubin A: Birth injuries: incidence, mechanism and end results. *Obst and Gyn* 1964;23:218–221.
58. Salomonsen L: Føtal og neonatal mortalitet: Tidsskrift for Den Norske Lægeforening 1928;157.
59. Schrager GO: Elevation of depressed skull fracture with a breast pump. *Pediatr* 1979;77:300–301.
60. Specht EE: Brachial plexus palsy in the newborn. *Clin Orthop and Related Research* 1975;110:32–34.
61. Stern L, Salle B, Friis-Hansen B: *Intensive Care in the Newborn* III. New York: Masson, USA, 1981;253–262.

62. Sørensen S: Pathogenesis of brain ventricle hemorrhage in newborns. *Ind J Pediatr* 1966;33:73.
63. Takagi T, Nagai R, Wakabayashi S, Mizawa I, Hayashi K: Extradural hemorrhage in the newborn as a result of birth trauma. *Child's Brain* 1978;4:306–318.
64. Takagi T, Fukuoka H, Wakabayashi S, Nagai H, Shibata T: Posterior fossa subdural hemorrhage in the newborn as a result of birth trauma. *Child's Brain* 1982;9:102–113.
65. Tan KL: Elevation of congenital depressed fractures of the skull by vacuum extractor. *Acta Pediatr Scand* 1974;63:562–564.
66. Tank ES, Davis R, Holt JF, Morley GW: Mechanisms of trauma during breech delivery. *Obst and Gyn* 1971;38:761–768.
67. Towbin A: Cerebral intraventricular hemorrhage and subependymal matrix infarction in the fetus and premature newborn. *Am J Path* 1968;52:121–140.
68. Volpe JJ: *Neurology of the Newborn*. Philadelphia, WB Saunders, 1981.
69. Volpe JJ, Herscovitch P, Perlman JM, Raichle ME: Position emission tomography in the newborn: extensive impairment of regional cerebral blood flow with intraventricular hemorrhage and hemorrhagicintracerebral involvement. *Pediatr* 1983;72:589–601.
70. Wickstrøm J: Birth injuries of the brachial plexus. *Cli Orthop* 1962;23:187–196.
71. Wise BL, Ballard R: Hydrocephalus secondary to intracranial hemorrhage in premature infants. *Child's Brain* 1976;2:234–241.
72. Aaslid R, Huber P, Nornes H: Evaluation of cerebrovascular spasms with transcranial Doppler ultrasound. *J Neurosurg* 1984;60:37–41.

CHAPTER 8

Germinal Matrix Hemorrhage (GMH) Syndrome and Intraventricular Hemorrhage (IVH) Syndrome in the Newborn

Jens Haase

Introduction

Autopsy studies have revealed intracranial hemorrhage to be the most common injury to the central nervous system of the premature child.[7,8] The term "intraventricular bleeding" was first applied in a broad sense for those newborn with bloody CSF and signs of cerebral irritation.[1,7,8] Since the introduction of ultrasound and CT scanning, the pathoanatomical basis of the clinical syndrome, often named the intraventricular hemorrhage (IVH) syndrome, was defined.* CT scanning and careful autopsy studies have shown that cerebral bleeding in premature children with IVH originates from the germinal matrix,[13,20] which is located beneath the ependyma in the lateral walls of the anterior part of the lateral ventricles. This is the location of neuroblasts and is largest at 24 to 32 weeks' gestation.[3] Germinal matrix bleeding may spread into the cerebral parenchyma or rupture into the ventricles.[20] As this bleeding is noted only among premature children or mature children in whom the germinal matrix is still present, renaming the IVH syndrome the *germinal matrix hemorrhage* (GMH) syndrome seems justified.[13] However, other names, such as the subependymal hemorrhage (SEH) syndrome[1,10,15] and the periventricular intracranial hemorrhage (PIH) syndrome,[20] are still found in the literature.

The GMH syndrome may be defined as a clinical and pathological syndrome characterized by hemorrhage into the cerebral white matter—the germinal matrix—in premature children. This bleeding may disperse within the brain parenchyma or through the ependyma into the ventricular system.[20] On the basis of this definition, it is evident that the diagnosis of the GMH syndrome may be made only using cerebral imaging techniques such as ultrasound, CT, or magnetic resonance (MR) scanning.[1,8] This is the main reason why different incidence rates have been published; most researchers base their diagnosis only on clinical grounds, ventricular taps,

---

* References 1, 4, 7, 9, 12–14, 18.

or lumbar punctures. The percentage of the GMH syndrome among 7000 premature live-born British children is 1.1, whereas more recent investigations of premature children show the percentage in this group to range between 25 and 75.[1,3,18] A recent review even states that premature children born vaginally at less than 34 weeks' gestational age have a 90% chance of having GMH.[8]

Etiology

Factors responsible for the GMH syndrome among premature newborn have been widely discussed.* There is no explanation for why this syndrome is more common among boys than girls (the ratio is 2 : 1).[4] Theories concerning mechanical factors in connection with birth through vaginal route, pathological pregnancies, change of intracranial/extracranial pressures and variations among these, neuroinfections, and hemorrhagic diathesis have been proposed.[4,7] The trauma theory, based on the assumption that certain types of vaginal or prolonged delivery are the reason for the bleeding, is now rejected.[18] Using radioactive isotope studies with marked erythrocytes, researchers have documented that most GMH bleedings develop during the first, second, or third day after birth. Thus, 60% of suffering infants bleeds between 15 and 48 hours after birth, and multiple bleeding episodes may be expected.[18]

Of pathophysiological interest is the fact that among stillborn premature infants, the percentage of the GMH syndrome is as low as 5.[1] The only possible traumatic GMH bleeding may be a compound complication of the infrequent posterior fossa hemorrhage.[6] If GMH occurs because of a gestational complication, it is always in connection with placental disruption or pre-eclampsia.[4] Neuroinfections and hemorrhagic diathesis may lead to intracranial bleedings, but not to GMH.[4,7]

It is evident that symptomatic GMH is common among children with respiratory distress syndrome (RDS),[1,4,7,8] premature children born with congenital heart disease, and children who aspirate or are asphyxic with a prolonged low Apgar score.[4,20] The incidence of intraventricular bleedings seems greatest among children with a birthweight below 1000 g, whereas combined bleedings in the parenchyma and ventricles are more common among older premature neonates.[14] It must be emphasized that although term newborns with intraventricular or cerebral bleeding have a similar frequency of asphyxic complications and lung disease, they are, in contrast to premature newborn, burdened with 40% congenital CNS malformations of the central nervous system or hemorrhagic diatheses. Their bleedings are derived from the choroid plexus unless remnants of the germinal matrix are found.[9]

---

* References 1, 4, 7, 8, 14, 17, 20.

Pathophysiology

During the growth of the fetal brain, the major cerebral venous drainage is central, through the vein of Galen and its tributaries; the superficial cortical veins are insufficiently developed.[9] The highly vascularized germinal matrix around the caudate nucleus area is drained through thin-walled terminal branches of the striothalamic vein in the direction of the foramen of Monro, from whence the flow is into the internal cerebral vein and the vein of Galen.[15,17] With maturation of the brain a gradual reduction of the germinal matrix, and thereby of vascularization, occurs in these areas. At the same time the cortical areas develops faster, and venous drainage shifts to the cortical veins and superior sagittal sinus. The subependymal zone close to the germinal matrix has virtually no supportive tissue, which is why thrombosis or stasis in the germinal matrix veins may lead to disruption of the thin-walled vessels and bleeding in the brain substance. The bleeding is subependymal, along the caudal thalamic sulcus. It gradually progresses through the germinal matrix and eventually ruptures into the ventricles[15] (see Fig. 8.1). Subsequent infarction in the germinal matrix leads to late leucomalacia.[20] Seventy percent of the bleedings are unilateral.[15]

Thrombosis or venous stasis seems closely linked to ischemia and/or hypoxemia.[11,19] With hypoxemia, a change to anaerobic metabolism results in subsequent lowering of the pH (lactate production). This leads to local vasodilatation, increased cerebral blood flow (CBF) with diminished autoregulation.[5,11,19] It is important to note that the germinal matrix seems to change from aerobic to anaerobic metabolism at a significantly higher arterial PO_2 than other cerebral structures.[5] In case of ischemia the early increase of lactate may be combined with the no-reflow phenomenon. Although it may be expected that CBF is high before the GMH syndrome, it could subsequently drop as a result of diminished reperfusion. As arterial PCO_2 is high during asphyxia and this is coupled with an increase in CBF, the presence of a low CBF before the hemorrhage extends into the brain parenchyma supports the theory that the primary lesion is hypoxic/ischemic.[5] Measurements of CBF with the intravenous xenon-133 clearance technique using either a computerized tomographic technique (Medimatic®) or conventional detector technique (Novo Cerebrograph 10a®) have shown extremely low CBF values, down to 20 ml per 100 g of tissue per minute or less.[5,11]

If the subependymal hemorrhage breaks through the ependymal wall into the ventricular system, impairment of CSF circulation may occur, thereby leading to communicating hydrocephalus.[1,8,12,13] Acute hydrocephalus may develop, usually in connection with clot formation in the IV ventricle.[1]

In conclusion, trauma seems not to play a major role in the development of the GMH syndrome. The bleeding is secondary to ischemia/

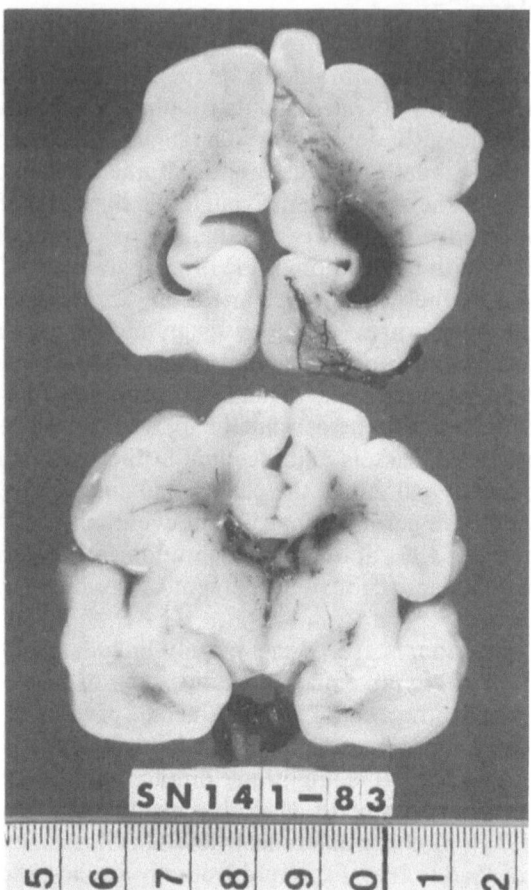

Figure 8.1. Autopsy: premature child with classic intraventricular hemorrhage from bleeding into the subependymal germinal matrix. The extension of intraventricular bleeding from its site of origin close to the foramen of Monro into the occipital horn is demonstrated.

hypoxia and leads to local—often unilateral—leucomalacia and, possibly, late onset of communicating hydrocephalus.

Symptomatology

Among preterm children with the GMH syndrome, few or no symptoms may guide the physician to a correct diagnosis. The often-noted signs—for example, bradycardia, apnea, hypotension, hyperactivity, seizures, drop of hematocrit, hyperbilirubinemia, severe acidosis, hypercalcemia, and low Apgar scores—are, of course, diagnostic criteria seen with a certain frequency among children with intracranial bleeding.[8,19,20] A sudden drop in hematocrit in connection with the rupture of blood from the germinal matrix into the ventricles, with subsequence bradycardia and development of acute hydrocephalus, should suggest the correct diagnosis.[1,10,20] Based on the above-mentioned high incidence of GMH among preterm children, physicians in the neonatal unit should consider the diagnosis of the GMH syndrome among all children with such symptoms unless faced with a premature child with normal Apgar scores, normal neurologic status, and absence of seizures.[8] The diagnosis must be confirmed or rejected using neuro-imaging techniques such as ultrasound, CT, or MR scanning.

The continuous clinical evaluation of many of these children is difficult because, as a result of RDS, they are often treated with artificial ventilation.[8] GMH syndrome children are difficult to wean from the ventilator, and increased frequencies of bradycardia and apnea are evident.[8] It is advisable to follow all suspect children clinically or with ultrasound scannings during the first 2 or 3 days—through which the GMH syndrome always develops.[1]

The diagnosis of hydrocephalus is difficult: "normal" ventricular size among preterm children is not known, and in a series of children "diagnosed" as having hydrocephalus, 77% showed spontaneous normaliza-

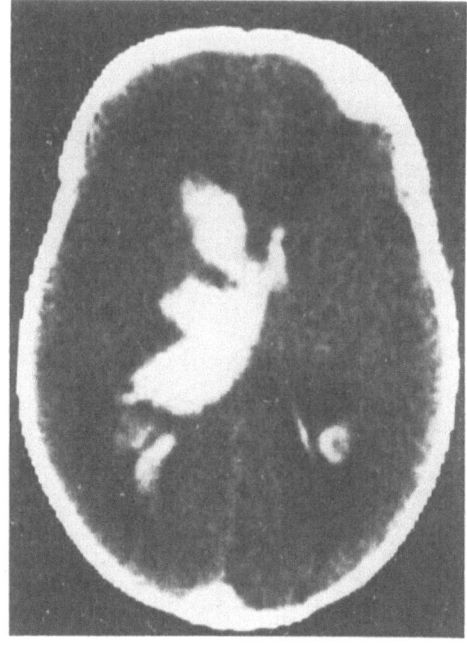

Figure 8.2. CT scan demonstrating severe intraventricular hemorrhage. The bleeding emerges from the germinal matrix and blocks the left ventricle and foramen of Monro.

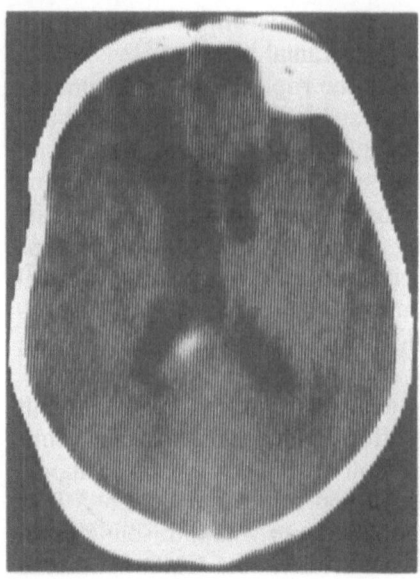

Figure 8.3. CT scan of same patient (Fig. 8.2), 1 month later, demonstrating that almost all the blood has been absorbed. A moderate left-side hemiatrophy, with loss of brain parenchyma around the left anterior ventricle, is clearly seen; there are no signs of hydrocephalus.

tion of their ventricles.[10] Increased head circumference and tense fontanel are not conclusive because of the low elastance of the brain parenchyma in the premature child. Only acute hydrocephalus provoked by a blockage of the aqueduct of Sylvius or a bleeding in the posterior fossa may be suspected on clinical grounds: opisthotonus, tense fontanel, bradycardia, and apnea.[8] It must be emphasized that the degree of bleeding does not

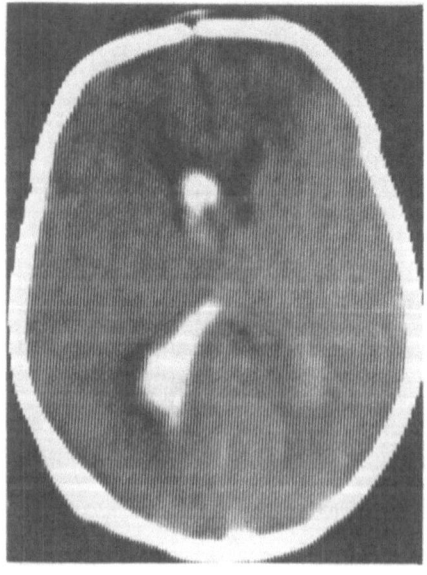

Figure 8.4. CT scan demonstrates minor, left intraventricular bleeding.

Figure 8.5. Same patient as in Figure 8.4, 3 weeks later. Blood is absent; however, severe hydrocephalus has developed.

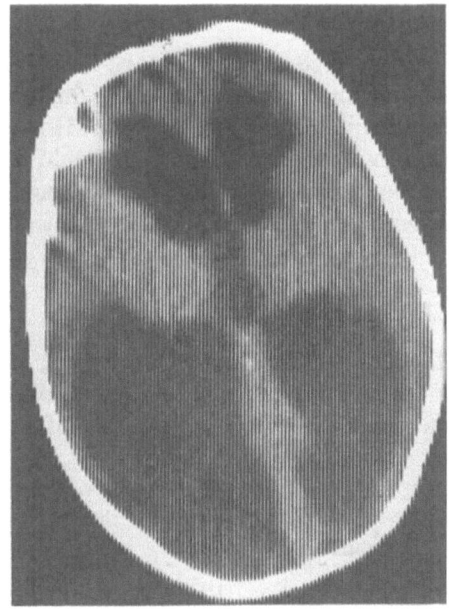

determine whether the child will develop hydrocephalus. This is demonstrated in Figures 8.2 and 8.3, where a severe intraventricular hemorrhage on a CT scan leads to a moderate left-sided hemiatrophy and no signs of hydrocephalus. In Figures 8.4 and 8.5 the minor intraventricular bleeding in another patient leads to a severe hydrocephalus 3 weeks later.

Diagnostic Methods

Ultrasonography (Ultrasound Scanning)

Ultrasonography is currently the diagnostic method of choice, an easy diagnostic tool that can be used at cribside without disturbing the child.[8] However, cranial ultrasonography introduces certain quantities of energy into the brain and may thus not be totally innocuous. Ultrasound produces biological effects by thermal, mechanical, and cavitational mechanisms.[2] Whether low-intensity ultrasound will lead to functional changes in the developing brain over the next 50 years has, of course, not been tested. However, using ultrasound in a preterm child does expose the *immature* brain to a potentially destructive energy force. The U.S. Bureau of Radiation and Health of the U.S. Department of Health and Human Services states that "although the body of current evidence does not indicate that diagnostic ultrasound represents an acute risk to human health, it is insufficient to justify an unqualified acceptance of safety."[2]

CT Scanning

Computerized Tomography (CT) scanning is an excellent way of demonstrating anatomical structures, including intracranial hemorrhages, as demonstrated in Figures 8.2–8.5. However, it should not be the first study used to diagnose GMH,[8] nor should it be used routinely. Its advantages are that it demonstrates clear anatomical changes around the ventricular system, especially the development of porencephaly (leucomalacia).

MR Scanning

Magnetic Resonance (MR) scanning may lead to a deeper understanding of the GMH syndrome but has no place today as a diagnostic tool since one cannot be sure the preterm infant will remain immobile throughout the scanning.

PET Scanning

Positron emission (PET) scanning has also been used to demonstrate biological features of the GMH syndrome. However, because of its high costs, it is not of practical use in routine diagnosis of the syndrome.

Lumbar and Ventricular Punctures

The demonstration of blood in the CSF is evidence only that erythrocytes are present in the CSF, not that they are caused by the GMH syndrome or that they result from a normal delivery.[1,8]

Intracranial Pressure Monitoring

Intracranial pressure (ICP) monitoring—by the intraventricular, subarachnoid, or epidural route—or through fontanel pressure monitoring, may be of interest.[8] Increased CBF and increased cerebral blood volume may be the first factors leading to the GMH syndrome.[5,11] Increased intracranial pressure in the presence of low arterial blood pressure results in reduced cerebral perfusion pressure, which may in turn lead to ischemia. However, ICP monitoring is still an experimental diagnostic tool; it may become a supplementary *monitoring* tool when the neurosurgeon treats children with developing hydrocephalus.[8]

CBF Measurements

Intravenous xenon-133 clearance techniques for measuring CBF are applicable today to preterm children, but their actual diagnostic use has not been documented.[5]

Table 8.1. Grading of germinal matrix bleeding.

Grade	Condition
1	Subependymal hemorrhage
2	Intraventricular hemorrhage without ventricular dilation
3	Intraventricular hemorrhage with ventricular dilation
4	Intraventricular hemorrhage with parenchymal hemorrhage

Source: Papile L-A, Burstein J, Burstein R, Koffler H: Incidence and evolution of subependymal and intraventricular hemorrhage: A study of infants with birth weights less than 1500 gm. *J Ped* 1978;92:529–534.

Electroencephalography (EEG)

Electroencephalography is the only way of monitoring electric cerebral activity and thereby demonstrating either reduced cerebral metabolism or continuous seizures.[18] Especially when treating sedated children in a respirator, the diagnosis of continuous seizures cannot be made unless EEGs are used.[8,18]

Grading

Grading of GMH is usually done according to Papile[14] (see Table 8.1). A practical protocol for the diagnosis of the GMH syndrome and subsequent hydrocephalus is illustrated in Table 8.2.

Early Treatment

Surgical removal of supratentorial germinal matrix hematomas in preterm children is usually not feasible.[1] The bleeding is parenchymatous "oozing," not a well-formed clot.[20] Theoretically, a situation where the child develops signs of a "mass" lesion resulting from a progressive hematoma, as demonstrated on ultrasound or CT scans, may warrant emergency craniotomy and removal of the hematoma. However, on the basis of a literature review, the rare, localized, hematoma in the posterior fossa, which leads to progressive hydrocephalus and clinical deterioration, seems to represent the only situation in which removal of the clot has proved of value.[6]

With intraventricular extension of the hematoma (as shown in Fig. 8.2), another form of active treatment with removal of bloody CSF through ventricular taps has been proposed.[1,8,12] Porencephaly usually follows ventricular punctures and may, thus, result in delayed neurodevelopment and clinical deficits.[8] The usual complications of ventricular punctures, such as lesions of cortical or subependymal veins or infection with subsequent necrotizing ventriculitis, must be borne in mind. Intracranial hemorrhage may lead to a transient ventriculomegaly, usually lasting less than a couple of days.[10] This condition needs no treatment. However, especially in children in Grades 3 and 4 of the GMH syndrome (see Table 8.1),

Table 8.2. Suggested protocol for diagnosis and treatment of the GMH syndrome and its complications.

	Day 1	Day 2–3	Day 7–14–21	Day ≥ 28
All Premature	All investigated with ultra-sound sonography	All with Neurological deficits Epilepsy GMH syndrome RDS syndrome are reinvestigated with ultrasound sonography If hemorrhage, CT scan is performed	All with Neurological deficits Epilepsy GMH syndrome are reinvestigated with ultrasound sonography If change in ultrasound sonography, CT scan is performed	All premature with GMH syndrome and/or hydro-cephalus, investigates with CT scan to confirm degree of leucomalacia and hy-drocephalus
Treatment	If GMH syndrome: Respirator treatment, anticonvulsant medication	If GMH syndrome or clini-cal deterioation Respirator treatment Anticonvulsant medication If Hydrocephalus alternative treatment No shunt	If hydrocephalus alternative treatment No shunt	Definite treatment of hydro-cephalus with ventriculo-peritoneal shunt (papile: grade 3 and 4)

ventriculomegaly usually progresses. Treatment with intermittent lumbar puncture has been advocated.[1,8,10,19] Although the hydrocephalic state may be temporarily controlled, a literature review indicates that no firm conclusion on the positive value of this treatment has been reached.[10]

In addition to ventricular and lumbar punctures, the use of a subcutaneous reservoir placed on an indwelling ventricular catheter has recently been advocated.[12] However, percutaneous puncture of the reservoir carries the risk of introducing bacteria into the reservoir and resulting in iatrogenic ventriculitis.

External ventricular drainage for control of progressing hydrocephalus seems dangerous because of the high infection rate (much higher than among adults) within the GMH population.[8] External ventricular drainage is preferable as a preoperative treatment in cases of posterior fossa tumors or subarachnoid hemorrhage with secondary hydrocephalus; however, preterm children thus treated suffer infections within a couple of days, probably as a result of their inferior immunoresponse. Acute ventriculo-peritoneal shunting (cribside shunting) has been sporadically used, but with a high frequency of obstruction because of blood and brain debris or infection.[8] Although not commonly accepted, head wrapping, as proposed by Epstein,[1] has in our experience been effective for temporary control of acute progressive hydrocephalus until definite treatment with ventriculo-peritoneal shunting can be established. Medical reduction of CSF production with glycerol, diuretics, or isosorbide has never been effective among children with the GMH syndrome.[1,8]

As the GMH syndrome results from cerebral hypoxia/ischemia, active treatment of the lung disease (e.g., respiratory distress syndrome) to maintain a high arterial pO_2 and a normal arterial pCO_2 is advocated.[5,8,11,20]

The GMH syndrome develops during the first few days after birth. Preliminary studies indicate that immediate ventilator treatment decreases the number of subsequent GMH's in these preterm newborn,[11] but it is not known for how long the treatment shall be continued. The possibility of hydrocephalus or significant hemorrhages exists, especially if it is difficult to wean the infant from the respirator.[8] With children who are heavily sedated and relaxed, continuous EEG monitoring is mandatory as a tool for diagnosing seizures.[8,18] Continuous seizures lead to increased local CBF and thus to a possible worsening of the GMH syndrome.[11] They should be prevented, by all means either by phenobarbital or other anticonvulsive agents.[18]

Late Treatment

The development of hydrocephalus within the first 3 weeks should be considered a possibly treatable condition. Although still debated, the thickness of the brain mantle seems statistically related to the neurodevelopmental character of the child.[8] With progressive ventricular dilation, shunting procedures (as in other causes of hydrocephalus) are indicated.[8] The complication rate with the ventriculo-peritoneal shunting procedure is higher among these premature infants than among older children; but the use of simple shunting devices like a one-piece shunt (Unishunt®) permits easy control of the hydrocephalus. Our morbidity rates are close to those in the older-child group.* One must not underestimate the significance of epilepsy and infantile spasms,[21] so they should be treated medically as early as possible, as described elsewhere. For a more detailed discussion of surgical and medical treatment of the GMH syndrome, the reader may review Chapters 13, 18, and 19 and Figure 8.6 in this volume.

Outcome

Using the grading system of Papile et al. (Table 8.1), children in Grades 1 and 2 generally survive, whereas the majority of those in Grades 3 and—mainly—4 die shortly after birth.[4,8,15,18] The surviving children in Grade 1 never develop hydrocephalus; 25% of those in Grade 2 become hydrocephalic.[8,12] The majority of children in Grades 3 and 4 suffer severe hydrocephalus and/or porencephaly.[8] Curiously, development of hydrocephalus is only mild among extreme preterm children with a birth weight of less than 1000 g.[16]

Cerebral palsy, usually in the form of spastic diplegia, is common following periventricular leucomalacia and is most severe in the lower extremities.[19] If the child presents with spastic quadriplegia, intellectual deficits are always found.[19,21] Roughly 70% of children with Grade 3 and 4 GMH develop major handicaps.[8,21] The poorest outcome is related to extreme prematurity, the outcome in infants with hydrocephalus appears more related to gestational age than to the grade of hemorrhage.[21]

Care of infants in an Intensive Care Unit seems not to have led to an increase in the number of children with severe mental retardation and multiple handicaps. Children in Grades 1 and 2 (who are the most common among survivors) have not been demonstrated to differ in outcome from other preterm children without hemorrhage.[8,16] It seems evident that the child with Grade 1 bleeding always develops normally.[8,21]

The literature review, however, permits no firm conclusions regarding outcome. As James and his co-workers[8] have said, because we cannot predict the limitations of brain development (which is a consequence of a multiplicity of pathologic mechanisms), a decision to withhold treatment

---

* Gjerlø I, Haase J, Bang F: Treatment of neonatal hydrocephalus with a single shunt. ICNA 3rd World Congress, Copenhagen, 1982.

from a child with the GMH syndrome should not be made only on clinical grounds or on the basis of neuro-imaging techniques.

References

1. Ahmann PA, Lazzara A, Dykes FD, Brann AW Jr, Schwartz JF: Intraventricular hemorrhage in the high-risk preterm infant: incidence and outcome. *Ann Neurol* 1980;7:118–124.
2. Bergman I: Questions concerning safety and use of cranial ultrasonography in the neonate. *J Ped* 1983;103:855–858.
3. Burstein J, Papile L-A, Burstein R: Intraventricular hemorrhage and hydrocephalus in premature newborns: A prospective study with CT. *Am J Roentgen* 1979;132:631–635.
4. Fedrick J, Butler NR: Certain causes of neonatal death: II. Intraventricular hemorrhage. *Biol Neonate* 1970;15:257–290.
5. Greisen G: CBF in the newborn infant: Issues and methods with special reference to the intravenous 133-Xenon clearance technique. *rCBF Bulletin* 1984;7:134–139.
6. Grunnet ML, Shileds WD: Cerebellar hemorrhage in the premature infant. *J Ped* 1976;88:604–608.
7. Gröntoft O: Intracranial haemorrhage and blood-brain barrier problems in the new-born. *Act Path et Microbiol Scand* 1954;suppl C; 8–92.
8. James HE, Bejar R, Merritt A, Gluck L, Coen R, Mannino F: Management of hydrocephalus secondary to intracranial hemorrhage in the high-risk newborn. *Neurosurgery* 1984;14:612–618.
9. Lacey DJ, Terplan K: Intraventricular hemorrhage in full-term Neonates. *Dev Med Child Neurol* 1982;24:332–337.
10. Liechty EA, Gilmore RL, Bryson CQ, Bull MJ: Outcome of high-risk neonates with ventriculomegaly. *Dev Med Child Neurol* 1983;25:162–168.
11. Lou HC, Lassen NA, Friis-Hansen B: Impaired autoregulation of cerebral blood flow in the distressed newborn infant. *J Ped* 1979;94:118–121.
12. McComb JG, Ramos AD, Platzker ACG, Henderson DJ, Segall HD: Management of hydrocephalus secondary to intraventricular hemorrhage in the preterm infant with a subcutaneous ventricular catheter reservoir. *Neurosurgery* 1983;13:295–300.
13. Ment LR, Duncan CC, Scott DT, Ehrenkranz RA: Posthemorrhagic hydrocephalus. *J Neurosurg* 1984;60:343–347.
14. Papile L-A, Burstein J, Burstein R, Koffler H: Incidence and evolution of subependymal and intraventricular hemorrhage: A study of infants with birth weights less than 1500 gm. *J Ped* 1978;92:529–534.
15. Ross JJ, Dimmette RM: Subependymal cerebral hemorrhage in infancy. *Am J Dis Child* 1965;110:531–542.
16. Stewart AL, Reynolds EUR, Lipscomb AP: Outcome for infants of very low birthweight: Survey of world literature. *Lancet* 1981;1:1038.
17. Towbin A: Cerebral intraventricular hemorrhage and subependymal matrix infarction in the fetus and premature newborn. *Am J Pathol* 1968;52:121–133.
18. Tsiantos A, Victorin L, Relier JP, Dyer N, Sundell H, Brill AB, Stahlman M: Intracranial hemorrhage in the prematurely born infant. *J Ped* 1974;85:854–859.

19. Volpe JJ: Perinatal hypoxic-ischemic brain injury. *Ped Clin N Am* 1976;23:383–397.
20. Volpe JJ: Neonatal intracranial hemorrhage: Pathophysiology, neuropathology and clinical features. *Clin Perinatol* 1977;4:77–102.
21. Williamson WD, Desmond MM, Wilson GS, Andrew L, Garcia-Prats JA: Early neurodevelopmental outcome of low birth-weight infants surviving neonatal intraventricular hemorrhage. *J Perinat Med* 1982;10:34–41.

CHAPTER 9

Epidemiology and Etiology of Craniocerebral Trauma in the First Two Years of Life

Concezio Di Rocco and Francesco Velardi

Introduction

Death records, hospital admissions records, accident and emergency department data, and surveys (family, social service agencies, office based physicians, etc.) constitute the customary sources from which estimates of the incidence of head injuries in children and adults have been made. Reported figures, however, indicate only a fraction of the actual incidence rate, which in effect remains unknown. This is not surprising, considering that the pathology of head injury ranges from the simple evidence of a bruised scalp to severe brain damage resulting in death. Furthermore, the distribution pattern of head injuries as reported by the above-mentioned sources, may misrepresent the epidemiology for a given population. Also, the lack of standardized definitions and the problems inherent in identifying and classifying pediatric craniocerebral injuries account for some of the obvious difficulties in planning effective measures to prevent head injuries and to reduce their medical, social, and economic impact.

Identification of these factors and limitations in this introduction have the purpose of alerting the reader to content and limitations. Many considerations must be made when undertaking a study of both epidemiology and etiology of craniocerebral injury in the pediatric category, since one may not transfer willynilly observations and concepts from the adult population. Limits are also evident when comparing epidemiologic studies performed in different areas, which reflect influence of several factors, such as: socio-economic and cultural levels of the families, local healthcare facilities and medical policies, degree of urbanization, criminality, climate and seasonal variations, and strategies of primary prevention (seat belt or safety helmet legislation, speed limits, extent of product liability for toys, furniture design). An overall review of published data on where, when, and how head injuries occur provides some information that differentiates children from adults, especially in light of the fact that the head is most frequently involved in injuries for which medical care is sought in children, especially those in preschool groups.[14,27] Very young children may have the lowest injury rate, but also the highest case : fatality ratio (4 : 30). Children are exposed to environmental risks first because of their absolute dependence and second because of their unwary mobility during the creeping and toddling stages of development. Most injuries in children under 2 years old take place at home or in familiar surroundings. Compared with accidental causes, nonaccidental causes of head injuries are relatively rare in this age group; the distinction, however, is not always easily made.

This chapter focusses on a variety of head injuries in infants and small children. It concludes with some perspectives on the prevention of such injuries.

Head Injuries in Children Under 2 Years of Age

Data on the actual incidence of head injury in children under 2 years old (calculated on the basis of the total number of children surviving to their second birthday and of those who died before the end of their second year) are unavailable. Some information can be drawn from reports dealing generally with accident rates in this age group; for example, a study by McCormick et al.[35] of 4989 infants under 1 year old shows that 8.6% suffered injuries requiring medical treatment. About one-sixth of these children were hospitalized, almost half of them because of head (or neck) injuries.

Another study[10] reports that of 8363 children up to 3 years of age who were hospitalized over a 5-year period, 3% suffered head injury. This trend seems to increase progressively.

The relatively large size of an infant's head compared to the rest of the body has been hypothesized to account for the preponderance of head injury over trunk and extremity injuries in this age group.[11,31,44] Parental anxiety leading to a request for medical care following an accident involving an infant's head may be regarded as an alternative explanation for this peculiar hospitalization distribution pattern.[35]

Most of the known data are obtained from family surveys or, more often, from hospital sources. Family surveys, which are almost always retrospective, are greatly limited by the general tendency of parents to remember serious accidents requiring hospital and medical care more clearly than minor injuries not involving professional treatment. Furthermore, parents' incidence of recall, especially for minor head injuries, appears to us to be inversely related to the length of time between the event and the interview. Consequently, it is quite possible that family surveys give inaccurate incidence rates—that is, lower than actual rates—at least for slight head trauma. Hospital sources, in contrast, seem to us to provide more reliable information. They also provide figures showing an excessive proportion of serious accidents. Admission, in fact, depends directly on the accessibility of a given hospital and the apparent severity of the injury, factors which may prevent hospitalization for minor head injuries especially when they occur far from a medical facility. Admission rates are further influenced by the habits of parents with regard to consulting doctors, the attitude of the emergency room's admitting physician, of the hospital's medico-legal responsibilities. [An obvious example of the implications of these responsibilities in many countries is the number of (relatively unnecessary) admissions determined solely by the radiological demonstration of skull fractures, which is particularly frequent in children under 2 years old (see Figs. 9.1 and 9.2).] According to various reports, the percentage of children under 2 years old admitted to hospital because of head injury ranges from a minimum of 5.5% to a maximum of 25% (Figure 9.3).

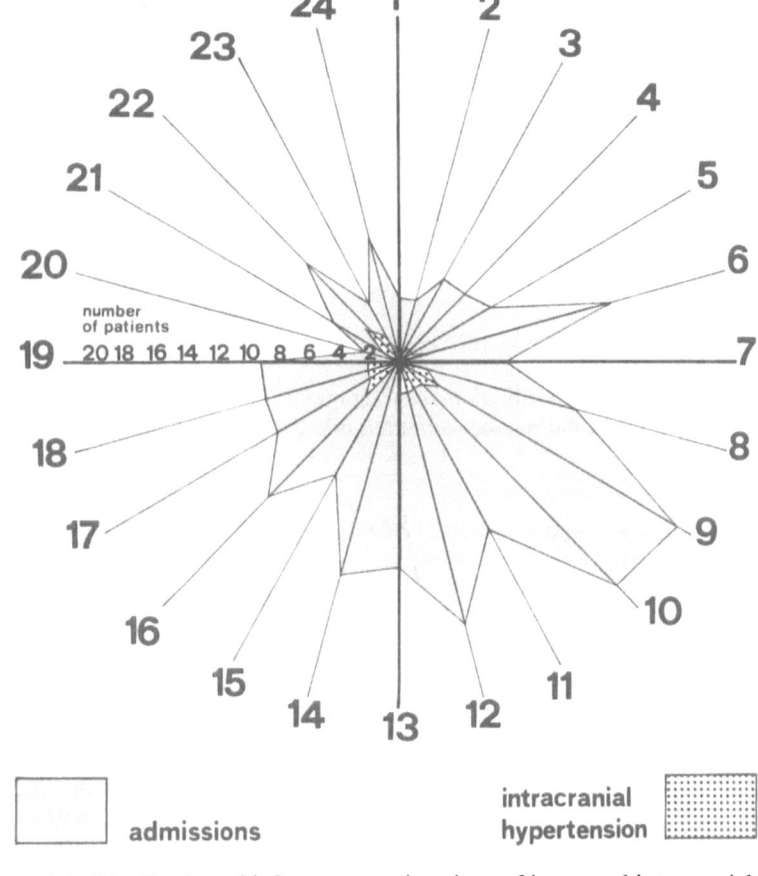

Figure 9.1. Distribution of infants presenting signs of increased intracranial pressure compared to the total number admitted because of head injury.

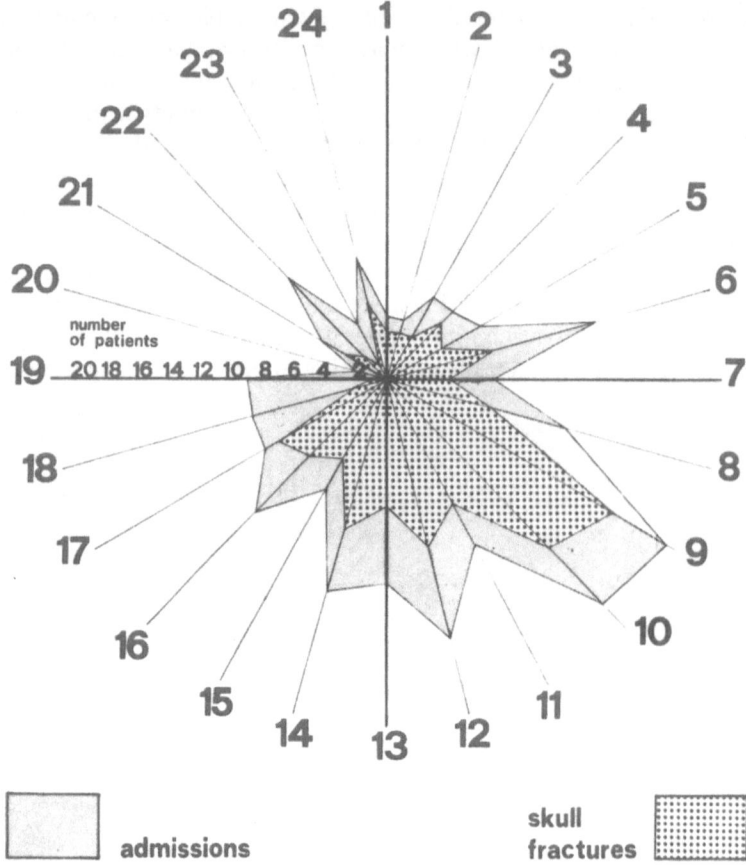

Figure 9.2. Distribution of infants presenting radiological evidence of skull fracture compared to the total number admitted because of head injury.

Falls, which are a major cause of head injury, are grouped in two main categories: falls from cots, cribs, prams, high chairs, and so on (i.e., due to insufficient supervision), and those against or from furniture and down steps (i.e., related to independent ambulation). Abuse, falls from heights, and traffic accidents constitute the three other major causes of head injuries (excluding perinatal brain damage) in children under 2 years old (Fig. 9.4). It is worth noting that each cause of injury, with the exception of falls from cots or prams, seems to become more common when the child begins sitting up and, even more, when it begins to walk. A decline is evident at the end of this age range, when the child becomes steadier and better able to evaluate risk. Poor balance and insufficient muscular coordination, typical of this period of life, are thus the main causes of accidents—and of the frequent injury of the head.

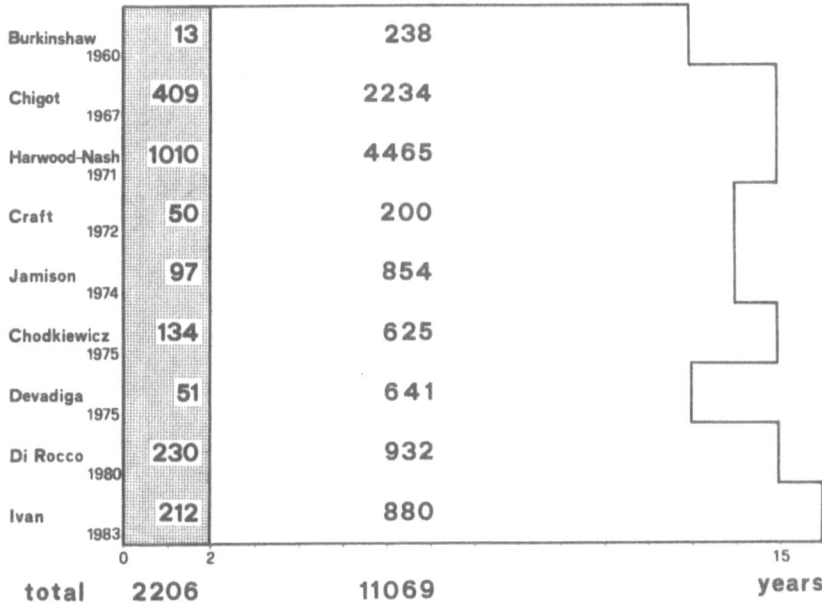

	0	2	15
Burkinshaw 1960	13	238	
Chigot 1967	409	2234	
Harwood-Nash 1971	1010	4465	
Craft 1972	50	200	
Jamison 1974	97	854	
Chodkiewicz 1975	134	625	
Devadiga 1975	51	641	
Di Rocco 1980	230	932	
Ivan 1983	212	880	
total	2206	11069	years

Figure 9.3. Age distribution of head injuries in children admitted because of head injury (dotted area: 0-2 year age group).

The distribution of head injuries by sex shows that they occur predominantly in males, even in the first months of life[13,19,21,37] (see Fig. 9.5). This predominance, however, is not obvious in all reports,[14,31,32,35] nor is a clear relationship between injury and socioeconomic level. The major incidence in head injury rates in children of the lower-income families, described in some papers published in the past,[31] has been denied in more recent surveys.[35] The characteristics of the developmental stages through which the infant passes in the first months of life seem, in effect, to suggest that home conditions are not terribly important. In the first months, when infants are immobile and sleeping for most of the day, they

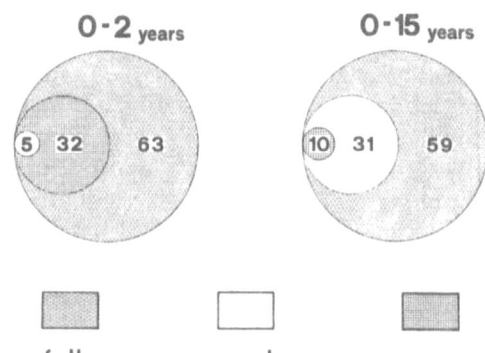

0-2 years   **0-15** years

5	32	63	10	31	59

Figure 9.4. Percentage distribution by etiology of head injuries in children.

falls   road   miscellaneous

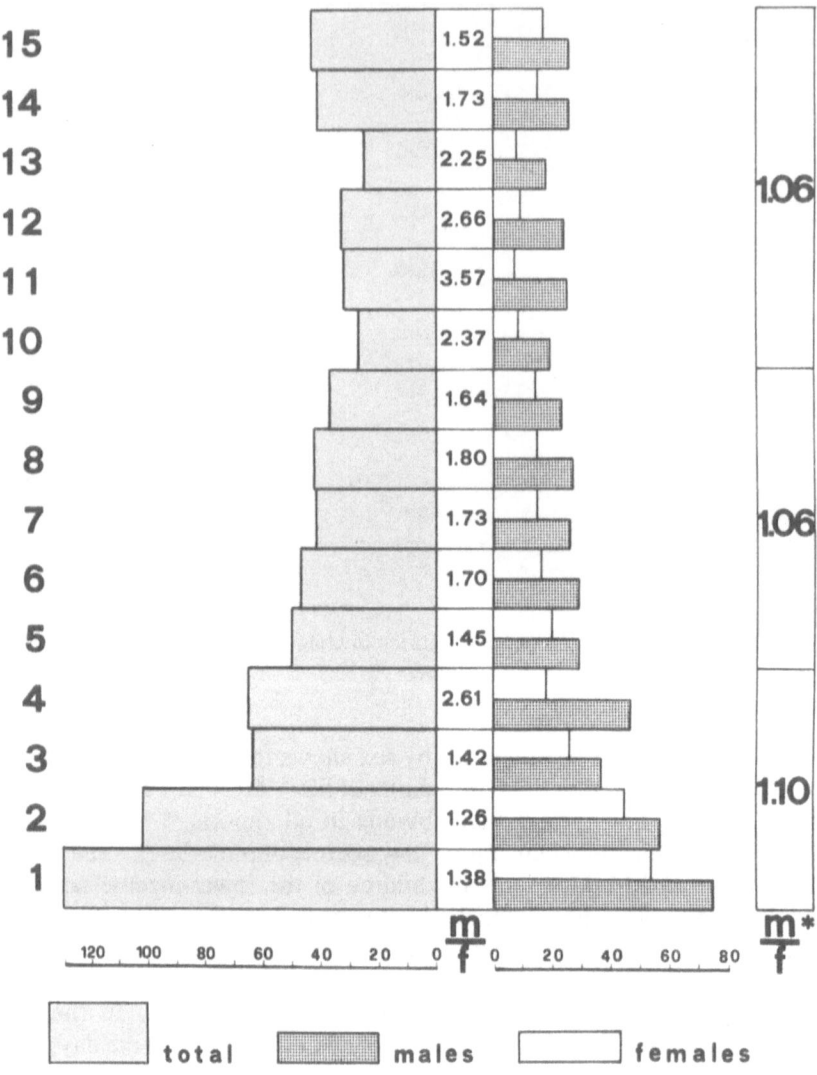

Figure 9.5. Male/female distribution of head injuries in children requiring hospital admission (authors' series) compared to the male/female ratio (*) in groups of children from 1 to 4, 5 to 9, and 10 to 15 years old. (*Source:* the Italian Statistics Institute, 1980.)

are at lower risk than whey they begin to, sit up and to walk—regardless of the kind of home in which they live.

Perinatal Head Injuries

Fetal and neonatal head injuries result almost exclusively from pressure applied to the head *in utero* or during the birth process. Their severity may vary considerably. Damage of the central nervous system resulting from direct obstetrical trauma or because of a difficult delivery account for a significant number of deaths. The Italian Statistics Institute review of 1980 reports that about 2.7% of total child deaths in 1975, occurring during the first 12 months of life, were directly related to obstetrical trauma. The incidence of less severe head injuries compatible with postnatal life is obviously more difficult to ascertain. Soft tissue damage or skull fracture suggest externally induced *noxae,* but the incidence, especially of such well known depressed fractures as the "ping-pong ball" variety, is unknown.[40,42] Relatively high figures have been reported for infants suffering head injuries during birth, and quite low percentages are reported for the general neonatal population.[3,36] Skull molding and depressions may occur during the birth process from pressure exerted on the calvarium by the last lumbar vertebra, the sacral promontory, the symphysis pubis, or the ischial spines, even in deliveries that are apparently uneventful.[22,40,47] More often, however, neonatal depressed skull fractures are the result of mechanical pressure exerted by the application of forceps during delivery. The introduction of vacuum-extraction deliveries has been reported to have decreased the number of these fractures and diminished the gravity of cerebral lesions with which they may be associated.[39]

Falls

In the first 2 years of a child's life, falls are the leading cause of head injury (Fig. 9.3). They occur as a result of circumstances peculiar to the life of the infant or toddler. In most cases infants fall from furniture—that is, from a height of about 90 cm or less. Despite parental concern, most of these accidents do not result in observable injuries.[24,32] Infants who cannot yet walk depend entirely on the supervising adult for protection from accidental falls. Thus, it is not surprising that breakfast and suppertime[32] or the hours around noon[31] constitute the peak periods for such falls; these accidents are clearly related to the infant's handling at feeding times. After the first 5 months of life, when the infant begins to roll from the prone to the supine position and to sit and stand, parental failure to attend to the infant is the largest contributing factor in this type of fall (see Figs. 9.6 and 9.7).

Dressing (and, in the hospital, examining) tables also constitute danger-ous places for infants, accounting for about 11% of falls.[31,32] Similar obser-vations may be made about infant seats; this suggests the possible contrib-uting role of poor equipment design. It is worth noting that slipping from adults' hands accounts for only a small number of head injuries (from 1.9% to 4%).[31,32]

Infant "walkers" also constitute a health hazard in the first months of life, being directly related to falls in about 2% of reported cases. Head injuries and skull fractures have been observed in 10.6% of 47 infants

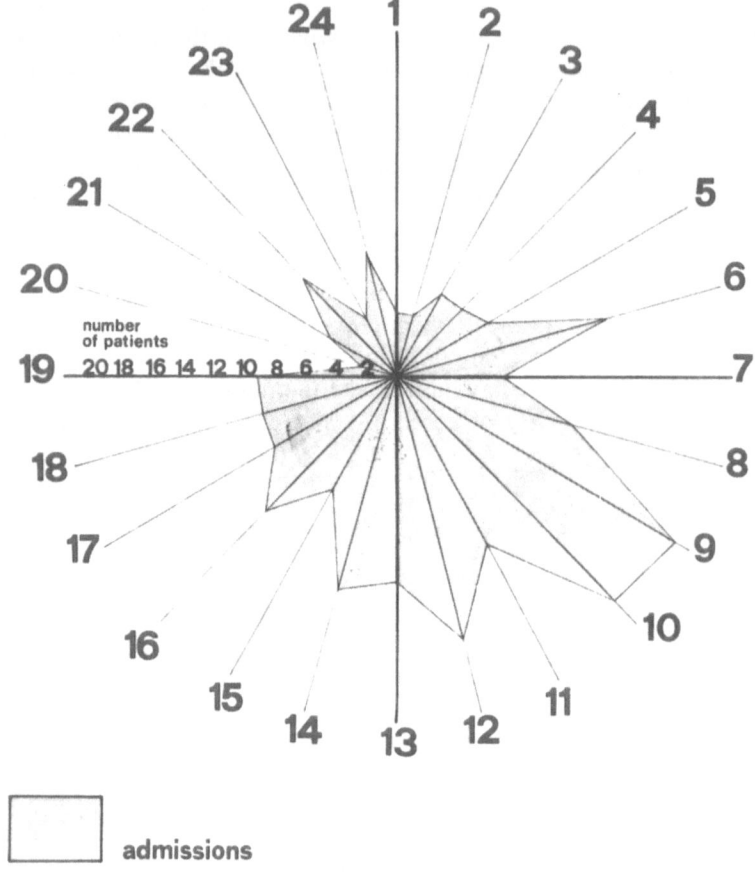

admissions

Figure 9.6. Distribution by age (in months) of infants admitted because of head injury.

suffering mishaps in a group of 150 infants using walkers, as described by Kavanagh and Banco.[29] Walkers tipping over on a flat surface or tipped over by a sibling, as well as walkers falling down stairs, constitute the principal modalities of accidents.

Vertical falls are a significant cause of death in children in major urban areas. Most cases occur in children less than 5 years old,[46] with a peak incidence near 2 years of age.[46] Thirty-three percent of the victims of window falls, as reported by Police Precincts and Hospital Emergency Rooms in New York City (February–October, 1973–1975) involved children under 2 years of age.[46] Summer months, afternoon hours, the lack of parental supervision, and the absence of apartment window guards constitute the main predisposing factors.

The frequency of skull fractures in such accidents is second only to that of fractures of the radius; however, head injuries without fractures, associated with eventual intracranial hematomas, appear to be the most common pathology in accidents of this type.[44]

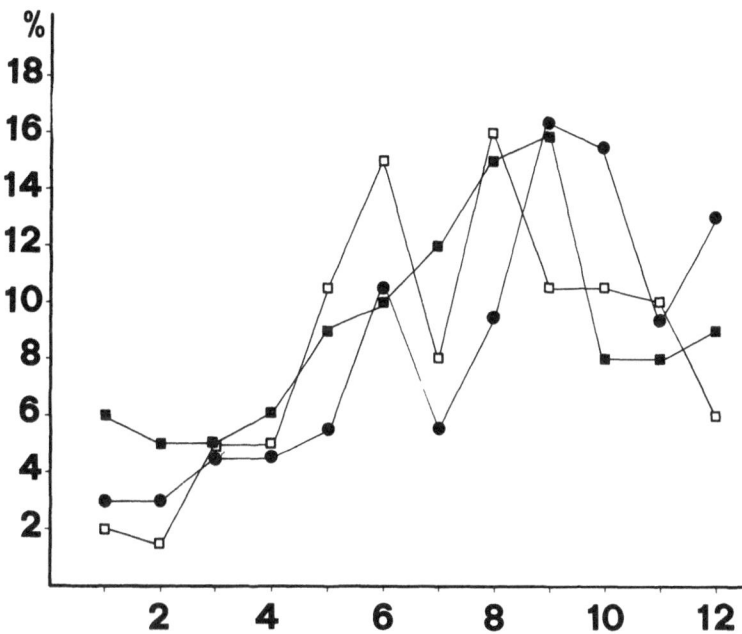

Figure 9.7. Percentage distribution of subjects under 1 year old admitted because of head injury (●: authors' series) compared to those not requiring hospitalization (■: Kravitz et al., 1969; □: Levin, 1972). (*Note:* the incidence peaks at 6 and 9 months.)

Road Accidents

Motor-vehicle related events are the leading cause of death and injury among children after the neonatal period. Mild and severe head injuries with or without skull fractures are present in about one-fourth of children involved in road accidents.[25] Larger figures (from 59% to 79%) are reported in studies concerning children injuried in automobile crashes.[45]

Rarely, children less than 2 years old may be victims of traffic accidents as pedestrians or struck by motor vehicles while in their strollers. The majority of head injuries in this age group occur during automobile rides. In other words, car occupant deaths and injuries largely exceed pedestrian death and injury rates.

The alarmingly high death rate of car occupants in the first year of life—especially of infants less than 6 months old (three times more than for children older than 6 years)—has been stressed by Baker.[14] In her study, the peak for car-occupant deaths was, in fact, at 1 to 2 months, with a median age at death of 5 months. This high death rate for infants has been related to two factors:

1. The particular characteristics of the brain and skull in the first few months of life, which predispose them to trauma induced cerebral tears.[33]
2. The greater likelihood of infants' being in the front seat and/or in someone's arms.[4,43]

Strong evidence for the need for some sort of restraint for child passengers in motor vehicles is given by the figures provided by Scherz[43] in his review of data collected from Washington State Seat Belt. The author, in fact, found that deaths of children of up to 4 years old travelling unrestrained were 10 times higher than those of children wearing some sort of restraint. Almost 80% of the deaths considered by this author involved children less than 2 years old.

Although head trauma as a result of crash events are more frequent and severe, noncrash events may still result in head injuries in child passengers. Those injuries seem more easily preventable by using appropriate child restraint systems. Injuries from noncrash events, in fact, result mainly from movement of the child within the vehicle (61%), sudden stops (22%), and swerves or turns (17%).[1]

Child Abuse

Medical and public awareness of the extent of the problem of child abuse has increased in recent years. Child abuse may be regarded as the main cause of nonaccidental head injury in children under 2 years old. Nonaccidental injury refers to injury caused by deliberate acts of (an)other per-

Table 9.1. Percentage distribution of abused children according to age.

Author(s)	No. of cases	% distribution of cases by age			
		6 mo.	9 mo.	12 mo.	2 yr.
McHenry et al.*	50		60		
Schloesser*	85	32			
Kroeger*	52			33	
Simons et al.*	313			28	
Illinois Central Registry	483	15		25	40
New York Central Registry	201			27	
McClelland et al. (34)	21			71	

* From: Gil, D.G.: Incidence of child abuse and demographic characteristics of persons involved in The Battered Child. R.E. Helfer, H. Kempe (Eds.) The University of Chicago Press, Chicago and London, 1968, pp. 19–40.

son(s). The term "deliberate act" does not exclude acts of deliberate omission, the importance of which is difficult to assess. Deliberate omission, however, should be distinguished from omission through ignorance. Even though these considerations suggest caution in evaluating the actual incidence of head injuries resulting from voluntary damage, many investigators agree that children involved in incidents of abuse tend to be very young (see Tables 9.1 and 9.2). Infants are more frequently involved in whiplash shaking than children. Examples are such playful practices as tossing a baby into the air and "horse riding," which are unintentional causes of brain damage by jolting. In the absence of actual head impact, whiplash and rotational displacements account for findings such as those experimentally demonstrated by Ommaya, et al.[37]

The very young age of most abused children accounts for the usual alleged causes of injury (falls from cribs, furniture, or down stairs); these causes obviously do not correspond to the most frequently confessed actual methods (striking with hands, fists, or weapons). The frequent occurrence of skull fracture in battered children contrasts sharply with

Table 9.2. Distribution by age and etiology of head injuries in children under 2 years old.*

Age		Etiology	
0– 2 months	4%	Falls	79%
2– 6 months	17%	Road accidents	8%
6–12 months	31%	Battered child	2%
12–18 months	22%	Others	10%
18–24 months	26%		

* Data from a series of 1719 cases observed at the Hôpital de La Timone, Marseille, France, over a 13-year period.

the relatively low incidence of such pathology (about 1%) in cases of simple falls from cribs and other furniture.[24]

Caffey[8,9] is said to be the first to have introduced the radiological recognition of the "battered-child syndrome" by calling attention to multiple fractures, of unknown origin, of the long bones; such factors accompanied cases of subdural hematomas. In abused children, the presence of subdural hematomas may be suggested by radiological demonstration of separated cranial bones and widened sutures (diastasis) or obvious fractures of the skull. This is especially true when they are not linear, but comminuted, resembling the multiple irregular fractures of an eggshell. In a recent study of 145 children admitted because of skull fracture, 31 were under 18 months of age; of these, 29% were instances of child abuse.[21] In only one case was there an associated fracture of the long bones; this called into question the diagnostic value of associating these two lesions (as had often been done in the past) and highlighted the importance of skull fractures, even if isolated.

In recent years, the introduction of the CT scan has made an enormous contribution to the recognition of brain injury in abused children by demonstrating a large range of lesions, including subdural and subarachnoid hemorrhages, intraparenchymal bleeding, parenchymal swelling, and brain lacerations even in patients without apparent evidence of head injury.[20,34]

Perspectives on Prevention

In recent years, and as a result of increased knowledge about the high vulnerability of newborn and young infants to trauma, the prevention of head injuries in the first months of life has become an issue of extreme importance. The neonate's brain is particularly susceptible to bleeding and the infant's brain to whiplash injuries. These result from the peculiar combination of incomplete myelinization, a relatively heavy head, and weak neck musculature. Consequently, educational programs for motivating parents have been developed. Their impact has proved to be effective, although to a lesser extent than hoped.[2,6,15,28] These programs (almost always for pregnant or postpartum women) have been designed mainly to increase the crash protection of infants in cars. In spite of this increased awareness—evident, for example, in the widespread use of infant carriers to transport babies in cars—the appropriate use of protective measures such as fastening infant carriers by car seat belts for crash protection has remained low[41] (see Fig. 9.8). Bass and Mehta[5] have identified extraordinary deficiencies in parental care and in the reported practice of basic household accident prevention throughout all social and ethnic groups. Furthermore, these deficiencies seem not to be significantly reduced by health education efforts.[17]

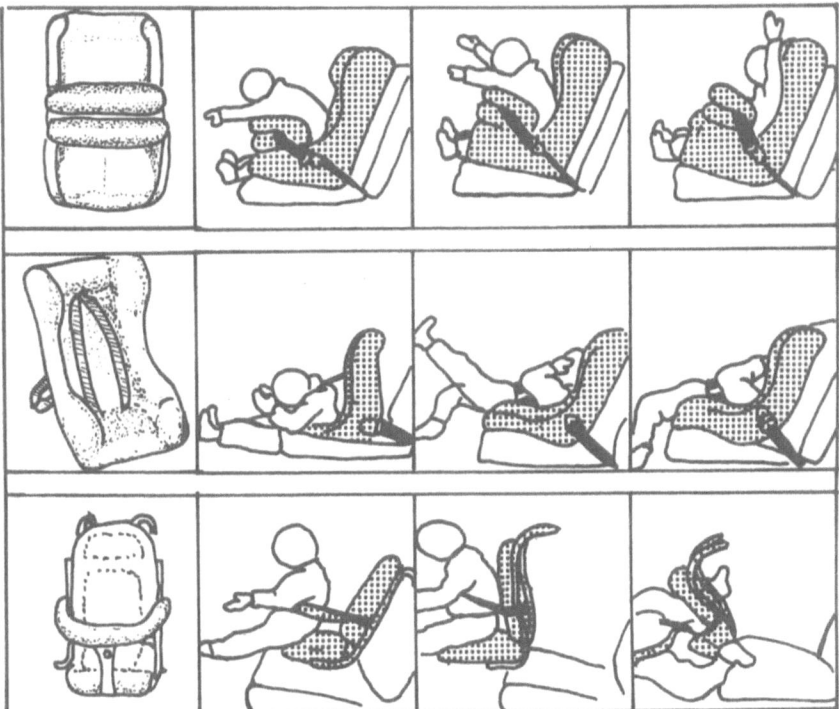

Figure 9.8. Reliability of different automobile child-restraint crash systems.

Even though the demonstrated limits should prompt us to develop more effective educational programs for the future, at the present time these observations indicate the obvious importance of passive techniques for the protection of infants. Reduction of the child's environmental hazards is crucial and can be effected by such measures as better safety standards for child passengers, restraints, protection from injury during crashes as well as from interior impact in cars,[4,41,45] window guards to prevent free falls in apartments,[46] and modifications in furniture design and toy manufacturing methods.

References

1. Agran PF: Motor vehicle occupant injuries in noncrash events. *Pediatrics* 1981;67:838–840.
2. Allen DB, Bergman AB: Social learning approaches to health education: Utilization of infant auto restraint devices. *Pediatrics* 1976;58:323–328.
3. Axton JHM, Levy LF: Congenital moulding depressions of the skull. *Br J Med* 1965;1:1644–1647.

4. Baker SP: Motor vehicle occupant deaths in young children. *Pediatrics* 1979;64:860–861.
5. Bass JL, Mehta KA: Developmentally oriented safety surveys. *Clin Pediat* 1980;9:350–356.
6. Berger LR: Childhood injuries: Recognition and prevention. *Curr Probl Pediatr* 1981;12:1–59.
7. Burkinshaw J: Head injuries in children: Observations on their incidence and causes with an enquiry into the value of routine skull x-rays. *Arch Dis Child* 1960;35:205–214.
8. Caffey J: Multiple fractures in the long bones of infants suffering from subdural hematoma. *Am J Roentgen* 1946;56:163–173.
9. Caffey J: The whiplash-shaken infant syndrome: Manual shaking by the extremities with whiplash-induced intracranial and intraocular bleedings, linked with residual permanent brain damage and mental retardation. *Pediatrics* 1974;54:396–403.
10. Canestri G, Monzali GL: Traumi cranici nell'infanzia. *Min Ped* 1970;22:1687–1689.
11. Chamberlain RN, Simpson RN: The Prevalence of Illness in Childhood. London, Pitman Medical Publishing Co Ltd, 1979.
12. Chigot PL, Esteve P: Traumatologie Infantile, ed. 2. Paris, L'Expansion Editeur, 1967.
13. Chodkiewicz JP, Redondo A, Merienne L, Cioloka C, Terrazas F: Pediatric head injuries (follow-up study of 625 cases). *Adv Neurosurg* 1975;3:390–400.
14. Choux M, Grisoli F, Baurand C, Vigoroux RP: Les hématomes extra-duraux traumatiques de l'enfant. *Neurochirurgie* (Paris) 1973;19:183–197.
15. Christophersen ER: Children's behavior during automobile rides: Do car seats make a difference? *Pediatrics* 1977;60:69–74.
16. Craft AW, Shaw DA, Cartlidge NEF: Head injuries in children. Br J Med 1972;4:200–203.
17. Dershewitz RA, Williamson JW: Prevention of childhood household injuries. *Am. J. Pub Health* 1977;67:1148–1153.
18. Devadiga KV: Head injury in children. *Indian J Pediat* 1975;42:291–297.
19. Di Rocco C, Stefanini MC, Velardi F: Traumi cranio-encefalici del periodo neonatale e della prima infanzia. *Min Ped* 1980;32:927–934.
20. Ellison PH, Tsai FY, Largent JA: Computed tomography in child abuse and cerebral contusion. *Pediatrics* 1978;62:151–154.
21. Girardet D: Etude épidémiologique des fractures du crâne chez les enfants de moin de 18 mois. *Helv Ped Acta* 1982;37:35–47.
22. Guha-Ray DK: Intrauterine spontaneous depression of fetal skull: A case report and review of literature. *J Reprod Med* 1976;16:321–324.
23. Harwood-Nash DC, Hendrick EB, Hudson AR: The significance of skull fractures in children: A study of 1187 patients. *Radiology* 1971;101:151–155.
24. Helfer RE, Slovis TL, Black M: Injuries resulting when small children fall out of bed. *Pediatrics* 1977;60:533–535.
25. Illingworth CM: 227 road accidents to children. *Acta Paediatr Scand* 1979;68:869–873.
26. Ivan LP, Choo SH, Ventureyra ECG: Head injuries in childhood: A 2-year survey. *J Can Med Assn* 1983;128:281–284.

27. Jamison DL, Kaye HH: Accidental head injury in childhood. *Arch Dis Child* 1974;49:376–381.
28. Kanthor HA: Car safety for infants: Effectiveness of prenatal counseling. *Pediatrics* 1976;58:320–322.
29. Kavanagh CA, Banco L: The infant walker. *Am J Dis Child* 1982;136:205–206.
30. Klauber RM, Barrett-Connor E, Marshall LF, Bowers SA: The epidemiology of head injury: A prospective study of an entire community—San Diego County, California, 1978. *Am J Epid* 1981; :500–509.
31. Kravitz H, Driessen G, Gomberg R, Korach A: Accidental falls from elevated surfaces in infants from birth to one year of age. *Pediatrics* 1969;44(suppl):869–876.
32. Levin S: Infant fall-out. *S Afr J Med* 1972;46:586–588.
33. Lindenberg R, Freytag E: Morphology of brain lesions from blunt trauma in early infancy. *Arch Pathol* 1969;87:298–305.
34. McClelland CQ, Rekate H, Kaufman B, Persse L: Cerebral injury in child abuse. *Child's Brain* 1980;7:225–235.
35. McCormick MC, Shapiro S, Starfield BH: Injury and its correlates among 1-year-old children. *Am J Dis Child* 1981;135:159–163.
36. Natelson SE, Sayers MP: The fat of children sustaining severe head trauma during birth. *Pediatrics* 1973;51:169–174.
37. Ommaya AK, Faas F, Yarnell P: Whiplash injury and brain damage. *J Am Med Ass* 1968;204:285–289.
38. Pellerin D, Rigault P, Fekete CN: Aspects chirurgicaux des accidents de l'enfant: 13,433 cas. *Rev. Pédiatrie* 1971;7:403–416.
39. Plauche WC: Fetal cranial injuries related to delivery with the Malmström vacuum extractor. *Obst Gynec* 1979;53:750–757.
40. Putet G, Lapras C: Les traumatismes crâniens et les lésions nerveuses en rapport avec les applications de forceps. *Rev Fr Gynécol Obstét* 1981;76:125–128.
41. Reisinger KS, Williams AF: Evaluations of programs designed to increase the protection of infants in cars. *Pediatrics* 1978;62:280–287.
42. Saunders BS, Lazoritz S, McArtor RD, Marshall P, Bason WM: Depressed skull fractures in the neonate. *J Neurosurg* 1979;50:512–514.
43. Scherz RG: Fatal motor vehicle accidents of child passengers from birth through 4 years of age in Washington State. *Pediatrics* 1981;68:572–575.
44. Smith MD, Burrington JD, Woolf AD: Injuries in children sustained in free falls: An analysis of 66 cases. *J Trauma* 1975;15:987–981.
45. Snyder RG, O'Neill B: Are 1974–1975 automotive belt systems hazardous to children? *Am J Dis Child* 1975;129:946–949.
46. Spiegel CN, Lindaman FC: Children can't fly: A program to prevent childhood morbidity and mortality from window falls. *Am J Pub Health* 1977;67:1143–1147.
47. Tan KL: Elevation of congenital depressed fractures of the skull by the vacuum extractor. *Acta Paediat Scand* 1974;63:562–564.

CHAPTER 10

Clinical Criteria—Children's Coma Score and Outcome Scale—for Decision Making in Managing Head-Injured Infants and Toddlers

Anthony J. Raimondi and Jeffrey Hirschauer

Introduction

Younger children suffer much greater damages than older children or adults from such deceleration-impact injuries as falls and from such acceleration-burst injuries as blows to the head. Approximately 50% of those children whose fontanels have not closed suffer skull fractures from either acceleration or deceleration injuries, whereas only 29% of children with closed fontanels and sutures suffer fractures.[5] Similarly, children less than 6 months of age suffer the highest death rate among motor vehicle occupants (9 per 100,000); 1-year-old children suffer the second highest rate (4–5 per 100,000); and children between the ages of 6 and 12 suffer the third highest (3 per 100,000).[1]

The age demarcation between good and poor outcomes in morbidity and mortality resulting from head injuries in childhood is sharp, occurring at the time of fontanel closure.[16] If one studies age distribution histograms of children with open and closed fontanels, it becomes apparent that fontanel closure occurs at approximately 1 year of age. This finding allows the clinician to superimpose the closed-fontanel population upon children greater than 1 year of age and the open-fontanel population upon children younger than 1 year of age. The higher incidence of skull fracture in children with open sutures and fontanels,[11] along with greater morbidity and higher mortality rates in the same population,[17] suggest that infants are more vulnerable to blunt trauma than toddlers in that they suffer more craniocerebral damage and a much higher incidence of neurological deficit.[16] Whether the primary impact itself, or a delayed cerebral response to this primary impact—one resulting from very different cerebral anatomy and physiology—are the causative factors is not possible to ascertain at this time.[9] The facts, however, are that infants have fewer chances of good recovery after blunt head injury than do children older than 1 year of age: 13.4% of children less than 1 year old, versus 4.9% of those between 1 and 3 years old, have a poor outcome.[11,16] Similarly, the highest incidence (18%) of hospital admissions for head injuries in children occurs during the first 3 months of postnatal life.[5] The incidence rate then falls off in an almost linear fashion to its lowest point (3%) between the 18th and 21st months of life, before leveling off at a plateau of 7% during each trimester between the 21st and 36th months of life.[16]

These very significant differences in age-incidence and hospital-admission epidemiology cannot be attributed exclusively to noxae characteristic of individual trimesters during the newborn, infant, and toddler ages of life: passage through the birth canal, falls in the delivery room, slippage from the parents' arms during feeding, falls from a high-chair or bassinet, crawling over the side rails of the crib, running and playing, and so forth. The corollary of these observations—one which may explain why the rule "the younger the child the greater the damage to the brain from blunt trauma" applies: it may be that open fontanel and sutures predispose a child to a higher possibility of subdural hematoma. It has been observed that 32% of the open-fontanel population suffer subdural hematoma as a consequence of blunt head injury, whereas only 5% of the closed-fontanel population suffer this complication.[16] In fact, in this review of our work, we observed that 79% of all posttraumatic intracranial mass lesions occurred in infants and that 93% of these were subdural hematomas.[46] Moreover, 7.5% (4 of 53) of these patients were toddlers, mostly suffering an admission Children's Coma Score (CCS) of 11 and none below 8.

Newborn and infants suffering subdural hematomas are generally admitted into hospital late, at a time when they are symptomatic (experiencing failure to thrive, seizures, vomiting, or lethargy) with clinical evidence of increasing intracranial pressure (split sutures, bulging fontanel, "sunset" phenomenon, etc.). Toddlers and older children, however, most often present immediately after a head injury significant enough to cause a subdural hematoma. Their long-term symptoms and signs are expressive of either the postconcussion syndrome (irritability, diminution of academic performance, headache, behavior change, etc.),[6] or of severe cerebral damage.[8] One may only hypothesize the reasons for the protection afforded by closed sutures and fontanels against the formation of a subdural hematoma. Among the possibilities are the following:

1. The clot formation may more easily assume a clinically significant volume within an expansile skull.
2. The absence of Pacchionian granules and arachnoidal adhesions to the dura both predispose the bridging cortical veins to tearing and blood to accumulate along the vertex.
3. The malleability of the skull permits more severe compression and distortion injury to the brain.

In any event, the occurrence of the subdural hematoma (whether acute or chronic) is responsible for the extreme difference in outcome between open- and closed-fontanel populations. This is evidenced by the fact that the exclusion of all subdural hematoma patients (83 of 462 in those studied) results in a drop in poor outcomes from 4.9% to 2.8% in the closed-fontanel population and from 13.9% to 4.6% in the open-suture population. (However, children under 1 year of age still suffer a higher incidence of poor outcome after head injury than older children.)

Development of the Child's Brain

A series of dilemmas confront investigators of craniocerebral trauma in children. It is often assumed that "children" include all those under legal voting age. The anatomical, physiological, developmental, and social differences among different age categories of children are enormous, however, and the clinician must separate one group from another when studying or treating head-injured children. The child evolves through very different structural and functional conditions as he or she ages.

During the first 3 years of a child's life, the central nervous system (CNS) continues to mature at almost the same rate as during the intrauterine period. Progression from the newborn existence (approximately 22 hours of sleep, with the waking intervals being limited almost entirely to feeding) to the 30-month-old child (who speaks, obeys commands, engages in meaningful play activities, and solves problems) is an infinitely greater change than those which occur over any other period in a lifetime. At birth, indeed, the brain's neuronal population is the same as in adult life, but glial cell proliferation, synaptic connections, and dendritic arborization have only begun. They progress almost logarithmically throughout the first 2 years of life; myelinization of the CNS, in contrast, begins within the first year of life but continues progressively through the 10th year. By 4 years of age, the child's brain weighs approximately 75% of the adult brain, although it is only 25% of that weight at birth: the result of glial growth, increased volume of neurons and axons, and myelinization. In fact, cerebral volume is not expressive of greater amounts of brain water, since there is a rapid decline in brain water during the first 2 years of life, during which time the child's brain is hydrated to the same extent as that of the adult. These structural factors are the basis for the characteristic pathoanatomical brain injuries characteristically suffered by infants less than 3 months of age—tears of the corpus callosum (the midbrain at its junction with the cerebral hemispheres), subcortical white matter, and the temporal and orbitofrontal lobes. The anatomical factors causing these lacerations are the malleability of the skull; the quasi-gelatinous consistency of a brain composed almost entirely of cells and without myelinated axons; small subarachnoid spaces; and large basal cisterns. (In contrast, older infants suffer tears at the pontomedullary junction, diffuse petechial hemorrhages, and cellular necrosis.) Along with the changes in cerebral structure of the infant brain, there are significant alterations in mesenchymal anatomy (skull, periosteum, sutures, and dura). The floating squamous bones of the calvarium first approach and then join one another; the fontanels become obliterated as membranous bone forms between the two layers of the periosteum; the sutures lose their anatomical definition as a mesenchymal bridge between outer layer of the dura (endosteum) and the periosteum; the tables of the skull thicken; and the diplöe convert from sinusoidal chambers to an irregular mass of channels running perpendicular to the surface of the skull. Thus, by one year of age—the clinically evident cutoff point between high and low incidence of subdural hematoma—the sutures have closed and the skull has become solid.

It is precisely this anatomical maturation, in which the child's brain progresses from a heavily hydrated mass of developing cells covered by pliable and isolated plates of membranous bone tethered at the sutures into a mass of solidly protected, highly specialized nuclear aggregates with myelinated axons, which makes it impossible to use constant clinical criteria to evaluate the nature, severity, and course of craniocerebral injury in children of different ages. These anatomical, physiological, and developmental factors have been too often ignored by investigators of pediatric head trauma. In fact, neonates, infants, toddlers, juveniles, adolescents and even young adults have frequently been considered a homogenous group. Of especial significance is the fact that, with only one exception, the subject of these patients' differences has never been reported chronologically—that is, by analyzing clinical observations in monthly or yearly age increments—in the critical first 3 years of life.

The efficacy of surgical or medical management (e.g., the use of Decadron),[7] as well as intensive care management with the use of bartiturate coma,[4] have been measured with the use of the Glasgow Coma Scale (GCS)[12,13] and evaluated in children of all ages. This has resulted in imprecise reporting of the incidence of subdural hematoma, intracerebral hematoma, cerebral laceration or contusion, brain swelling, cerebral vascular dilation, and alterations in the volume of circulating cerebral blood. The GCS is a standardized and generally accepted convention for evaluating the severity of head injury in adults, but it is not useful when applied to infants or toddlers. It is a grading system in which varying degrees of higher integrative functions (obeying commands, being oriented, spontaneous eye opening) are interpreted. Such a system permits disarticulation and resolution of individual integrative functions, but does not allow one to interpret functional alterations at subcortical and brain stem levels, which are the normal performance levels for newborn and infants. In fact, "a normal infant would not score better than 4 (of 6) on the motor exam (flexor withdrawal) or 2 (of 5) of the verbal exam (incomprehensible sounds)" on the GCS. Also, the interpretation of any eye opening other than spontaneous might be misguided, as newborn and infants generally close their eyes when feeling pain.

In addition to these obvious inadequacies of the GCS in evaluating craniocerebral injury in childhood, one must consider the fact that the time necessary to evaluate the effects of cerebral damage is not known. Some forms of damage become less noticeable over the years, and others remain obscure until a later age when more demands (motor and intellectual) are put upon the brain.[2,3] "Moderately" brain-injured infants and toddlers very often appear to recover soon after the injury and do not show signs of sensory, motor, cognitive, or behavioral impairment for many years. This is as true for cerebral injury as it is for hydrocephalus, meningitis, porencephaly, vasospasm, and the dysraphic state. Very severe neurological deficits are the rule when porencephaly or meningitis occur in the neonatal period; moderate deficits are much more common when meningitis and encephalitis occur during the first 2 years of life. One cannot accept anecdotal reports that less damaging long-term effects result from injuries suffered in the early years of life, or that young children "outgrow," or are more resistent to, cerebral damage. Approximately 20% of head-injured children suffer hyperkinesis, difficulty in anger control, impaired attention, and headache—the "post-traumatic syndrome."[6] Also, studies of delinquent children with psychiatric problems reveal that a statistically significant number of them suffered head or face injuries in childhood.[15] Therefore, normal neurological or IQ examinations of children who have suffered head injuries are no assurance that permanent and significant brain damage has not occurred.

The Children's Coma Score and Outcome Scale

In a previous publication the authors reported on a study of 462 head-injured children (between 1 and 36 months of age) in whom the head injuries ranged from trivial to deep coma.[16] Neither penetrating head injuries nor birth injuries were considered in this study. The results permitted the categorization of a Children's Coma Score (CCS) and the preparation of a Children's Outcome Scale (COS), both predicated entirely upon direct observations of injured infants and toddlers.

The three elements of the neurological examination that forms the basis of the CCS are motor, ocular, and verbal. The total score is the sum of the three subscores, as shown in Table 10.1. Since infants are unable to speak and injured toddlers generally neither obey commands nor respond appropriately to verbal stimuli, no points were allocated to responses requiring such complex behavior as speech or stimulus localization. Five COS categories were designated:

I—excellent recovery
II—moderate, but nondisabling deficit
III—either a severe motor or cognitive deficit
IV—vegetative
V—death

Table 10.1. Children's Coma Score (CCS) subscores.

Ocular response: maximum score = 4
    4 pursuit
    3 extraocular muscles (EOM) intact, reactive pupils
    2 fixed pupils or EOM impaired
    1 fixed pupils and EOM paralyzed

Verbal response: maximum score = 3
    3 cries
    2 spontaneous respirations
    1 apneic

Motor response: maximum score = 4
    4 flexes and extends
    3 withdraws from painful stimuli
    2 hypertonic
    1 flaccid
      Total maximum score = 11
      Total minimum score = 3

Categories I and II are considered good outcomes, and III to V are considered poor outcomes.

A comparison of the GCS and the CCS shows that the maximum score on the GCS is 15, whereas it is only 11 on the CCS. In addition to this, the former examination permits good discrimination of higher integrative functions, whereas the latter provides only for evaluation of subcortical and brain stem functions. In fact, comparing the GCS to the CCS for higher integrative functions reveals that in the GCS, a score of 12 to 15 is awarded when the patient is either "normal" or, at the very least, able to open his or her eyes to command. The score is lowest when the patient is not responding (in terms of either motor or cognitive responses) to verbal command or pain.

None of these higher integrative functions are testable in infants and toddlers. Cortical functions are expressed by a score of 9 to 11 on the GCS, but infants and toddlers must get the highest score, 11, on the CCS—the score of a normal child in this age range. Subcortical functions score out at 5 to 8 on the GCS and at 8 to 10 on the CCS, which illustrates that the CCS is more sensitive for appraising subcortical function. Adults who are functioning at the brain stem level score from 3 to 4 on the GCS, whereas infants and toddlers score from 3 to 7 on the CCS.

Despite the fact that seizures, split sutures, a bulging fontanel, and a high-pitched cry are the common presenting signs of increases in intracranial pressure in infants—signs that result in a much higher percentage of head-injured infants brought to the hospital early and treated early—infants suffer greater cerebral damage and do not recover as well as toddlers. Infants do not have a greater incidence of seizures, lateralizing signs, or skull fractures than toddlers, and vice versa. Neurologically intact children with open sutures at the time of hospital admission are more likely to have a poor outcome; this observation applies across the full range of CCSs at admission right down to a score of 3. The single most reliable examination for evaluating outcome in children is the ocular one, since it is most consistent at both the high and low ends of the scale: 100% of closed suture and 94% of open suture children enjoyed "good" recovery at ocular level 4, while no patient with an ocular level of 1 survived. In the verbal exam, 98% of the closed-fontanel children and 92% of the open-fontanel children with a score of 3 had "good" outcome; in contrast, the percentages for children with a score of 2 were 56% and 8%, respectively. The p number for "good" outcome at motor level 4 is 0.0005, with only 6% suffering a "poor" outcome; at motor level 3, 19% suffered "poor" outcomes.

Radiographic evidence of posttraumatic splitting of the sutures is indicative both of a poor outcome and a higher incidence of posttraumatic seizure. Palpation of the open fontanel provides good evidence regarding outcome, as only 5% of children with a soft fontanel suffered a "poor" outcome. Of those with a full fontanel, 16% suffered a "poor" outcome; and 50% of those with a tense fontanel suffered a "poor" outcome. Only 12% of those children with a soft fontanel had subdural hematomas, whereas the percentages rose to 71% and 83%, respectively, for those with full and tense fontanels. The presence of a linear skull fracture may not be correlated with outcome unless it is bilateral. Seven percent of those children without and 4% of those with linear fractures had a "poor" outcome, whereas 26% with bilateral fractures suffered a "poor" outcome. One must also distinguish between linear and diastatic fractures, as 33% of children with diastatic fractures suffered poor results. Posttraumatic seizures occurred in 10% of those children with depressed fractures and in 7% of those without such fractures.

Regardless of whether a child's sutures and fontanel are open or closed, ocular deviation and hemiparesis may not be correlated with a "poor" outcome; in contrast, simple hemiparesis (in the absence of ocular deviation) was significantly associated—in 26% of the cases studied—with a "poor" outcome. The presence of an extensor plantar response did not alter these relationships. In fact, a unilateral Babinski sign, along with hemiparesis and ocular deviation are indicative of a benign course in 97% of head-injured children under 3 years old. Whether the coexistence of this triad is expressive of a seizure rather than of discrete neurological destruction is not known, although approximately 62% of children with this triad may be expected to suffer focal motor seizures sometime during their hospital stay, and 23% remain permanently epileptic. When these numbers are compared to the incidence of posttraumatic seizures in the general population (only 3%), this correlation becomes quite meaningful. It is also important to realize that such hard evidence of neurological deficit as an extensor plantar response, ocular deviation, and hemiparesis are actually indicative of a benign course.

Given the possibility that the triad (extensor plantar response, ocular deviation, and hemiparesis) may be a seizure equivalent and that it may be correlated with a benign course, the examiner must immediately separate this clinical picture from tonic–clonic posttraumatic seizures, whether focal or generalized. Of the children with focal seizures 14% suffered poor outcomes and another 14% had recurrent seizures; 69% of the posttraumatic seizure patients were less than 1 year old. Of the children with generalized seizures, 27% suffered a poor outcome, and 10% had recurrent seizures; 76% of the patients were less than 12 months old. Late seizures occur more commonly in children who suffer early focal seizures, and 66% of the patients who developed late seizures were expected to suffer a poor outcome. The incidence of posttraumatic seizures was higher in infants than in toddlers (26% versus 10%), and there is evidence that the toddler has the same incidence of posttraumatic epilepsy as does the adult. A comparison of percentages in the age categories— 26% of the newborns, 18% of the children between 1 and 12 months of age, and approximately 10% of the patients older than 1 year—indicates that the seizure rate drops after the first month of life, remains high during the first year, and levels off thereafter.

Bilateral retinal hemorrhages correlate directly with poor outcome, whereas a unilateral retinal hemorrhage is of no significance at all. Split sutures and bilateral retinal hemorrhages often coexist; both indicate a sudden and severe rise in intracranial pressure. In fact, 65% of those children with bilateral retinal hemorrhage had extra-axial hematomas. Such signs indicate to the clinician that immediate surgery is essential, especially in light of the fact that timely removal of the clot is associated with a good outcome in exactly the same percentage of cases as subdural hematoma alone without split sutures or retinal hemorrhages (69% had good outcomes in both groups). Two conclusions may thus be reached:

1. Unilateral retinal hemorrhages are qualitatively and quantitatively different from bilateral hemorrhages—they are less severe, occur in older children, and are less often associated with extra-axial hematoma.
2. Bilateral hemorrhages are a reliable signal of the need for emergency treatment. They are a result of an acute increase in intracranial pressure, as are split sutures and diastatic fractures.

In fact, however, retinal hemorrhages are more reliable as an indicator of an increase in intracranial pressure than a bulging and tense anterior fontanel because an expanding extra-axial hematoma does not invariably cause a tense or bulging fontanel.

Of the children studied who were suffering intracranial mass lesions, 79% were less than 1 year old; subdural hematoma was the pathological lesion in 93% of the cases, with the chronic variety occurring in two-thirds of the children studied. There was no difference in the outcomes of children with subdural hematoma treated with burr holes, subdural puncture, or subdural peritoneal shunts. In fact, in these children the subdural fluid continued to reaccumulate even if all three forms of treatment were employed. The children treated with craniotomy and evacuation of the hematoma did enjoy a much better outcome: 73% of the open-fontanel children and 62% of the closed-fontanel children had good outcomes. If "hanging veins"[18] were present in cerebral angiography, lowering of the superior sagittal sinus was an effective treatment in 90% of the children.[8] Epidural hematoma and intraparenchymal edema are most unusual in open-fontanel children, though they represent 25% and 12%, respectively, of intracranial clots in toddlers. An epidural hematoma in a toddler is normally associated with a "good" outcome if treated before pupil changes occur; with a "poor" outcome if treated after pupil changes have occurred; and with either a vegetative state or death if the pupils are fixed and dilated. In contrast, regardless of the status of the pupils, intraparenchymal mass lesions are always associated with severe edema and a "poor" outcome.

References

1. Baker S: Motor vehicle occupant deaths in young children. *Pediatrics* 1979;64:860–871.
2. Black P, Blumer D, Wellner A, Walker A: The head-injured child: Time-course of recovery, with implications for rehabilitations, in *Proceedings of the International Symposium on Head Injuries, Edinburgh 1971*. Edinburgh, 1971, Churchill Livingstone, pp 131–137.
3. Black P, Blumer D, Wellner A, Shepard R, Walker E: Head trauma in children: Neurological, behavioral, and intellectual sequelae, in Black P: Brain Dysfunction in Children: Etiology, Diagnosis & Management. New York, Raven Press Publishers, 1981.
4. Bruce D, Schut L, Bruno L, Wood J, Sutton L: Outcome following severe head injuries in children. *J Neurosurg* 1978;48:679–688.
5. Craft A, Shaw D, Cartlidge N: Head injuries in children. *Br Med J* 1972; 4:200–203.
6. Dillon H, Leopold R: Children and post-concussion syndrome. *JAMA* 1961; 175:80–92.
7. Gobiet W, Bock W, Liesengang J, Grote W: Treatment of acute cerebral edema with high dose dexamethadone, in Mario Brock: *Intracranial Pressure*, ed 3. Berlin, Springer-Verlag, 1976, pp 231–235.
8. Gutierrez FA, McLone DG, Raimondi AJ: Physiopathology and a new treatment of chronic subdural hematoma in children. *Child's Brain* 1979;5:216–232.
9. Heiskanen O, Kaste M: Late prognosis of severe brain injury in children. *Dev Med Child Neurol* 1974;16:11–14.
10. Hendrick E, Harris L: Post-traumatic epilepsy in children. *J Trauma* 1968; 8:547–566.

11. Jennett B: Head injuries in children. *Dev Med Child Neurol* 1972;14:137–147.
12. Jennett B, Bond M: Assessment of outcome after severe brain damage. *Lancet* 1975;1:480–484.
13. Jennett B, Teasdale G, Braakman R, Minderhoud J, Heiden J, Kurze T: Prognosis of patients with severe head injury. *Neurosurgery* 1979:4:283–289.
14. Jennett B, Teasdale G, Galbraith S, Pickard J, Grant H, Braakman R, Avezaat C, Mass A, Minderhoud J, Vecht J, Heiden J, Small R, Caton W, Kurze T: Severe head injuries in three countries. *J Neurolog Neurosurg Psychiat* 1977;40:291–298.
15. Lewis D, Shanok W: Medical histories of psychiatrically referred delinquent children: An epidemiologic study. *Am J Psychiat* 1979;136:231–233.
16. Raimondi AJ, Hirschauer J: Head injury in the infant and toddler—coma scoring and outcome scale. *Child's Brain* 1984;11:12–35.
17. Raimondi AJ: Pediatric Neuroradiology. Philadelphia, WB Saunders and Company, 1972.
18. Raimondi AJ, Cerullo LJ: *Atlas of Cerebral Angiography in Infants and Children*. Stuttgart, Georg Thieme Verlag, 1980.

CHAPTER 11

Medical Management of Head Injuries in Neonates and Infants

Marion L. Walker and Bruce B. Storrs

Introduction

The medical management of children with head injuries is often the most important aspect of their treatment. Children have a much lower incidence of surgical mass lesions (25%)[4,5,19,20] than adults (50%)[1,2,9] They also suffer an 80% incidence of increased intracranial pressure following severe head injuries.[15] Thus, the medical management of their injuries has an increased importance. The age of the patient has a profound influence on the type of injury sustained and the ultimate outcome. It appears that a child under 2 years old is at the highest risk for significant complications and sequelae following a severe head injury. Many of these complications are related to the secondary injury of the brain[6,19,20] such as edema, hyperemia, hypoxia, and so on, and thus are managed medically.

The medical management of head injuries can be conveniently divided into three areas: emergency-department, intra-operative, and intensive-care management. This chapter discusses the types of medical therapy to be given and the timing of such therapy in the severely injured infant and neonate.

Medical Management in the Emergency Department

Emergency department management includes prehospital status of the severely injured child. There is no question that the active involvement of trauma personnel in the prehospital care of such a child contributes significantly to the patient's improved outcome. This involvement should begin with the provision of emergency care at the accident scene and should be appropriate to the needs of the infant. Provision of an adequate airway, prevention of hypoxia and hypercapnia, administration of appropriate intravenous fluids and blood, aggressive treatment of hypotension, temperature control, assessment and management of other injuries, and rapid transport to appropriate neurosurgical care facilities are all imperative prehospital activities.

Hypoxia, hypotension, and/or hypercapnia are serious complications which often follow severe head injury.[6,19] Since these factors are frequently present soon after the injury, it is important that the trauma personnel, especially the first ones to see the patient, do everything possible to eliminate or minimize such complications. The first step in the medical management of the severely head injured infant, therefore, is to assure an adequate airway for the child. Oxygen should be given as soon as possible either by mask or endotracheal tube. Spontaneous breathing must be sufficient, or else respirations should be controlled. In the event it is necessary to control the respirations, hyperventilation should be initiated with the intent of keeping the PCO_2 in the range of 25 to 35 torr. This is easily accomplished in the infant by providing a symmetrically full chest wall rise with the inspiration of air and by increasing the inspiratory rate to the range of 30 to 40 breaths per minute. Circulation should be normal, and appropriate intravenous fluids administered as required (see Table 11-1).

All this treatment may be initiated prior to the patient's arrival in the emergency department. In the seriously head injured child, especially one with respiratory compromise, it is imperative that these measures be undertaken immediately. Indeed, it is the obligation of all personnel involved in the care of head injured children to be aware of the importance of prehospital management and to be actively involved in such care.

After arriving in the emergency department, the patient is again evaluated for the presence of any evidence of hypoxia, hypotension, and/or hypercapnia. Blood gases should be drawn immediately. The PO_2 values may have been corrected by the administration of oxygen, but the presence of acidosis strongly suggests that serious hypoxia has been present. The patient must have a complete examination for other injuries as well as an evaluation of the central nervous system (CNS). Multiple trauma has a very negative impact on the outcome of the head injured patient.[11-14,19,20], so that treatment of other injuries must begin concurrently with the management of the head injury.

Table 11.1. Intravenous fluid therapy.

For normal fluid maintenance:
   First 10 kg: 100 cc/kg/day
   Second 10 kg: 50 cc/kg/day
   Thereafter: 20cc/kg/day
If shock is present:
   Start 2 intravenous lines
   Pump in 20 cc/kg Ringer's lactate solution
     If blood pressure remains below 70 mm Hg
   Repeat the bolus of Ringer's lactate solution
     If blood pressure remains below 70 mm Hg,
   Transfuse 20cc/kg packed red blood cells

Laboratory examination of the blood and urine should begin while the examination and initial treatment of the patient are proceeding, in order to facilitate a rapid return of this vital information. We use a standard trauma laboratory protocol for all seriously traumatized patients (see Table 11-2). This ensures that important lab values will not be forgotten, and saves the time consumed with decisions regarding which lab values are essential to managing the child during a most critical time in the patient's care.

One of the most important aspects of the medical management of the head injured child is appropriate intravenous fluid therapy and fluid resuscitation. Two routes of venous access are required. The intravenous catheters must be at least 22 (or preferably even larger) so that blood can be given if necessary.

Children have much lower blood volume than adults, and a child's blood volume constitutes a larger portion of his or her body weight.[17] Loss of relatively small amounts of blood can produce dramatic changes in circulation. It should also be remembered that a child can lose significant amounts of blood intracranially, into the scalp, or into the soft tissue spaces around long bone fractures—in an insidious manner. Particularly in the neonatal period and early infancy, profound circulatory collapse can occur from a combination of intracranial and scalp bleeding with no evidence of external hemorrhage.[18] Accordingly, appropriate fluid and blood resuscitation should always be available. Children in this age group with skull fractures may frequently suffer dramatic decreases in the hematocrit and will, thus, occasionally require blood transfusions.

Early signs of shock should be treated with 20cc/kg of lactated Ringer's solutions to maintain the blood pressure at 80 mm/Hg, + 2 times the age in years, e.g., 88 mm Hg for a four-year-old child. If hypotension persists, another bolus of 20 cc/kg of lactated Ringer's solution should be given. Profound shock should be treated with 20 cc/kg of whole blood. It is advisable to keep universal-donor, low-titer whole blood available at all time for the serious trauma victim. Should a patient's shock not allow

Table 11.2. Laboratory protocol for severe trauma victims.

Complete blood count with differential:

Electrolytes
Amylase
Creatinine
Blood urea nitrogen
Prothrombin time
Partial thromboplastin time
Platelets
Type and cross-match two units of whole blood
Arterial blood gases

time for formal typing crossmatching of blood, this universal-donor blood is immediately available and can be life-saving.

The early post-injury initiation of anticonvulsant therapy can be important. Any patient with a penetrating brain injury, a significantly depressed skull fracture, any type of intracranial bleeding, or a Glasgow Coma Scale (GCS) score of 5 or less should be considered a candidate for anticonvulsant therapy. Initiation of this therapy at an early stage will often prevent further complications. In the seriously head injured child, the objective of therapy is prevention of any secondary brain injury. Seizures dramatically increase intracranial pressure and may cause further neurological deterioration. This becomes important when one remembers that seizures may increase intracranial pressure to unacceptable levels. Seizures must not be awaited; therefore, anticonvulsant medications should be administered immediately. It may then be discontinued when no longer indicated. There is disagreement regarding the appropriate length of prophylactic anticonvulsant therapy in those children who have shown clinical evidence of convulsions. We advise treating a patient for 6 to 18 months unless the electroencephalogram shows continuing evidence of seizure risk.

Phenytoin (Dilantin) is the author's drug of choice to control seizures. Phenytoin has less sedative effect than phenobarbital. Rapid therapeutic levels can usually be achieved by the intravenous route. A loading dose of 15 mg/kg given intravenously is followed by a daily maintenance dose of 5 mg/kg/day. Should the patient arrive at the hospital in status epilepticus, intravenous diazepam (Valium), 0.10mg/kg to 0.25mg/kg, is a good choice for controlling the seizures. Caution, however, should be exercised with use of intravenous diazepam; always be prepared to intubate and to control respirations if necessary.

Phenytoin is often poorly absorbed from the gastrointestinal tract in neonatal and early infant populations. Thus, when changing from intravenous to oral phenytoin therapy, serum levels should be monitored carefully. If phenytoin cannot be maintained in the proper range by oral administration, the patient should be changed to phenobarbital or another anticonvulsant medication.

There is still some controversy regarding the use of steroids in the treatment of head injuries.[7,8,16] Evidence suggests that steroids are not effective in treating acute brain injuries; accordingly, we do not use them in our patients.

Osmotic diuretics have a limited place in the prehospital and emergency department management of head injuries. This is especially true for children. There is no doubt that in a patient who is rapidly deteriorating from an expanding intracranial hematoma, osmotic diuretic therapy may indeed be lifesaving. However, there are many reasons not to use osmotic diuretic therapy in a child. First, and perhaps most important, children have a significant incidence of hyperemia in injured brain areas.[3] Since blood occupies space, there may also be a significant increase in intracranial pressure. The diuretic agent, mannitol, causes an increase in cerebral blood flow, which may be enough to cause further neurological deterioration. Second, the injudicious use of osmotic diuretics may confuse the clinical picture. Should the patient have a small expanding intracranial hematoma (not yet clinically apparent), osmotic diuretic therapy may allow enough brain shrinkage to keep the bleeding clinically silent until there is sudden deterioration from a large intracranial hematoma. This condition can truly be catastrophic. It is therefore always important to exercise extreme caution before administering osmotic diuretic therapy. This should be given only after a neurosurgeon approves. Yet another consideration when using osmotic diuretics in small children is the potential for producing shock. If the blood volume of the patient is even moderately decreased, continued loss of fluid may further lower the blood pressure and affect oxygen concentrations.

Antibiotics are indicated for all open brain injuries. Ampicillin (200 mg/kg/day) and methicillin (200 mg/kg/day) are recommended; however, we do not use antibiotics for closed head injuries or for basilar skull fractures. There is evidence to suggest that the prophylactic use of antibiotics in basilar skull fractures does not decrease the incidence of meningitis.[10] Moreover, should meningitis occur, a resistant organism is usually encountered when antibiotics have been used.

Other important considerations in the emergency department management of the seriously head injured child include raising the head, neck position, treatment of pain, and recognizing and treating other injuries. It has been demonstrated that raising the head can significantly lower intracranial pressure.[6] This simple maneuver should be used in all seriously injured patients unless the patient's cardiovascular status would be compromised. The neck should be positioned in the midline.[6] Turning the head too far to the right or left can cause jugular occlusion and diminished venous drainage on one side, sometimes dramatically increasing intracranial pressure.

Pain should be treated if the patient's response to that pain is muscle tension, which increases intracranial pressure. Occasionally, more than just neuromuscular paralysis is necessary. The judicious use of analgesics can be an important part of intracranial pressure management.

As noted earlier, multiple trauma is a serious complicating factor of head injuries which should never be overlooked.[20] An important part of medical management is making certain that all other injuries are being appropriately treated.

Intra-Operative Medical Management

Although the neurosurgeon is often preoccupied with the surgical management of trauma while in the operating room, it should never be forgotten that medical management is equally important in ensuring a good outcome. Much of medical management is a continuation of the appropriate therapy initiated in the emergency department.

Again, it should be noted that intravenous fluids and appropriate blood resuscitation are important. An important concept to remember is that there is a physiologic response to the sudden release of intracranial pressure that is peculiar to patients in the neonatal and infant age groups. During a surgical procedure, the sudden release and evacuation of a subdural or epidural hematoma often precipitates an immediate and profound shock, sometimes followed by cardiac arrest. This is related entirely to a sudden collapse of the vascular system, which occurs upon release of the increased intracranial pressure that has been maintaining increased vascular tone. With the vasuclar tone relaxed, there is pooling of blood into the periphery of the vascular system. In some circumstances the result is profound cardiovascular collapse.

The surgeon and anesthesiologist must be prepared to treat this emergency. The best treatment is prevention. Surgery should never be started before blood is running into the patient through large bore intravenous catheters. At least two routes of intravenous access are mandatory. If blood is given at the beginning of the procedure, the possibility of sudden vascular collapse is often either eliminated or kept minimal. If such precautions for blood transfusion are not followed, cardiac arrest is likely to occur, and the patient may die.

During the intra-operative phase, the patient should be continued on any anticonvulsants and antibiotics that may have been started prior to his arrival in the operating room. Anesthetic management of the severely injured neonate and infant is also a vital part of intra-operative therapy. The anesthetic agent chosen should minimize any increased intracranial pressure that may already be present.

Medical Management in the Intensive Care Unit

It has been noted by many authors that secondary injury to the brain is often the most significant determinant of the eventual outcome.[4,5,6,9] Many patients with severe primary head injury either do not survive long enough to reach hospital or do not live beyond the first few hours following their injury. Those patients who do survive their primary injury can be expected to continue improving in a high percentage of the cases, barring secondary complication.[5,19]

Intensive care unit (ICU) management of the seriously head injured neonate and infant is designed to minimize secondary complications and to provide an adequate environment for recovery. Therapy is directed toward maintaining normal cerebral blood flow (CBF), normal cerebral metabolism, and normal intracranial pressure (ICP).

Maintenance of normal CBF is obviously an important part of the ICU

Table 11.3. ICP monitor protocol.

Indicator	ICP monitor required
GCS 3–5	Yes
GCS 6 or 7	
with *abnormal* CAT scan	Yes
with *normal* CAT scan	No

management.[6] The patient's blood pressure should be kept in the normal range (i.e., blood pressure > 80 mm/Hg plus two times the age in years). If there is serious concern about the possibility of increased ICP, consideration should be given to keeping the cerebral perfusion pressure greater than 50 torr. Because at present there are few practical and readily available methods of measuring CBF rapidly in most intensive care units, it is appropriate to place an ICP monitor for observing cerebral perfusion pressure.

A special type of injury seen in young children is the "malignant edema" or cerebral hyperemia syndrome.[33] It causes a dramatic increase in ICP as a result of increased CBF. These patients generally arrive at the hospital with low GCS scores. They improve dramatically, however, if monitored in the ICU with respirations and if their ICP is controlled over a 2- to 3-day period.

Efforts should also be made to maintain normal cerebral metabolism. Blood glucose levels should be kept well within the normal range. It is also important to maintain the PO_2 at 100 torr or slightly above.

Much intensive care effort is directed toward control of ICP. It should be remembered, however, that not all patients require ICP monitoring. Early in the patient's course, a decision should be made as to whether he is an appropriate candidate for ICP monitor placement (see Table 11.3). Patients who are not candidates should be observed closely for any signs of neurological deterioration.

Figure 11.1 presents a protocol for determining which children should receive ICP monitoring. Patients with GCS scores of 5 or less should be considered candidates for ICP monitoring. (Exceptions might be patients with brain death.) Patients with GCS scores of 6 or 7 and normal CT scans are generally observed in the ICU without ICP monitoring. An abnormal CT, however, is an indication of the need for intracranial pressure monitor placement and appropriate therapy. Patients with GCS scores of 8 or above are generally observed and do not require intracranial pressure monitoring unless there is neurological deterioration. Any patient who is able to cry is given a full verbal score for GCS scoring purposes.

It has been our experience that a normal CT scan generally translates into normal intracranial pressure. For this reason, we often observe the patient with a GCS of 6 or 7 without monitoring unless deterioration

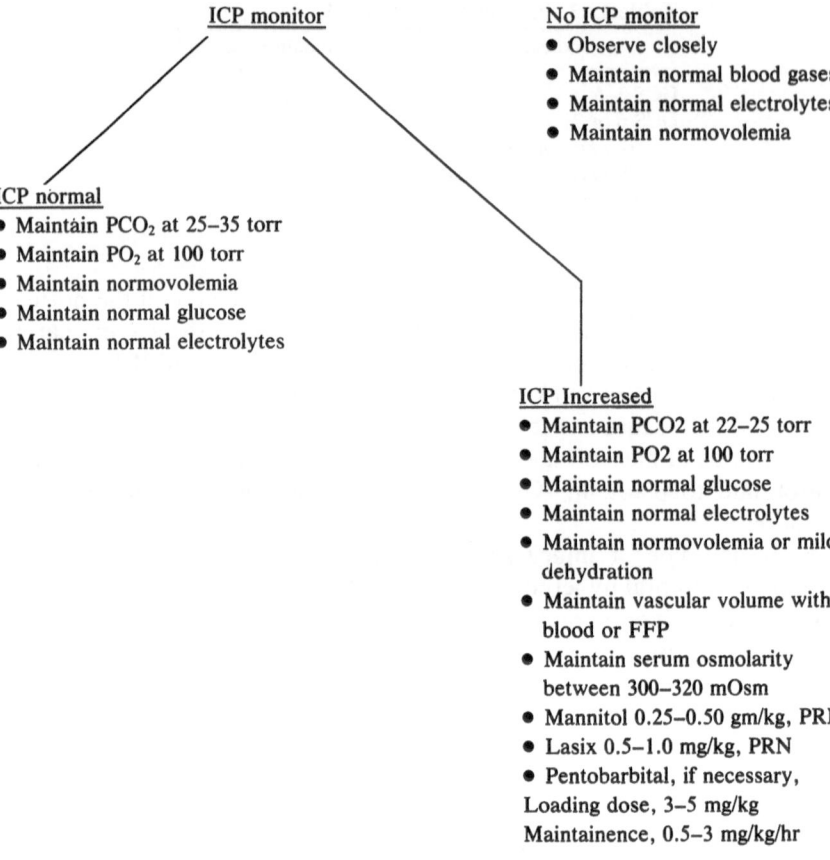

ICP monitor

No ICP monitor
- Observe closely
- Maintain normal blood gases
- Maintain normal electrolytes
- Maintain normovolemia

ICP normal
- Maintain PCO_2 at 25–35 torr
- Maintain PO_2 at 100 torr
- Maintain normovolemia
- Maintain normal glucose
- Maintain normal electrolytes

ICP Increased
- Maintain PCO2 at 22–25 torr
- Maintain PO2 at 100 torr
- Maintain normal glucose
- Maintain normal electrolytes
- Maintain normovolemia or mild dehydration
- Maintain vascular volume with blood or FFP
- Maintain serum osmolarity between 300–320 mOsm
- Mannitol 0.25–0.50 gm/kg, PRN
- Lasix 0.5–1.0 mg/kg, PRN
- Pentobarbital, if necessary, Loading dose, 3–5 mg/kg Maintainence, 0.5–3 mg/kg/hr

Figure 11.1. Head injury protocol: Intensive-care management flow sheet.

occurs. However, in the severely injured patient with a GCS of 3 or 4, an intracranial pressure monitor is often desirable even though the CT scan may be normal. This patient may be expected to remain unconscious for several days following injury, and to develop cerebral edema because of the serious nature of the brain injury.

Care should be exercised in selecting the appropriate intracranial pressure monitor for the infant and neonate. A ventricular catheter is often easiest because of the baby's thin skull and the difficulty of keeping a subarachnoid bolt in place. If it is anticipated that the ICP monitor will be needed for an extended period, it should be remembered that there is an increased risk of infection with an indwelling ventricular catheter. We have successfully used a three-way stopcock inserted through a twist drill hole in the skull of neonates and infants for ICP monitoring. This works quite well under most circumstances.[18] For the infant, the Philadelphia bolt has modifications that keep the bolt rigidly fixed to the skull.

Although approximately 80% of children with serious head injuries do develop increased intracranial pressure, not all such patients will have increased intracranial pressure at the time of placement of the ICP monitors. This may be because cerebral edema has not yet begun or because initial therapy has effectively lowered the pressure to the normal range. Normal intracranial pressure should be maintained with as little treatment as possible.

The patient should always have an arterial line for easy access to arterial blood gases.[6] The PO_2 should be kept at approximately 100 torr or slightly higher. If the ICP is normal, the PCO_2 can be kept in the 25 to 30 torr range. If the ICP later rises to unacceptable levels, the PCO_2 may be lowered to the 21 to 25 torr range. Lowering the PCO_2 to 21 torr in the absence of increased intracranial pressure eliminates one treatment option that might be used at a critical time.

Neuromuscular paralysis may sometimes be used to control ICP.[6] Residual muscle tone can dramatically increase intracranial pressure by reducing cerebral blood flow in patients who have already moved to the right hand portion of the cerebral compliance curve.

Seizure activity in a patient who is paralyzed with neuromuscular paralysis and is being maintained on a respirator may also cause a sudden rise in ICP.[18] The seizure activity will not be clinically apparent because of the neuromuscular paralysis. Treatment of these patients with intravenous diazepam (0.25–0.5 mg/kg) may dramatically lower the ICP to normal. The ICP of such patients can suddenly rise from 20 torr to 90 torr only to respond immediately to intravenous diazepam. (An EEG will confirm the presence of seizure activity.)

Osmotic diuretics are also effective in the treatment of increased intracranial pressure.[6] Mannitol is used in doses of 0.25 to 0.5 g/kg and can be repeated every 4 to 6 hours as needed. Furosemide (lasix) in a 1 mg/kg dose will also help in the treatment of cerebral edema and tends to enhance the action of mannitol.[18] When frequent doses of osmotic diuretics are used to control ICP, the serum osmolarity should be watched closely.[6,18] It should be checked every four hours and kept between 300 and 320 mOsm. Although dehydration has long been considered important in controlling ICP, it should be remembered that a child, especially a neonate or infant, can quickly become seriously dehydrated. Therefore, normovolmeia should be maintained. Should fluid restriction be essential for management of ICP, it is best to do this with great caution. Packed red blood cells and fresh frozen plasma may be used to maintain physiologic blood volume.[18]

In the seriously injured child, it is prudent to have some measure of monitoring central venous pressure for assistance in fluid management. Either a pulmonary capillary wedge pressure (PCWP) or a central venous pressure (CVP) line should be placed.[18] In most neonates and infants, the CVP accurately reflects left heart function and fluid status. The CVP measurements should be kept on the lower side of normal.

Barbituates have long been known to be effective in the treatment of increased ICP[16] because of their vasoconstrictive action and their reduction of the cerebral metabolic requirements resulting in reduced cerebral blood flow.[18] However, patients who are selected for barbituate therapy are generally those who have not responded to more conventional therapies in the intensive-care unit. For this reason, they are the patients at the highest risk for poor outcome. Pentobarbital is generally used when barbiturate coma is needed. It has a relatively short period of action and is cleared from the body within 1 to 2 days. If long-acting barbiturates such as phenobarbital are used, it may be a week or more before the blood levels allow appropriate testing of brain function after the barbiturates are discontinued. Rapid acting barbiturates require large volumes of medication and thus are not as practical as pentobarbital.

Pentobarbital is given in a 3- to 5-mg/kg loading dose and thereafter at 0.5 to 3.0 mg/kg/hr. A blood level of 35 to 50 mg/ml is maintained. An EEG will identify burst suppression as the endpoint for pentobarbital therapy. If the patient has not received significant reduction of ICP by the time burst suppression appears on the EEG, he is not likely to benefit from such therapy. In approximately 15% of patients thus treated, barbituate therapy will not reduce ICP; these patients are obviously doomed to poor outcomes.

Many patients with severe head injury experience the onset of the syndrome of inappropriate secretion of antidiuretic hormone (SIADH) early in their clinical course,[6] which sometimes results in low serum sodium and seizure activity. These patients should be closely observed for just such an occurrence. Electrolytes should be checked daily during the first 48 hours of their ICU stay. Decreasing urine output and falling PO_2 levels are other clues to the development of SIADH. Intravenous fluids should maintain sodium level in the therapeutic range, and solutions that contain too much free water should be avoided.[6]

Summary

Medical management plays an important role in the overall management of patients with head injuries. Because children have fewer surgical mass lesions and a higher incidence of increased intracranial pressure, medical management assumes an increased importance for patients in this age group. The infant and neonate require even more specialized care because of their small blood volume and their more fragile brain substance. Medical management begins in the prehospital phase and continues through the emergency room, operating room, and intensive care unit. When appropriately provided, such management may be expected to reduce the rates of morbidity and mortality of seriously head injured infants and neonates.

References

1. Becker DP, Miller JD, Word JD et al: The outcome from severe head injury with early diagnosis and intensive management. *J Neurosurg* 1977;47:491–502.
2. Bowers SA, Marshall LF: Outcome in 200 consecutive cases of severe head injury in San Diego County: A prospective analysis. *Neurosurgery* 1980;6:237–242.
3. Bruce DA, Alavi A, Bilaniuk LT, Dolinskas C, Obrist WA, Zimmerman RA, Uzzell B: Diffuse cerebral swelling following head injuries in children: The syndrome of "malignant brain edema". *J Neurosurg* 1981;54:170–178
4. Bruce DA, Rapyaely RC, Goldberg AI et al: Pathophysiology, treatment and outcome following severe head injury in children. *Child's Brain* 1979;5:174–191.
5. Bruce DA, Schut L, Bruno LA et al: Outcome following severe head injury in children. *J Neurosurg* 1978;48:679–688.
6. Bruce DA: Clinical care of the severely head injured child, in Shapiro K (ed), *Pediatric Head Trauma*. New York, Futura Publishing Co Inc, 1983, pp 27–44
7. Cooper PR, Moody S, Clark WK et al: Dexamethasone and severe head injury: A prospective double blind study. *J Neurosurg* 1979;51:307–316.
8. Faupel G, Reulen HS, Miller D, Schurmann K: Double blind study on the effects of steroids on severe closed head injury, in Papius HM and Feindel W (eds), New York, Springer-Verlag New York Inc Publishers, 1976, pp 337–343.
9. Gennarelli TA, Spielman GM, Langfitt TW et al.: Influence of the type of intracranial lesion on outcome from severe head injury. *J Neurosurg* 1982;56:26–32.
10. Ingelzi RJ, VanderArk GD: Analysis of the treatment of basilar skull fracture with and without antibiotics. *J Neurosurg* 1975;43:720–721
11. Mayer T, Matlak ME, Johnson DG, Walker ML: The modified injury severity scale in pediatric multiple trauma patients. *J Ped Surg* 1980;15:719–726.
12. Mayer T, Walker ML, Clark P: Further experience with the modified injury severity scale. *J Trauma* 1984;24:31–34.
13. Mayer T, Walker ML, Johnson DG, Matlak ME: Causes of morbidity and mortality in severe pediatric trauma. *JAMA* 1981;245:719–721.
14. Mayer T, Walker ML, Johnson DG, Shasa I: The effect of multiple trauma on the outcome of pediatric patients with head injuries. *Child's Brain* 1981;8:189–197.
15. Mayer T, Walker ML: Emergency intracranial pressure monitoring: Management of the acute coma of brain insult. *Clin Pediatr* 1982;21:391–396.
16. Saul TG, Ducker TB, Salcman M: Steroids in severe head injury: A prospective randomized clinical trial. *J Neurosurg* 1981;54:596–600.

17. Steele MW: Plasma volume changes in the neonate. *Am J Dis Child* 1962;103:10–18.
18. Venes JL: Management of Pediatric Head Injuries. *Contemporary Neurosurg* 1984;6:15.
19. Walker ML, Storrs BB, Mayer T: Pediatric head injury: The role of early therapy to prevent secondary injury. *Conc Ped Neurosurg* 5, 1985 (in press).
20. Walker ML, Storrs BB, Mayer T: Factors affecting outcome in the pediatric patient with multiple trauma. *Child's Brain* 1984;11:387–397.

CHAPTER 12

Incidence, Diagnosis, and Management of Skull Fractures

Maurice Choux

Introduction

Skull lesions after head injuries in infants occur relatively frequently in comparison with adults and even older children. The flexibility of the bones of the infant's skull, as well as open sutures present in very young children, explain the main characteristics of fractures and, especially, their frequency. If a true fracture is a disruption of the bones of the skull as a result of head trauma, a lesion of a suture (localized dysjunction or disruption) must also be considered a traumatic lesion.

A fracture is sometimes the only proof of head injury because many bony lesions are present without clinical symptoms, especially in small children. Consequently, a fracture may be the main reason to hospitalize a baby for observation. It is impossible to determine whether all injured babies presenting with a fracture of the skull should be hospitalized, however, since the majority will experience the same benign evolution. In 2020 infants with head trauma treated in our department, 10% had a complicated evolution in the form of intracranial hematoma or brain damage. The proportion of fractures in this category of patients was the same as that in patients with benign head trauma. Harwood-Nash, in a series of 4465 children of all ages,[26] arrived at the same conclusion: children with simple fractures (excluding depressed fractures) and children without fractures have the same incidence (8%) of serious sequellae. In a series of 570 children Roberts and Shopfner[56] found a similar absence of clinically significant symptoms in the groups with and without fractures: 72% and 78%, respectively.

Practically, one may ask the following questions: What are the medical and legal indications for skull Röentgenograms in pediatric patients with head trauma? What triggers the necessity for detecting a skull fracture? Might the detection of such a fracture require hospitalization?

It is clear that the presence of a skull fracture per se can have little or no medical management. This is especially true in infancy. Consequently, an immediate skull film after a head injury is not necessary; the initial clinical evaluation and management are more important.

Fractures can now be evaluated by CT scans in the high-resolution thin section (especially fractures of the cranial base). The three projections that are necessary in infants are the straight posterior-anterior view, the anteroposterior (Towne) view, and the lateral view of the suspected injured side. A further lateral view of the opposite site can be taken. Because of the horizontal development of the occipital bone in neonates and infants, the anteroposterior view or a stereo(Towne) view is necessary to visualize a fracture around the foramen magnum or of the occipital bone. However, because of the rarity of fractures of the cranial base, the petrous or ethmoid bones in infants, tomography of the base of the skull is seldom indicated.

Most linear fractures in infants are more sharply visualized in the lateral view. In fact, it is common to see the fracture in only one projection. Hence, knowledge of the injured side is important for radiographic examination.

Particularly in infants, fracture may be confused with sutures, intrasutural bones, accessory sutures, or synchondrosis. False traumatic aspects may be observed in the occipital region or at the level of the parietotemporal suture. The symmetry of the suture is an element of correct diagnosis. Vascular grooves are seldom confused with fracture in small babies.

Incidence of Fracture

The incidence of skull fracture in children—of all ages—varies, as reported in the literature, from 7% to 40%. In many studies, all injured children are considered; in others, reported incidence rates are lower because only children admitted to the hospital are considered.

In a study by Matson of 3053 children hospitalized because of head injury,[43] 1253 (41%) presented with skull fracture (simple, depressed, or compound). In the study by Harwood-Nash of 4465 children,[26] a skull fracture was present in 8% of all children and in 27% of hospitalized children. Jamison and Kaye, in a series of 857 children,[33] found 216 skull fractures (25%). In our department, among 8702 head-injured children 23% presented with skull fractures. Considering only children under 2 years old, the proportion of skull lesions is significantly higher in the majority of studies. In the study by Canestri and Monzali of 254 children under 3 years old,[12] 32.3% presented with fractures. In a study by Harwood-Nash of 1010 infants with head trauma, the incidence of fracture was 40%. Di Rocco and co-workers in a series of 230 infants with head trauma,[16] mentioned skull fracture in 132 cases (57%). In our study of 2022 head injured infants, 788 skull fractures were found (39%). We note that in many series the percentage of skull lesions in infants is nearly identical (about 40%).

Table 12.1. Incidence of head fracture in infants of different ages.

Age	Harwood-Nash	Choux
0–6 months ⎫ 6–12 months ⎭	30%	42% 42.8%
12–18 months ⎱ 18–24 months ⎭	37%	33.7% 20.2%

Age and Sex

The incidence of fractures in infancy at different ages in two studies is shown in Table 12.1, and the type of fractures at different ages of infancy is shown in Table 12.2. As the latter indicates, the percentage of fractures increases between 6 and 12 months.

In our study, as in that of Harwood-Nash,[26] the same percentage of boys and girls had fractures.

Types of Injury and Fracture

We have studied the incidence of fractures associated with the following types of injury:

	Linear fracture
Fall	86.1%
Traffic accident	6.3%
Impact	4.1%
Battered Children	3.5%

Four types of lesions are described: linear fractures, which are the most common; depressed fractures; open fractures; and those characteristic of infancy, growing fractures.

Linear Fractures

Linear fractures are the most frequent; they represent 88.38% of all fractures in our study, and 73% in that of Harwood-Nash.[26] A significant

Table 12.2. Distribution of head fractures in infants of different ages.

Age	Harwood-Nash (400 fractures)	Di Rocco (132 fractures)	Choux (788 fractures)
0–6 months ⎱ 0–12 months ⎭	43.5%	20% 43%	26.8% 37.6%
12–18 months ⎱ 18–24 months ⎭	56.5%	28% 9%	20.7% 14.9%

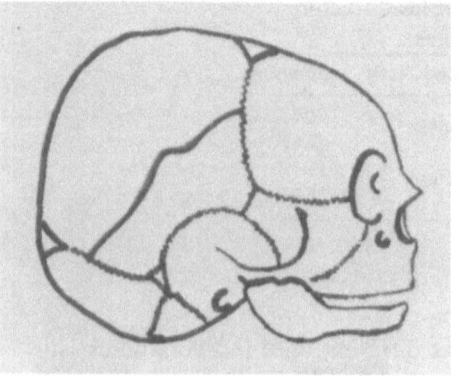

Type 1: straight fracture from suture to suture

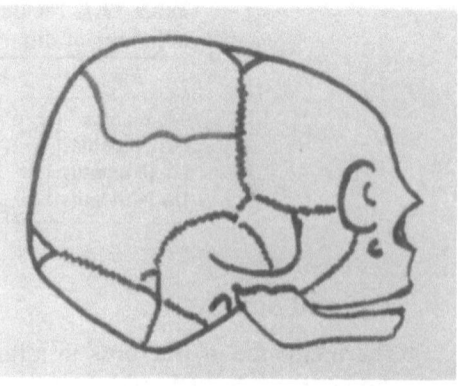

Type 2: right angle fracture from suture to suture

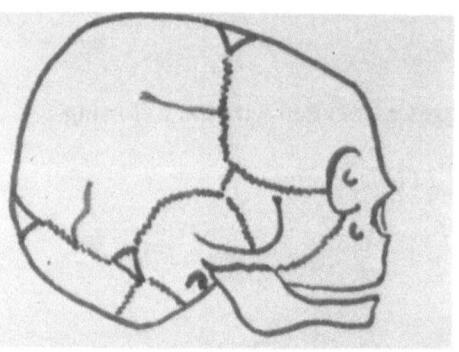

Type 3: small fracture ended at the suture

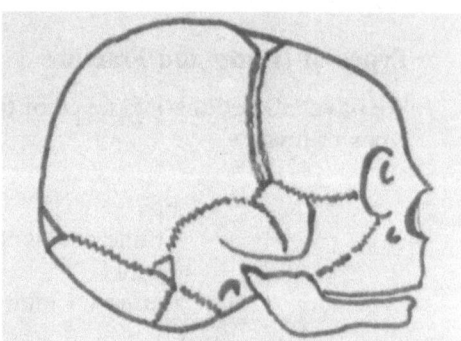

Type 4: diastatic suture fracture

Figure 12.1. Linear fractures: 4 types.

Figure 12.2. Linear fracture: Type 1. Parietal fracture extended from the coronal suture to the lambdoid suture.

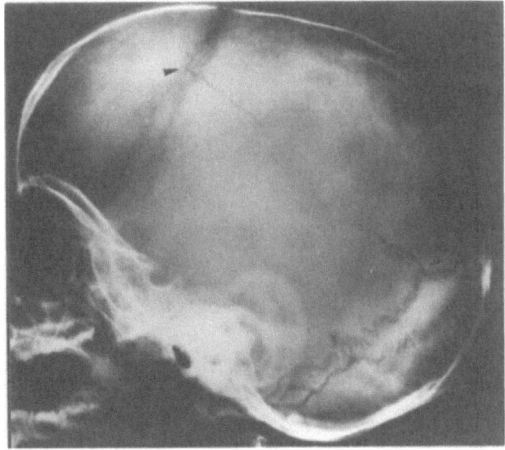

percentage of linear fractures (35.2%) are encountered in children between the ages of 6 and 12 months in our study.

We have distinguished four types of linear fractures in infants (see Fig. 12.1):

Type 1: This fracture extends from one suture to another, generally from the coronal to the lambdoid sutures (see Fig. 12.2).
Type 2: A right-angle fracture that extends from the coronal or the lambdoid suture to the sagittal suture (see Fig. 12.3).
Type 3: This fracture extends from a suture to a bone of the vault after a course of few centimeters (see Fig. 12.4).
Type 4: A traumatic (diastatic) suture separation.

As a rule, in infancy a linear fracture stops at the level of a suture. For example, in the case of head injury at the parietal level, the fracture will

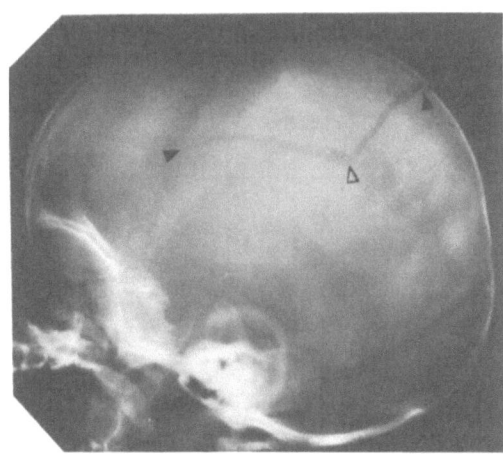

Figure 12.3. Linear fracture: Type 2. Right-angle parietal fracture extended from the coronal suture to the sagittal suture.

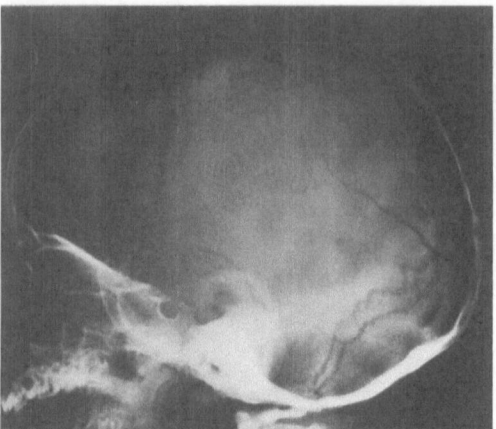

Figure 12.4. Linear fracture: Type 3. Partial parietal fracture ends at the level of the lambdoid suture.

extend to the coronal and lambdoid sutures (Type 1) without passing crossing them; if the impact is less severe, a fracture that begins at the center of the parietal bone extends to only one suture (Type 3). It is interesting to note that in infants, most linear fractures are horizontal except at the level of the occipital bone. When a vertical fracture is present, the clinical manifestations are generally more severe.

The localizations of linear fractures in our study are shown in Figure 12.5. The parietal bone is more frequently involved (in 536 cases, 76.3%), and the right side is more often involved than the left. The occipital bone is involved in 14.8% of the cases. The relative occipital bulging in young children, paucity of musculature, and the frequency of posterior falls in infants, explain the frequency of linear fractures of the occipital bone. Frontal localization is less common in infants (4.7%) than in older children (18% to 23%). Finally, we have only rarely noted fractures of the petrous bone (1%) nor have we seen a fracture of the anterior fossa of the

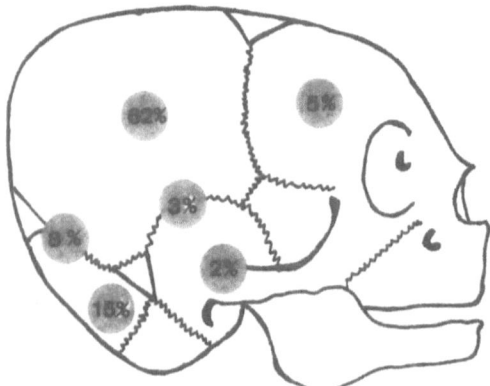

Figure 12.5. Localization of linear fractures in our series of 703 cases.

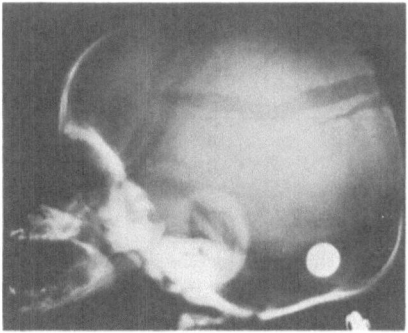 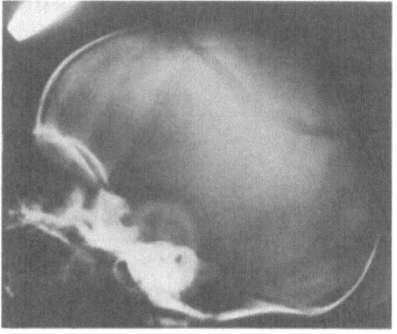

Figure 12.6. (A) Large parietal fracture in an 11-month-old child. (B) Large parietal fracture extending from the coronal to the lambdoid sutures in a 2-month-old child.

skull in living infants. Fractures were bilateral in 13% of our cases, multiple fractures were not rare, especially in battered children.

The aspects of a linear fracture are different according to the age. In neonates and infants under 6 months old, the fracture may be very large (2 to 6 mm) in the middle; the distance diminishes where the fracture ends at the level of the suture (Fig. 12.6). In these cases the fracture may enlarge significantly during the next days following the trauma, so we recommend, in cases of very large fractures, that skull x-rays be repeated two or three weeks later to detect the possible evolution of a growing fracture (see Fig. 12.7). In most cases, however, the fracture presents as a thin linear defect with the same spacing along all the trajectory. Healing of all linear fractures except the meningocele spuria in infants occurs quite rapidly, normally within 1 to 2 months.

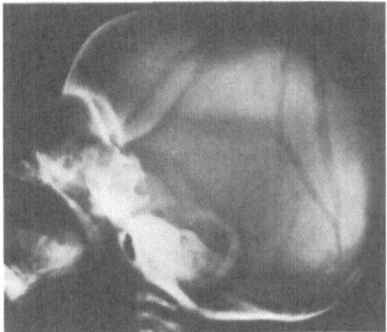 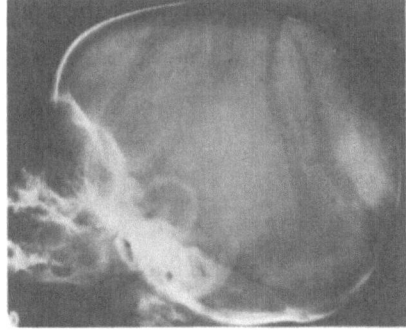

Figure 12.7. (A) Bilateral parietal fractures in a 2-month-old child. (B) 20 days later, enlargement of both fractures.

Table 12.3. Age distribution of children with
depressed skull fractures.

Age	Harwood-Nash (62 cases)	Choux (85 cases)
0–2 months ⎱ 3–6 months ⎰	32	16 8
7 months–1 year ⎱ 1–2 years ⎰	30	28 33

Depressed Fractures

Depressed fractures occurred in 7% to 10% of children admitted with a
head injury: 10% according to Matson,[43] 7% according to Harwood-
Nash,[26] and 9% in our study. In children with skull fractures, depressed
fractures represent 24.5% of the cases for Matson, 27% for Harwood-
Nash, 24.3% for Coulon,[15] and 25% for us.

In infants the frequency of fracture is lower than in older children, as a
great number of depressed fractures are caused by birth trauma. In the
study by Harwood-Nash,[26] of 400 skull fractures in children under 2 years
old, 62 (15.5%) were depressed fractures. In our series, among 703 skull
fractures in infants, 85 (12%) were depressed fractures.

In the Harwood-Nash series of 62 children with depressed fractures and
in our series of 85 children, the age distribution of patients is as given in
Table 12.3.

It is noteworthy that depressed fractures in infants between 3 and 6
months old are rare. Coulon,[15] in a series of 100 children with fractures,
found 15 cases of such fractures in children less than 2 years old. In our
series of 314 children with depressed fractures, 85 (27%) were infants.

Etiology

In comparison with linear fractures, the causes of depressed skull fractures are significantly different, as shown in Table 12.4. Note the relatively high incidence of depressed fractures after birth injury. A depressed fracture may appear and be diagnosed before birth, as we
observed in one case. The diagnosis was possible with echography and
was confirmed by abdominal x-rays at seven months' gestation. At birth,
a parietal depressed fracture was present. Alexander[2] has also docu-

Table 12.4. Causes of depressed versus linear head
fractures in children.

	Depressed fracture	Linear fracture
Falls	40%	82.4%
Traffic accident	22%	6.3%
Birth injury	16%	
Other	22%	11.3%

mented the intrauterine etiology of depressed fracture resulting from pressure on the fetal skull by the sacral promontory. In the majority of cases, depressed skull fractures in neonates are caused by forceps application or by the pressure of the obstetrician's hand. Axton[4] and Levy reported 31 cases, in an African population, which were the result of a difficult passage of the fetal skull through the birth canal.[4] In many cases, however, depressions occur in deliveries that were easy and not traumatic.

Clinical Aspects

An initial loss of consciousness does not occur in most cases of depressed fractures (90% in our series). In contrast to what happens in older children and in adults, depressed fractures in infants are generally asymptomatic. Consciousness is normal in more than 80% of the cases in our study. Only six patients were comatose; neurological examination revealed normal findings in 72 cases (87%). Motor deficit and seizures are rare. Subgaleal hematoma at the level of the depressed fracture is not rare in children older than 1 year. In newborn a "ping-pong ball" fracture may be clinically detected, as subperiosteal and subcutaneous hematomas are rare. Cutaneous lesions are also unusual at this age.

Radiological Findings

Three types of depressed fractures may be distinguished.

True Depressed Fractures. These fractures represent the majority of cases (45%). In this category the depressed bone remains connected with the cranial vault, but a break in the outer, or inner, or both tables may exist (see Fig. 12.8).

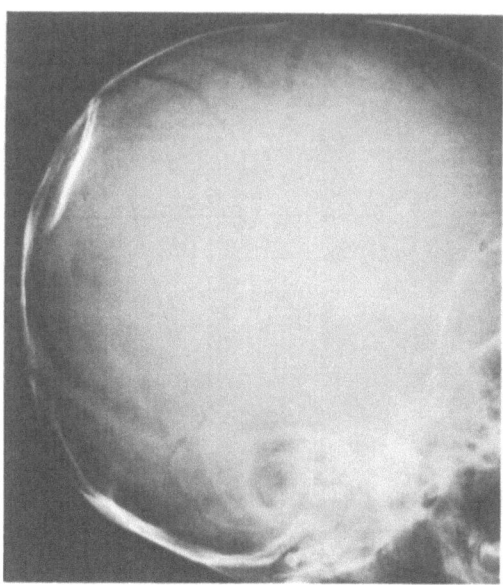

Figure 12.8. True depressed fracture.

"Ping-Pong Ball" Fractures. These constitute the second type, and represent the majority of depressed fractures in neonates (81%). It is comparable to the "greenstick fracture" of long bones in children and looks like a localized depression of the vault without a break in the continuity of the cranial bone (see Fig. 12.9).

Flat Depressed Fractures. These fractures are less frequent (15%). In this third type, a penetrating depressed bone fragment is disconnected

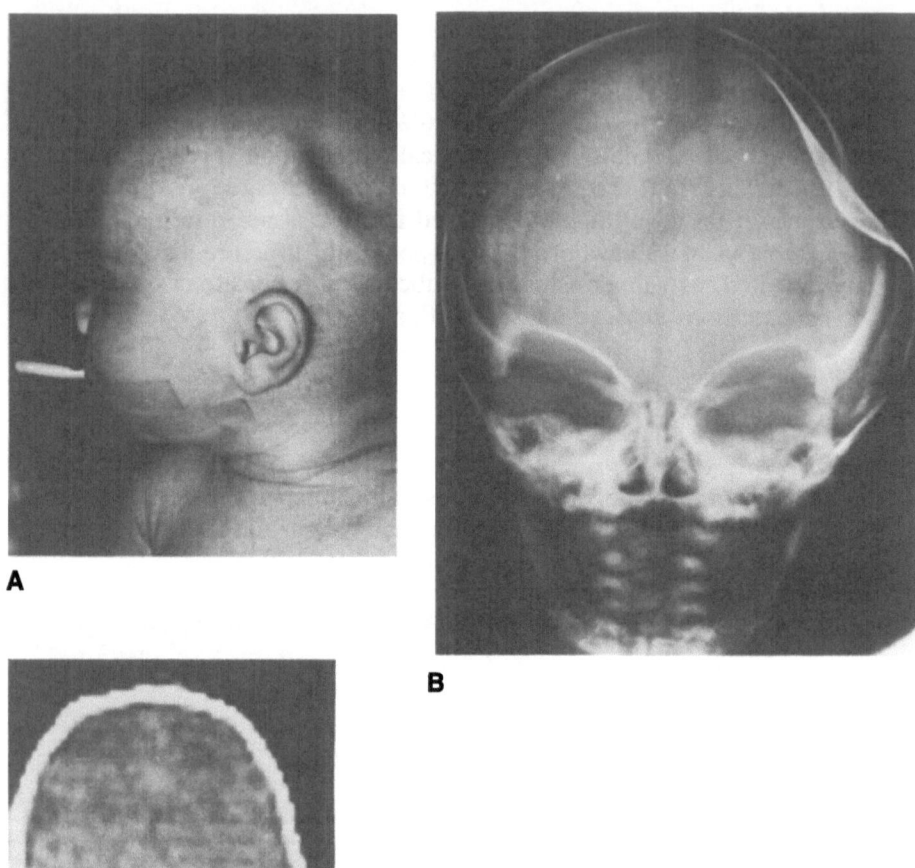

A

B

C

Figure 12.9. "Ping-pong ball" fracture of the parietal region. (**A**) Clinical aspect. (**B**) Radiological aspect. (**C**) CT scan aspect.

Figure 12.10. Flat, depressed fracture of the frontal region associated with a parietal fracture.

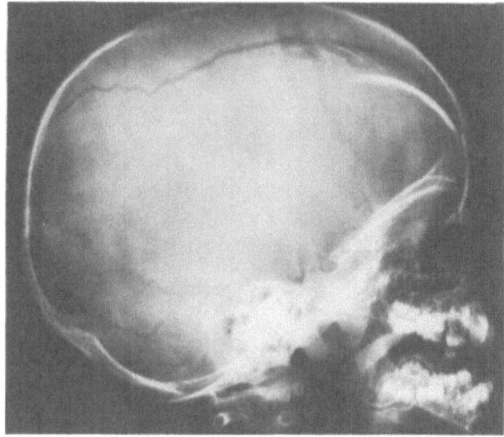

from the vault. The mechanism of such a depressed fracture is generally a local impact by an object (see Fig. 12.10).

The age distribution of these three types of depressed fractures is given in Table 12.5.

Location

Depressed fractures, like linear fractures, commonly involve the parietal bone (51% of the cases in our study) (see Fig. 12.11). In neonates the proportion increases to 75%. The frontal location represents 16% (15% in neonates). The third most frequent localization is the occipital bone (10%). Depressed fractures across the sutures are rare: Only 12 cases in our series (14%) had such fractures. They are usually located at the level of the parietotemporal or the occipitotemporal sutures.

The localizations of depressed fractures in infants and children of all ages are indicated in Table 12.6 for three studies.

Treatment

Surgical elevation of a depressed fracture is the most suitable treatment. In newborn with closed depressions, a burr hole or small craniectomy at the margin of the depression allows the fragments to be raised.

Table 12.5. Age distribution of three types of depressed skull fracture observed.

Type of fracture	0–60 days (16 cases)	2–24 months (69 cases)
True depressed	2 (12.5%)	37 (53%)
"Ping-pong ball"	13 (81%)	20 (30%)
Flat depressed	1 (6.5%)	12 (17%)

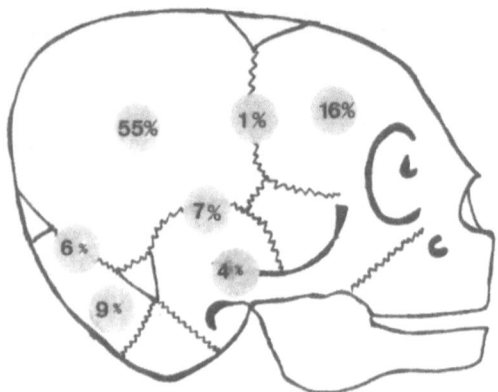

Figure 12.11. Localization of depressed fractures in our series of 85 cases.

Spontaneous elevation has been reported in the literature. Natelson[47] reported one case; Ross[57] presented the case of a 3 month old infant with a parietal depressed fracture that elevated itself spontaneously after a period of four hours. Loeser et al described three cases of neonatal depressed skull fracture treated without surgical elevation.[41] Raynor and Parsa[53] reported a case of a depressed fracture in an infant which was reduced by digital pressure on the skull. Schrager[60] discussed a case of elevation of a depressed fracture with a breast pump. Other authors[71,66,59] used the obstetrical vacuum extractor for the elevation of depressed fractures in neonates.

Loeser et al proposed five indicators for surgical treatment:

1. bone fragment in cerebral tissue;
2. associated neurological deficits;
3. signs of increased intracranial pressure;
4. evidence of cerebrospinal fluid beneath the Galea;
5. failure to elevate by nonsurgical means.[41]

We recommend surgical elevation in all cases. First, the exact extension of the depressed fracture and the severity of underlying lesions are not

Table 12.6. Localizations of depressed skull fractures in infants and children of all ages.

Location	Choux 0–2 years (85 cases)	Harwood-Nash 0–16 years (315 cases)	Coulon 0–16 years (100 cases)
Parietal	51%	40%	43%
Frontal	16%	27%	30%
Occipital	10%	7%	8%
Temporal	7%	7%	4%

easy to evaluate before surgery. Second, the incidence of secondary epileptic seizures is significantly lower in operated cases. The only time one is warranted to consider not operating a depressed fracture is when it is small and over a venous sinus. Dural tears are found at surgery in nearly 30% of the cases, in most studies. In a few cases, there is associated cerebral damage.

Open Fractures

The thinness of the vault in infants, especially in the temporal region, accounts for the accidental penetration of the skull with sharp instruments like scissors, knitting needles, or other tools (see Fig. 12.12). If a linear or depressed fracture is compounded by a scalp laceration or a rent in a paranasal sinus they must be explored to determine whether there is a dural tear. In such cases of open fractures with underlying dural and brain damage, the skull lesions are generally extensive and evident. The injured bone may be elevated or depressed and is often multi-fragmented.

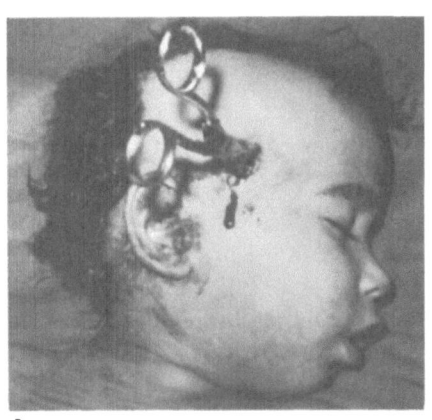
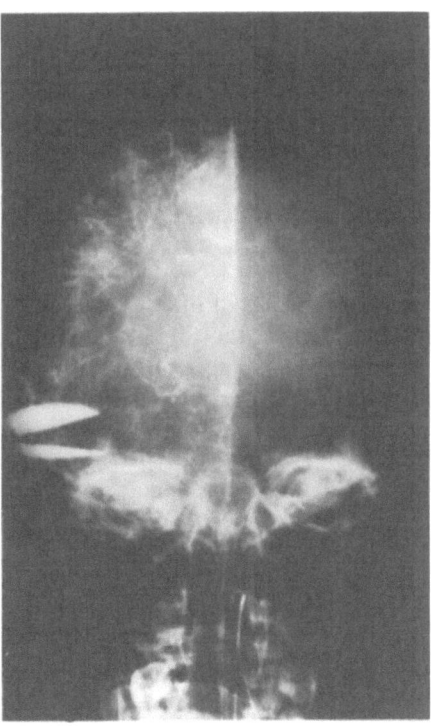

A   B

Figure 12.12. Open craniocerebral injury of the temporal region by scissors. (**A**) Aspect of the child. (**B**) Preoperative angiography.

Open fractures with lesions of the skin, the bone, the dural region, and the brain are rare in infants. In 2022 cases of head trauma in infants, we treated only six cases of penetrating fractures with cortical lesions.

Growing Fractures

In some cases, especially in infants, a linear fracture may enlarge progressively and produce a permanent skull defect. This state is known as a growing fracture (meningocele spuria). The first instance of such a fracture was described in 1816 by John Howship,[30] who noted "partial absorption of the parietal bone, arising from a blow on the head" in a child 9 months old. The first pathological description was by von Rokitansky[73] in 1856. Billroth,[8] in 1862, mentions a case of "spurium meningocele." Weinlechner[75] and von Winiwarter[74] in 1882 and 1885, respectively, stressed the importance of bone defect. In 1907 Ballance[5] described, for the first time, the surgical procedure in a case of "traumatic meningocele." The same year, Krauseon called this condition "circumscribed cystic arachnoiditis."[39] Dyke,[18] in 1937, called this lesion a leptomeningeal cyst. Pancoast, in 1940, used the term "fibrosin osteitis."[39] Schwartz,[61] in 1941, described the mechanism of the effects of the "leptomeningeal cyst." In 1949 Ombredanne[48] mentioned a lesion called "cephalhydrocele traumatique." In 1953 Taveras and Ransohoff,[67] studying seven cases treated surgically, suggested that the major factor is the dural tear. The same year Pia and Tonnis,[50] in a major study, called the lesion "wachsende Schädelfrakten," which can be translated as growing fracture. In 1961 Lende and Erikson[39] first reviewed the literature of "enlarging skull fracture" and described its four essential characteristics:

1. a skull fracture in infancy or early childhood;
2. a dural tear at the time of fracture;
3. a brain injury beneath the fracture;
4. a subsequent enlargement of the fracture to form a cranial defect.

Finally, in 1981, Lamesch and co-workers[38] proposed the French term "Fracture du crâne à l'écartement progressif."
Numerous cases have been reported in the literature.*

Incidence

The incidence of growing fractures varies in different studies from 1% to 15%. In our series of 1460 head traumas in infants, we treated only seven patients with this fracture.

---

* See the references at the end of this chapter, which include significant reports on growing-fracture studies.

Age

The majority of cases of growing fracture are encountered in children under 3 years old. The causal trauma generally appears during the first year of life (e.g., in 11 of the 17 cases of Matson,[43] the 4 cases of Sato,[58] 9 of the 11 cases of Ito,[32] and 16 of the 21 cases of Arseni[3]). In the series of 10 cases of Kingsley,[35] all but one sustained the injury within the first 18 months of life. After cranial trauma the development of a growing fracture may take months or years, only a few authors mention an interval of weeks.[70,42]

Clinical Findings

The most frequent sign of growing fracture is a palpable skull defect that is soft and pulsating. (The knowledge that the patient has a history of previous trauma with a fracture naturally facilitates the diagnosis.) This swelling of the vault, sometimes visible, gradually increases in size. The scalp overlying the skull fracture is rarely injured and never broken. Cerebrospinal fluid (CSF) beneath the scalp may be present but generally not diagnosed. It is important to note that initially a pulsation may not be present at the fracture site even if it is large. The onset of pulsations in the area of the skull defect, however, indicates the existence of a growing fracture.

Infrequently, the child presents with seizures that appear long after the trauma. Manifestation of epilepsy was mentioned by Gaist and Scarcella[20] in 1956 in their report of five cases and by Paillas and Darcourt[49] in 1959, in two cases. In 76 cases of the literature* and in our own work we have found 26 manifestations of epilepsy—that is, roughly 34% of all reported cases.

Neurological deficits may be present, but generally they appear later. Consequently, in the event of delayed appearance of clinical symptoms after an initial silent period, the presence of a growing fracture may be suspected.

Radiological Findings

X-rays reveal the bony defect to be of considerable size, elongated, and irregular. The edges of the defect are elevated and thickened. In follow-up x-rays, after the initial trauma, it is easy to see a gradual enlargement of the fracture line. This enlargement may begin a few weeks later without any modifications in the size of the fracture. After birth injury and especially after forceps delivery, the skull fracture may be quite large, but not expansive. Subsequently a round bone defect may appear with a crater-like deformity (see Fig. 12.13).

---

* References 40, 43, 52, 58, 32, 35, 3.

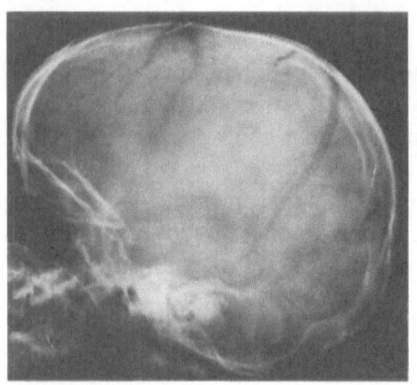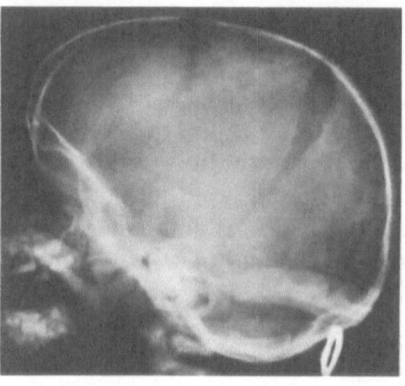

A   B

Figure 12.13. Growing fracture. **(A)** Initial aspect of parietal fracture. **(B)** Secondary enlargement of the fracture indicates growing fracture.

In a CT scan unilateral ventricular dilation is found in 70% to 80% of reported cases. In many cases it is an irregular dilation; on some occasions it extends outside the cranial defect. At this time, on examination the swelling pulsates and may be transilluminated. In other cases, porencephaly is present beneath the bone defect. It may appear to be separated from the enlarged ventricle. An arachnoid cyst is a less frequent finding; and all sizes may be present.

A CT scan will show the existence of CSF beneath the bone defect and also the presence of vessels and, more precisely, the venous sinuses.

Pathogenesis

The constant and main pathogenic factors in a growing fracture are a dural tear and the presence of pulsating CSF at the level of the fracture. Experimentally, Goldstein[21] has stressed the role of fluid pulsation into a cavity, a ventricle, or a cyst at the level of the fracture. Other authors emphasized the significance of brain injury; for Goldstein this lesion is of secondary importance. Kingsley[35] mentions the close relationship of the external layer of the dura with the periosteum. A diastatic fracture may cause tearing of the dura mater. Lende,[40] experimentally, has suggested that a bone defect does not heal when an underlying dural defect is present.

Accumulation of pulsating CSF at the level of the fracture explains the secondary enlargement, but it is difficult to explain why this enlargement stops after a few months of evolution.

Treatment

Ramamurthi[52] in one case and Rothman[55] in another, have mentioned spontaneous resolution of the lesion—but this is a rare occurrence. A surgical approach to this lesion remains imperative at the moment of the diagnosis in order to avoid subsequent enlargment of the fracture and extension of the often associated underlying porencephaly. Surgical treatment, however, permits only closure of the dura and a cranioplasty, with bone or acrylic. A CT scan is advisable before surgery to locate precisely the position of very large fractures and the dural sinuses. A large scalp incision is needed to completely visualize the bone defect. Very often the dural defect is larger than the bone defect; consequently, it is necessary to enlarge the fracture before closing the dura with a graft. The excision of the cyst is done first.

Summary

In conclusion, skull fractures in infants are common. Despite the high incidence of skull lesions, the clinical course of head trauma in infancy remains good in most cases. An initial loss of consciousness accompanying skull fractures is present in only 22% of reported cases. Only 5% of infants with linear fracture suffer coma (7% in the case of depressed fracture). Consequently, it appears that skull fractures in infants have a good prognosis and are not difficult to manage clinically or surgically.

References

1. Alajouanine R, Thurel R: Perte de substance crânienne consécutive à un traumatisme fermé. *Rev Neurol* 1945;77:71.
2. Alexander E, Davis CH: Intrauterine fracture of the infant skull. *J Neurosurg* 1969;30:446–454.
3. Arseni C, Ciurea AV: Clinicotherapeutic aspects in the growing skull fracture: A review of the literature. *Child's Brain* 1981;8:161–172.
4. Axton JHM, Levy LF: Congenital mouldery depression of the skull. *Br J Med* 1965;1:1644–1647.
5. Ballance CA: Some points in the surgery of the brain and its membranes, in MacMillan and Co, Ltd, *A Glimpse into the History of Surgery of the Brain. 15,* 405, 1907.
6. Bandi SK, Singh SD, Dwivedi MS: Traumatic leptomeningeal cyst: Report of a case. *Indian J Ped* 1969;36:447–451.
7. Bayerthal: Ueber die im frühesten Kindesalter entstehende Menin gocele spuria traumatica. *Brun Beitr klin Chir* 1891;7:367.
8. Billroth T: Ein fall von Meningocele spuria cum fistula ventriculi cerebri. *Arch klin Chir* 1862;3:398.
9. Brandesky G: Die wachsende Schädelfraktur im Säuglings und Kleinkinde salter, in Rehbein F: *Der Unfall im Kindesalter* (Suppl. zu Bd. 11, *Zeitschr f Kinderchir*). Stuttgart, Hippokrates-Verlag, 1972, p 381.
10. Brihaye JM, Locoge R, Potvliege, Mage J: Lacune osseuse de la voute du crâne avec kyste proencéphalique sous-jacent d'origine obstétricale chez un adulte. *Acta neurol belg* 1957;57:803.

11. Burkinshaw J: Head injuries in children. *Arch. Dis. Child* 1960;35:205.
12. Canestri G, Monzali CL: Trauma cranici nell'infanzia. *Min Pediatrica* 1970;22:1687–1689.
13. Coffin M, Bailleul: Perte de substance crânienne chez un nourrisson. *Bull Soc Péd* (Paris) 1936;34:278.
14. Cooperstock M: Leptomeningeal cyst associated with hemiplegia and skull defect of traumatic origin. *J Ped* 1946;28:488–492.
15. Coulon RA: Depressed skull fractures in children. *Concepts Pediat Neurosurg* 1984;4:253–263. Karger, Basel
16. Di Rocco C, Stefanini MC, Velardi F: Traumi cranio encefalici del periodo neonatale e della primo infanzia. *Minerva Ped* 1980;32:927–934.
17. Duez G: Les images lacunaires crâniennes. Thèse, Université de Lille, 1951.
18. Dyke CG: The roentgen X-ray diagnosis and treatment of diseases of the skull and intracranial contents, in Palmer WW, Nelson T. *Loose Leaf Medicine*. New York, *6*, 185, 1937.
19. Friedmann G, Krohm G: Aetiologie und Klinik der "wachsenden Schädel frakturen." *Kinderheilk* 1964;89:49.
20. Gaist G, Scarcella G: Erosioni craniche de ciste leptomeningea a cicatrice meningocerebrale in corso di epilepsia post traumatica. *Annali Ital Chir* 1956;33:585–604.
21. Goldstein FP et al: Experimental observations on enlarging skull fractures. *J Neurosurg* 1970;32:431.
22. Grob M: Ueber die Schadelfrakturen im Kindesalter. *Langenbecks Arch klin Chir* 1942;34:442.
23. Grubea FH: Post-traumatic leptomeningeal cyst. *Amer J Roentgen* 1969;105:305–307.
24. Guffa-May DK: Intrauterine spontaneous depression of fetal skull: A case report and review of the literature. *J Reprod Med* 1976;16:321–324.
25. Handa I: On the growing skull fracture. *Brain Dev* (Tokyo) 1969;1:61.
26. Harwood-Nash DC, Hendrick EB, Hudson AR: The significance of skull fracture in children: A study of 1187 patients. *Radiology* 1971;101:151.
27. Hendrick EB, Harwood-Nash DC, Hudson AR: Head injuries in children: A survey of 4465 consecutive cases at the hospital for sick children, Toronto, Canada. *Clin Neurosurg* 1964;II:46–65.
28. Higazi I: Post-traumatic leptomeningeal cysts of the brain: Report of unusual case. *J Neurosurg* 1963;20:605–608.
29. Hobbs G: Spontaneous elevation of a depressed skull fracture in an infant. *J Neurosurg* 1975;42:727.
30. Howship J: *Practical Observation in Surgery and Morbid Anatomy*. London, Longman, Hurst, Rees, Orme and Brown, 1816.
31. Ingraham FD, Matson DD: *Neurosurgery of infancy and childhood*. Springfield, Ill., Charles C Thomas Publishers, 1954, vol 17, p 456.
32. Ito H, Miwa T, Onodra Y: Growing skull fracture of childhood *Child's Brain* 1977;3:116.
33. Jamison DL, Kaye HH: Accidental head injury in childhood. *Arch Dis Child* 1974;49:376–381.
34. Keener EB: An experimental study of reactions of the dura mater to wounding and loss of substance. *J Neurosurg* 1959;16:424.

35. Kingsley D, Till K, Hoare R: Growing fractures of the skull. *B Neurol Neurosurg and Psych* 1978;41:312.
36. Kitamura K, Sawada T: Growing skull fracture and false meningocele of childhood. *Brain Nerve* (Tokyo) 1964;16:473–479.
37. Kravitz H, Driessen G, Gomberg R, Korach A: Accidental falls from elevated surfaces in infants from birth to one year of age. *Pediatrics* 1969;44:869–876.
38. Lamesch A, Conter C, Gose C, Riekel I, Mohn M: La fracture du crâne à l'écartement progressif du petit enfant. *Chir Pediat* 1981;22:231–236.
39. Lende R, Erickson T: Growing skull fractures of childhood. *J Neurosurg* 1961;18:479.
40. Lende RA: Enlarging skull fracture of childhood. *Neuroradiology* 1974;7:119.
41. Loeser JD, Kilburn HL, Jollet T: Management of depressed skull fracture in the newborn. *J Neurosurg* 1976;44:62–64.
42. Lye RH, Occleshaw JV, Dutton J: Growing fracture of the skull and the role of computerized tomography. *J Neurosurg* 1981;55:470–472.
43. Matson DD: *Neurosurgery of Infancy and Childhood.* Springfield Ill, Charles C Thomas Publishers, 1969.
44. Mealey JR: *Pediatric Head Injury.* Springfield, Ill, Charles C Thomas Publishers, 1968.
45. Mercier: Lacunes et images radiologiques lacunaiers du crâne. Thèse, Université de Marseille, 1939.
46. Moriyasu N: Enlarged skull fracture: A mechanism of its entity without treated dura in one case. *Neurol Surg* (Tokyo) 1972;2:153–159.
47. Natelson SE, Sayers MP: The fate of children sustaining severe head trauma during birth. *Pediatrics* 1973;51:169–174.
48. Ombredanne L: *Prècis Clinique et Opératoire de Chirurgie Infantile.* Paris, Masson Édit, 1949, p 327.
49. Paillas JE, Barcourt C: Epilepsie ultratardive et lacunes crâniennes consécutives à un traumatisme neo-natal: Deux observations. *Sem Hôp* (Paris) 1959;35:1965–1968.
50. Pia HW, Tönnis W: Die waschende Schädelfraktur des Kindesalters. *Zbl f Neurochir* 1953;1:1.
51. Piusson C, Risbourg B, Krim G, Herbaut C, Lenaerts C, Quintard JM: Fractures évolutives des os du crâne. *Ann Pédiat* 1979;26(5):289.
52. Ramamurthi B, Kalyanraman S: Rationale for surgery in growing fractures of the skull. *J Neurosurg* 1970;32:427–430.
53. Raynor RB, Parsa M: Nonsurgical elevation of depressed skull fracture in an infant: *J Pediat* 1968;72:262–264.
54. Rickham PP: Head injuries in childhood. *Helv Chir Acta* 1961;28:560.
55. Rothman L, Rose HS, Laster DW, Quencer R, Tenner M: The spectrum of growing skull fractures in children. *Pediatrics* 1976;57:26.
56. Roberts F, Shopfner CF: Plain skull roentenograms in children with head trauma. *Am J Roentgeno* 1972;114:230–240.
57. Ross G: Spontaneous elevation of a depressed skull fracture in an infant. *J Neurosurg* 1975;42:726–727.
58. Sato O, Tsugane R, Kageyama N: Growing skull fractures of childhood. *Child's Brain* 1975;1:148.
59. Saunders BS, Lazonitz S, McArtor RD: Depressed skull fracture in the neonate. *J Neurosurg* 1979;50;512–514.

60. Schrager GO: Elevation of depressed skull fracture with a breast pump. *J Pediat* 1970;77:300–301.
61. Schwartz CW: Leptomeningeal cysts from a roentgenological viewpoint. *Am. J. Roentgen, Radium Therm Nucl Med* 1941;46:160–165.
62. Shapiro K: *Pediatric Head Trauma.* New York, Futura Publishing Inc, 1983.
63. Simon PG: Les lacunes craniennes après traumatisme de la première enfance. Thèse, Université de Lyon, 1954.
64. Soul AB, Whitcomb BB: Extensive erosion of base of skull from leptomeningeal cyst: Report of case. *Arch Neurol Psychiat* 1946;55:382–387.
65. Stein BM, Tenner MS: Enlargement of skull fracture in childhood due to cerebral herniation. *Arch Neurol* 1972;26:137–143.
66. Tan KL: Elevation of congenital depressed fractures of the skull by the vacuum extraction. *Acta Paediatr Scand* 1974;63:562–564.
67. Taveras JM, Ransohoff EJ: Leptomeningeal cysts of the brain following trauma with erosion of the skull. *J Neurosurg* 1953;10:233.
68. Testa C, Nizzoli V: Fracture evolutive dans les traumatismes crâniens fermés de la première enface aboutissant à la constitution d'une lacune crânienne. *Neurochir* 1968;14:111–134.
69. Thompson JB, Mason TH, Haines GL, Cassidy MJ: Surgical management of diastatic linear skull fractures in infants. *J Neurosurg* 1973;39:493–497.
70. Twerdy K, Lugger JL: Problemative der Kindlicher Wachsenden Schadelfraktur. *Unfallheilkunde* 1977;80:101–106.
71. Van Enk A: Reduction of Pond fractures. *J Br Med* 1972;2:353.
72. Vas CJ, Winn JM: Growing skull fractures. *Dev. Med Child Neurol* 1966;8(6):735.
73. Von Rokitansky K: Lehrbuch der pathologischen, in *Ahatomia. Wien.* W. Braun-Müller, 1856.
74. Von Winiwarter A: Ueber einen Fall von defekt des Knöchernen Schadeldaches infolge einer während des ersten lebensjahres erlittenen Vereltzung. *Arch Klin Chir* 1885;31:135.
75. Weinlechner J: Ueber die im Kindesalter vorkommenden subkutanen Schädelfissuren und die damit zasammenhängenden Schädellücken mit anlagerndem Gehirn und falschen Meningocelen. *Mschr f Kinderheilk* 1882;18:367.
76. Yarzagaray L: Craniocerebral trauma in children. *Surg Clin N Am* 1973;53:59–71.
77. Zimmerman RA, Bilaniuk LT: Computed tomography in pediatric head trauma. *J Neuroradiol* 1981;8:257–271.
78. Zimmerman RA: The effectiveness of skull plain films in the evaluation of traumatic coma. *J Neurosurg* 1983;10:145–148.

CHAPTER 13

Cerebral Damage

Robert L. McLaurin and Richard Towbin

Introduction

The customary practice in studies of pediatric head trauma has been to lump together all injuries occurring beyond the immediate neonatal period. The implications of this practice are that these head injured children form a homogeneous group and that epidemiologic, pathologic, and prognostic generalizations can be made about their injuries. As further experience has been gained in studying and treating head injury in infants, however, it has become increasingly apparent that such homogeneity does not exist beyond the neonatal stage. The purpose of this chapter is to review certain aspects of brain damage resulting from pediatric head trauma, with an emphasis on those aspects unique to the infant up to 2 years of age.

Unique Characteristics of Brain Injury in Infants

It has been recognized that basic differences exist between the nature of tissue damage of craniocerebral trauma occurring in infants and that in older children and adults. Courville, on the basis of autopsy results, has described some of these differences.[4] Specifically, he noted the relative infrequency of contrecoup lesions in infancy, although he was definite in not denying (as had been previously claimed) that contrecoup injury never occurred in this age group. Indeed, he had recorded a typical contrecoup lesion in a 6-week-old infant.

Contrecoup lesions in fatal injuries have been recorded in about 85% to 90% of adult patients. In a group of 4-year-old children the incidence rate was only slightly less. In infancy, however, the incidence rate appears to be approximately 10%.

Courville analyzed a series of fatal head injuries in 48 patients below the age of 5 years.[4] The mechanism of injury was noted in each case, and the results in each of five locations of impact were compared with similar injuries in adults. Specifically, Courville noted that impacts received in the frontal region cause no contusion in any age group. By contrast, the incidence of coup and contrecoup lesions is high when the impact is received on the side of the head. In the infants and young children there were no coup injuries and a low incidence of contrecoup lesions. Similar differences were found in young patients receiving blows to the postero-lateral and posterior surfaces of the head, as well as to the vertex. In summary, the incidence of contrecoup lesions increased rapidly between infancy and 3 years of age and thereafter remained approximately at the same level.

The difference between the results of injury in infants and in older age groups may be related to several contributing factors. The skull of the infant is more plastic and probably permits some movement of the brain within it without damage. Also, convolutional markings of the inner skull table are fewer in infancy; such markings may contribute to bruising of the temporal and opercular areas. Finally, the softer texture of the infant brain probably minimizes superficial contusions that may be seen in adult brains.

These same factors are probably responsible for the unique character of cerebral lesions resulting from blunt trauma in infancy (Fig. 13.1). In contrast to the contusion that occurs in mature brains, similar trauma to the infant brain produces tears in the cerebral white matter, parallel to the surface, and similar (microscopic) tears in the superficial cortical layers (Fig. 13.2). The most common areas for such tears are the white matter of the frontal and temporal lobes.

Lindenberg and Freytag reviewed the brains of 16 infants who died as a

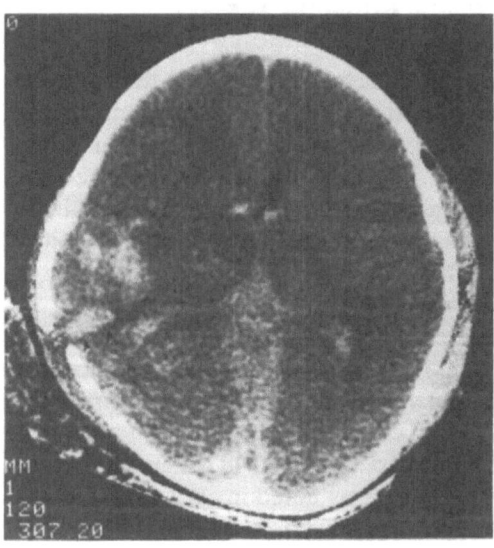

Figure 13.1. Eighteen-month-old child who fell from a fourth story window. Non-enhanced image demonstrates intraventricular, subarachoid, and intraparenchymal hemorrhage. A large right temporo-parietal hemorrhage with a linear component is present, as are presumed lacerations (at arrowheads) extending to the brain surface adjacent to a diastatic fracture.

Figure 13.2. Twenty-two-month-old child who fell 15 feet from a balcony, striking his head. He was unresponsive with left hemotympanum and decorticate posturing. A large focal hemorrhage with surrounding edema primarily involves the left centrum semiovale, but extends into the gray matter. A linear hemorrhage (perhaps a small laceration) is adjacent to the diastatic fracture.

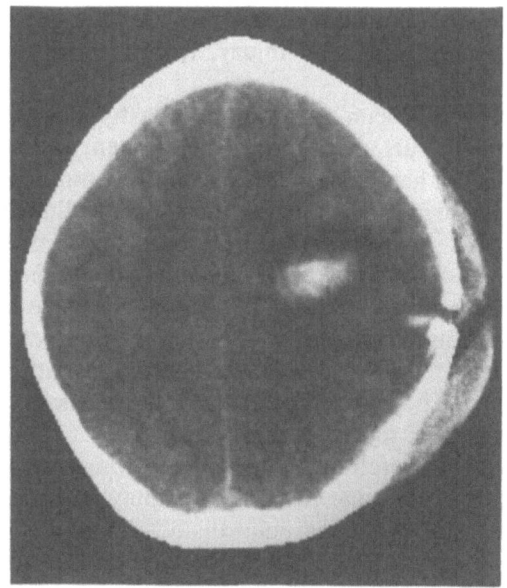

result of blunt head trauma.[15] The trauma included falls, abuse by parents, and blows to the head. In all cases the tears involved the white matter, with occasional extension through the cortex, the ventricular wall, or both. Depending on the age of the injury, blood may be present within the tear. It is noteworthy, however, that such tears occurred only in infants under 5 months of age, whereas older infants had areas of contusion and necrosis characteristic of the mature brain.

Restriction of the tear to early infancy suggests that factors similar to those responsible for the lack of contrecoup lesions are at work. The soft consistency of the poorly myelinated cerebrum must play a role, as well as the pliancy of the skull, which is more easily deformed by external forces than a more mature skull. The floors of the frontal and middle fossae are smoother and provide less resistance to movement of the adjacent brain. Finally, Lindenberg and Freytag believe that a shallow subarachnoid space contributes to the result of impact.[15] It must be concluded, therefore, that brain injury from external trauma is modulated by mechanical factors within the brain, the meninges, and the skull. This combination of modifying factors results in the different location and character of brain damage in the infant brain.

A unique type of brain injury infrequently seen after blunt trauma involves damage to the basal ganglia without associated cerebral injury. This may occur in infants who have fallen from modest heights and who have no indication of severe or extensive brain injury. Indeed, there may have been no external evidence of injury and no skull fracture. The characteristic clinical hallmark has been the occurrence of hemiparesis noted within an hour after injury, with no other signs of intracranial dysfunction.

The CT scan usually shows a hypodense area in the region of the caudate nucleus, (Fig. 13.3), putamen, and anterior levels of the internal capsule; hemorrhagic lesions more common in children than infants; persistence of the hypodense area despite clinical resolution of the hemiparesis. There are no long-term observations of the late effects of such injuries, as they have been recognized only since the use of CT scan. Older children with injuries to basal ganglia have been noted to have athetosis and tremor, but these have not been reported in infancy.

Maki et al. attempted to define the pathogenesis of basal ganglia injury.[16] They hypothesized, on the basis of the mechanism and lack of severity of injury in their patients, that rotational movements cause the greatest stretch to the lateral perforating vessels from the middle cerebral artery—the same vessels that supply the anterior basal ganglia. Infarction results from this vascular dislocation and stretching.

Injuries to the basal ganglia, hemorrhage, or necrosis are not uncommon in association with more generalized craniocerebral trauma. They have been reported by Jellinger to occur in 28% to 50% of injuries in the pediatric age group.[11] In autopsied series the hematomas were found

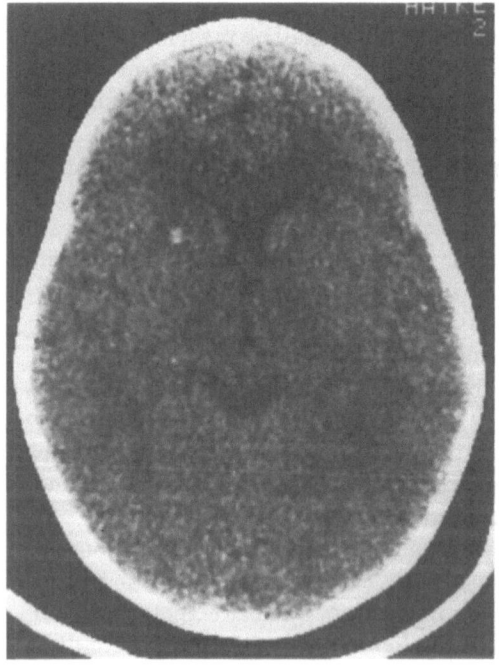

Figure 13.3. Twenty-two-month-old child struck by a car that rendered him unconscious and immediately epileptic. A small hyperdense lesion (blood) is present within the right lentiform nucleus. Minimal surrounding edema and frontal horn compression are present.

mainly in the anterior portion of the corpus striatum, between the lateral putamen and external capsule, in the thalamus, or in the pallidum. Autopsy examination of fatal injuries in infants and children has also demonstrated, in addition to more superficial injuries, damage to the corpus callosum.[11] The injury may result in partial or complete, unilateral or bilateral, tears of this structure. It has been postulated that the principal mechanism of injury is impact or whiplash movement in the sagittal plane, resulting in a shearing effect. It is noteworthy that the injury is usually localized to one or both sides of the midline rather than centrally located. The clinical effect of such an injury is not recognized, as it usually occurs in association with other cerebral damage. Nevertheless, infants have survived complete traumatic rupture of the corpus callosum for many years. Recognition by CT scan of localized injury to this structure is rare.

Cerebral Swelling After Trauma

Cerebral swelling following blunt trauma to the infant head is both the cause and the result of cerebral damage. There are certain features unique to this pathophysiologic event in this age group. Basically, traumatic cerebral swelling may be localized or diffuse; the latter is characteristic of the reaction seen in infancy and childhood.

Regional or focal edema occurs adjacent to areas of contusion, shearing injury, or hematomas. This edema is probably of the vasogenic type, predominantly seen in the white matter, and due to leakage of fluid from damaged vessels. It tends to spread from the area of injury through the white matter, and is similar in most respects to that occurring in adult brains after trauma.

Generalized swelling is a unique response of the young brain and has been studied rather intensively by Bruce and his associates.[1] On the basis of CT scans and measurement of cerebral blood flow, Bruce et al. concluded that swelling of this type was not due to edema but rather to hyperemia from cerebral vasodilation (Fig. 13.4). The pathophysiologic basis for the loss of vasomotor tone has not been defined. The implications of this mechanism are profound, however. Diffuse brain swelling, usually bilateral, may accompany relatively minor head injury. Clinically, this is characteristically seen in the young child who is lucid on admission to the hospital and then progressively deteriorates because of brain swelling and consequent intracranial hypertension. If the intracranial pressure problem is aggressively treated, the prognosis for satisfactory recovery is quite good and there is unlikely to be residual brain damage.

In contrast, the infant or young child who is comatose on admission (with a Glasgow Coma Score of less than 5) may develop delayed intracranial hypertension; in this instance, however, the hypertension is likely to

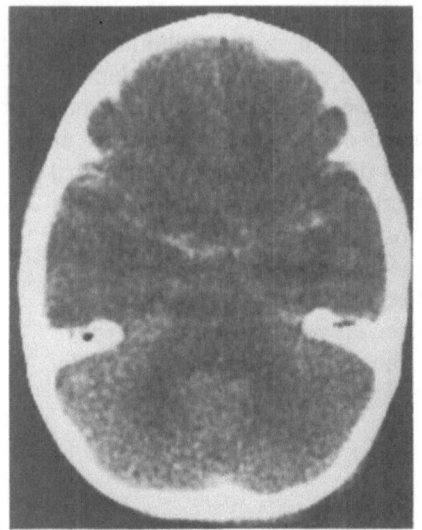
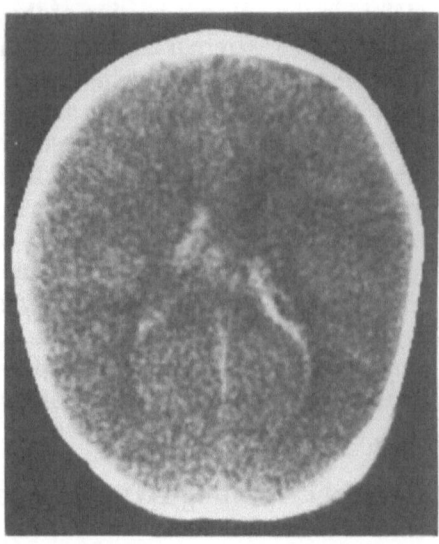

A   B

Figure 13.4. This eight-month-old infant was involved in an auto accident, not wearing a seat belt, and comatose on admission. (**A**) Blood in the suprasellar cistern. The temporal horns and IV ventricle are compressed, and (**B**) intraventricular hemorrhage is present. The ventricles are compressed and gray-white differentiation is poor, suggesting diffuse edema (hyperemic swelling?). The infant died four days later.

be a result of multifocal edema. The prognosis for cerebral recovery is correspondingly poor, and late CT scans show ventriculomegaly, areas of focal atrophy, and microcephaly. It is apparent, then, that the occurrence of persistent residual brain damage in this age group is largely dependent on whether cerebral swelling is due to edema or hyperemia.

It should be noted, however, that intracranial hypertension from any cause may in itself lead to brain damage if not aggressively controlled. Postmortem studies on infants have shown swollen and pale brains, flattened convolutions, small ventricles, and an early reactive gliosis. Hippocampal and tonsillar herniation may or may not be present.[11]

Infant Abuse

Intentional child abuse as a cause of craniocerebral and skeletal injuries in infancy has been recognized for several decades. The magnitude of the problem, however, has been increasingly appreciated because of enhanced awareness of the evidence of abuse and because of improved diagnostic techniques. The ultimate significance of this prevalent form of trauma is measured in terms of mortality, permanent neurologic handicap, and mental retardation.

Intracranial injury in the abused infant probably occurs through one of two mechanisms: direct impact or whiplash shaking. Direct impact is more likely to result in cerebral contusion. The pathophysiology of brain damage after abuse has been a matter of considerable interest to the clinician. Although subdural hematoma has been clearly recognized and often mistakenly assumed to be responsible for residual brain damage, the coexistence of underlying brain trauma has been increasingly appreciated. Indeed, the existence of parenchymal damage without subdural hemorrhage has been documented by CT scan (Fig. 13.5). Ellison et al. described the findings in four cases in which abuse was responsible for cerebral damage without surface hematoma.[5] Cerebral contusion occurred both with and without external evidence of injury. It seems likely that those without external trauma are the result of whiplash shaking. Three of the four children, on follow-up examination, showed evidence of developmental delay and permanent neurologic deficit.

In a more recent series of abused infants reported by McClelland et al., two of three patients with proven cerebral contusion succumbed, and the third was permanently damaged.[18] It must be concluded that contusion resulting from direct impact usually results in persistent cerebral dysfunction.

Caffey originally called attention to the *whiplash-shaken infant syndrome*.[2] The infant is manually shaken by the extremities; intracranial and intraocular bleeding are caused by the whiplash motion and result in permanent residual brain damage and mental retardation (Fig. 13.6). According to Caffey the most characteristic pattern of physical findings in the whiplashed infant was the absence of external signs of trauma to the head and soft tissues of the face and neck, as well as the facial bones and calvaria, but the presence of massive intracranial and intraocular bleeding. Necropsy in cases of whiplashed infants showed subdural, subarachnoid, and subpial hemorrhages as well as hemorrhage within the cerebral parenchyma. The walls of the inferior and superior sagittal sinuses were lacerated at the points of entrance of bridging veins. Ganglion cells were sparse and pyknotic, and blood covered parts of the falx.

The whiplash-shaken infant syndrome results from the severe stresses imparted to the intracranial structure as a result of the infant's relatively heavy head and weak neck muscles. The maximized stress is further amplified by the pliable sutures and larger fontanels that allow excessive motion of the brain and shearing forces applied to the bridging vessels. Finally, the infantile brain is unmyelinated and softer than older brains. The combination of these factors leads to permanent mechanical damage (contusion and shearing) and vascular insults to the brain.

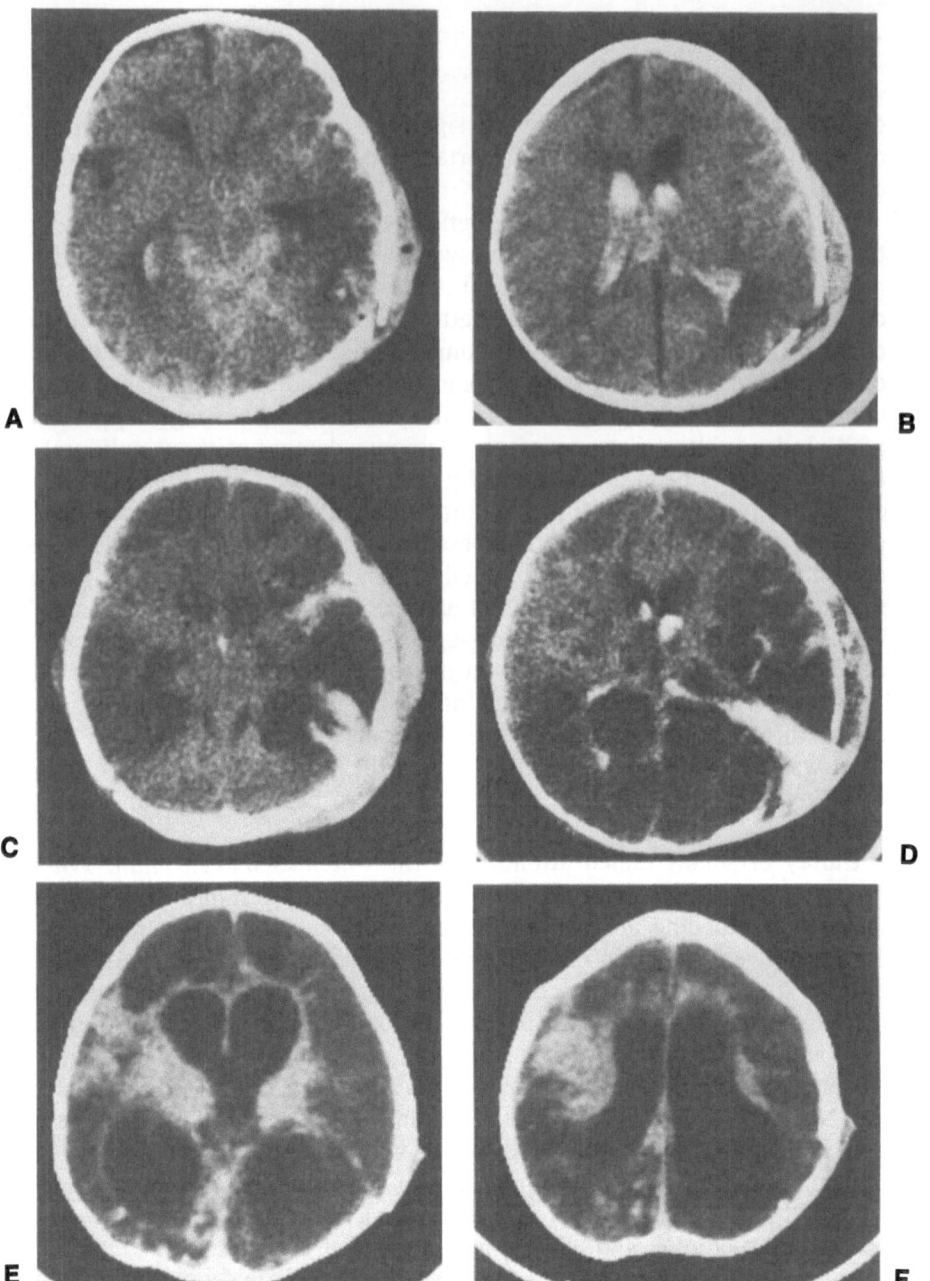

Figure 13.5. This is a 3-month-old, severely abused infant. (**A,B**) Admission CT shows diffuse left hemisphere injury with diffuse edema, effacement of the left frontal horn, subarachnoid hemorrhage, and intracerebral and intraventricular hemorrhage. A diastatic left posteroparietal fracture with adjacent calvarial hematoma is also present. (**C,D**) Two days later, the ventricles dilated (arrows). One notes generalized severe hypodensity involving the majority of both hemispheres with relative sparing (reversal sign) of the central structures. Resolving intraventricular blood is also noted, as is hemorrhage into a left posteroparietal laceration extending from left lateral ventricle is present. (**E,F**) Four months later, generalized severe encephalomalacia and atrophic hydrocephalus in an irreparably damaged brain developed.

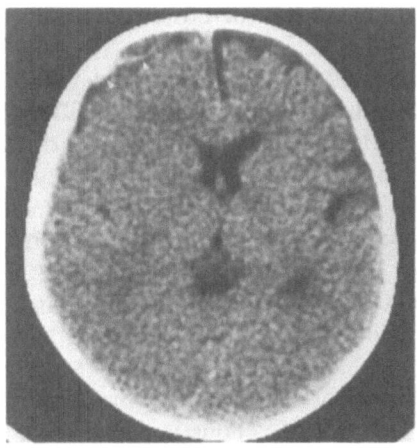
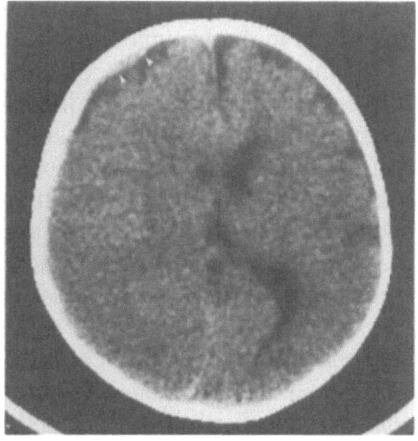

A   B

Figure 13.6. Five-month-old infant with seizures, apnea, retinal hemorrhages, and bruises. Suspected child abuse. (**A**) A small right frontal subdural hematoma (arrowheads) effaces the brain surface and causes right-to-left midline shift, which is out of proportion to the size of the collection. (**B**) Associated hypodensity (contusion) affects the right hemisphere; this effaces the lateral ventricle, flattens surface markings, and distorts gray-white interface.

Brain Damage Associated with Subdural Hemorrhage

The combination of surface hematoma and underlying brain damage is commonly present. Under these circumstances, brain damage may be secondary to the effects of the surface hematoma, by pathophysiologic mechanisms yet undefined, or to the initial trauma that led to the hematoma.

One such example of associated injury is that which occurs with acute subdural hematoma (Fig. 13.6). Most of the literature up to this time has been concerned with the recognition, treatment, and outcome of chronic subdural accumulation; nevertheless, acute hematomas do occur in infancy and childhood. The most extensive review of this problem was provided by Gutierrez and Raimondi.[9] These authors reviewed 27 cases of acute posttraumatic subdural hematoma, including 5 newborns, 18 infants, and 3 toddlers. They emphasized the frequent angiographic evidence of coexisting surface hematoma and intracerebral contusion and hematoma. The neurologic manifestations included an array of signs of brain damage (e.g., seizures, hemiparesis, spasticity), and the later psychometric evaluation clearly indicated permanent brain damage. Those infants who underwent surgical evacuation of the subdural hematoma had better long-term prognoses than those treated only by subdural tapping. This suggests that the brain damage was more effectively prevented by surgical treatment and that the residual damage was therefore not entirely due to the initial trauma.

The mechanism of development of the subdural hematoma is related to the residual brain damage. Since acute subdural hemorrhages in infants are frequently the result of tearing of bridging veins between the cortex and the dural sinuses, it is reasonable to believe that circulatory disturbances of the brain will contribute to the neurologic sequellae. Moreover, occasional subdural hematomas are secondary to hemorrhagic contusions that rupture through the pia-arachnoid. Finally, the rare acute subdural hematomas of the posterior fossa (from tear of the tentorium) may cause upward herniation of the cerebellum; this may lead to compression and sclerosis of the cerebellar cortex.[6]

Residual brain damage in acute subdural hematoma survivors—from whatever mechanism—is not entirely a result of venous impairment or associated cerebral contusion. The acutely expanding lesion causes intracranial shifts to occur rapidly with no chance for accommodation; consequently, brain injury results.[11] For example, the ipsilateral cingulate gyrus herniates beneath the free edge of the falx and may lead to hemorrhagic pressure, necrosis of the gyrus, or infarction in the pericallosal artery distribution. Also, transtentorial herniation of the uncus and hippocampal gyrus may lead to compression and infarction of the brain stem, herniating portions of the temporal lobe, the contralateral peduncle, and occlusion of the posterior cerebral artery. These effects are clearly seen in fatal head injuries and obviously may occur with lesser degrees of severity, thereby leading to permanent neurologic and developmental impairment.

Chronic subdural hematoma and effusion are commonly observed in infants, and probably no other posttraumatic complication has generated more diverse theories concerning etiology, pathophysiology, and treatment. Unfortunately, the condition is followed by permanent brain damage in a significant number of children.

Although effusion in the subdural space may follow meningitis, hematomas, and rarely as complications of coagulopathies, it is believed that the majority of hematomas and hydromas result directly from trauma. They are seldom due to birth trauma. Indeed, the traumatic event is frequently sufficiently mild that it is not recognized; this factor contributes to the difficulty in explaining the resulting encephalopathy.

The original theory regarding brain damage was that the membranes that developed in response to the hematoma prevented normal growth and development of the brain by mechanical constriction (Fig. 13.7). It was on the basis of this principle that earlier recommendations for treatment included extensive craniotomies to excise the membranes.[17] The initial phase of treatment consisted of removal of the fluid mass causing pressure on the cerebrum, usually bilaterally and symmetrically, and later excision of membranes to prevent long-term cerebral constriction. Despite these aggressive measures of treatment, however, a significant num-

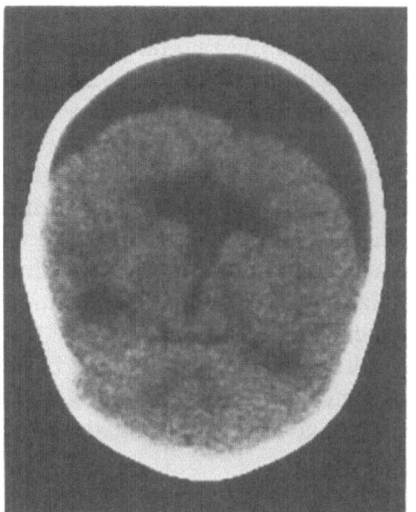
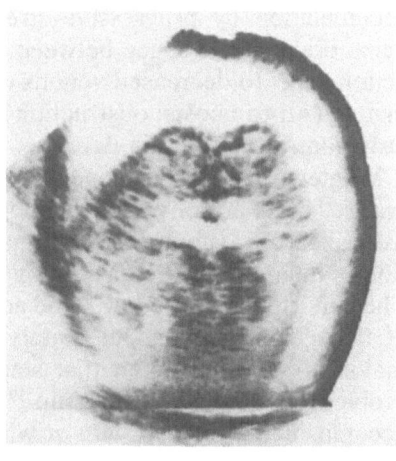

A

B

Figure 13.7. Two patients with traumatic deliveries causing intracranial hemorrhage. (**A**) CT (**B**) Ultrasound (different patient) demonstrate bifrontal chronic subdural collections. The CT reveals an enlarged, crescentic subdural space with flattening and loss of surface markings. The ultrasound was anechoic.

ber of infants suffered developmental delay, often accompanied by seizures. Moreover, it was then discovered by Collins and Pucci that the membranes, after the fluid had been shunted to the peritoneal cavity, progressively regressed in thickness, cellularity, and vascularity.[3] Finally, surgeons removing chronic membranes frequently observed that there was no apparent expansion of the "constricted" brain tissue. At present, therefore, there is little support for the theory of brain damage resulting from the presence of membranes.

The various methods advocated for treating chronic subdural hematomas in infants have noted a remarkably constant frequency of developmental retardation, which indicates that the method of management is probably less contributory to successful brain recovery and growth than other factors that cannot be defined.[20] The incidence of subnormal development among these infants remains at approximately 25%. The logical explanation for this statistic seems to be the effects of initial trauma. Unfortunately, as noted above, this finding is hardly·consistent with the lack of recognized severity of trauma in most infants.

An intriguing concept regarding the pathophysiology of head trauma has been put forth by Gutierrez and Raimondi.[9] It is based on the existence of a craniocerebral disproportion known to be present in many infants with chronic accumulations of subdural fluid. The authors also postulated that this disproportion leads to chronicity of subdural fluid accumulation by progressive stretching and narrowing of the cortical veins bridging the space between the cortex and the sagittal sinus. This action leads to decreased venous drainage from the hemisphere and ultimately to thrombosis; obstruction by narrowing and angulation may similarly contribute to brain damage.

Whatever pathophysiologic mechanism is involved, it is clear that generalized brain atrophy and dysfunction may be sequelae to recognized and treated chronic subdural hematomas in infants. Craniocerebral disproportion is thus due to a combination of macrocrania and cerebral atrophy. The persistence of subdural fluid accumulation may lead to mineralization of the membranes and ultimately to calcification and ossification. Removal of such lesions at that stage is not beneficial because the basic problem is in the damaged brain.[19] Pathologically, the cerebral atrophy is accompanied by gliosis with or without damage to the white matter and, occasionally, to polycystic changes.

Growing Skull Fracture

Growing skull fracture is characteristically a disease of infancy. The presenting feature is a cranial defect resulting from erosion of bone adjacent to a linear fracture, but the main pathology is intracranial. It seems appropriate, therefore, that this entity be included in a consideration of brain damage of traumatic origin in this age group.

Lende and Erickson originated the term "growing skull fracture" but later recommended that it be known as "enlarging skull fracture of childhood."[13] Unfortunately, the term "leptomeningeal cyst" was introduced, but the concept of pathogenesis suggested by this term has not been supported by autopsy or surgical findings. By contrast, the literature has consistently emphasized the significance of cerebral damage and herniation.

Experimental observations on infant animals demonstrated that a simulated skull fracture healed rapidly if the underlying dura was intact.[7] If the dural layer was opened beneath the fracture, however, a permanent bone defect resulted. These observations led to the conclusion that the significant pathology involved the meninges. Yet, though dural defect is an essential factor, the significance of growing fracture is the underlying cerebral damage that is always present and that includes a variety of late pathologic sequelae: local cerebral atrophy, cortical compression and scarring, porencephalic cavitation of the brain, focal ventricular dilation, and complex adhesive scarring between the scalp, meninges, and brain.

Several reports have verified the radiologic, electroencephalographic, and clinical manifestations of this lesion (see Fig. 13.8). Till reviewed ten cases of which only one was older than 16 months.[22] Two of the cases resulted from forceps delivery. The location, consistent with the observa-

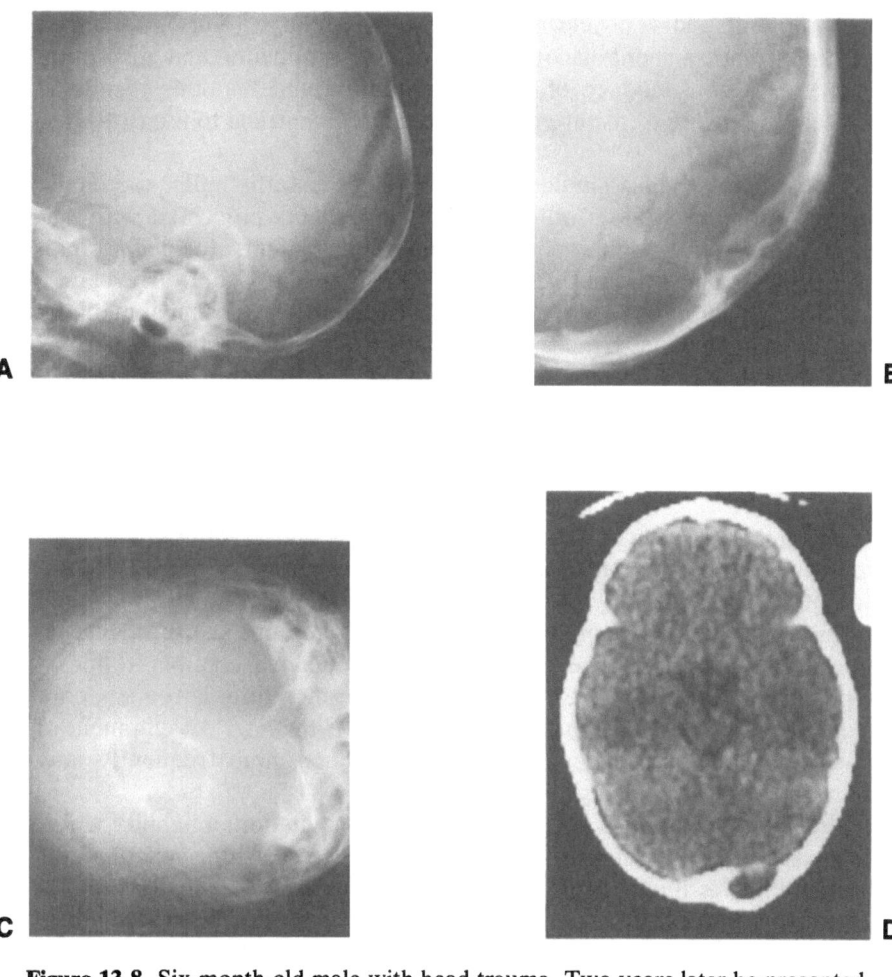

Figure 13.8. Six-month-old male with head trauma. Two years later he presented with head pain. (**A**) Lateral view of the skull demonstrated a diastatic parieto-occipital fracture. (**B, C**) Nineteen months later, multilocular lytic expansion of the occipital bone occurred because of an "intradiploic leptomeningeal cyst." (**D**) CT shows brain contents extending into the diploic space.

tions of all authors, was almost exclusively in the parietal region. Of the ten cases, eight had pneumoencephalograms, and each one demonstrated dilation of the ipsilateral ventricle, usually accompanied by displacement of the midline toward the affected side. In seven patients there were parenchymal cysts, some communicating with the ventricle and others with the surface lesion. A CT scan in one patient confirmed the finding of ventricular dilation and cystic cavity. Till proposed that the persistent dural and bone defects are related to enhanced transmission of pressure from the enlarged ventricle to the site of the injury.[22] This mechanism presumes that transient disequilibrium of CSF production and absorption occurs as a consequence of the initial trauma and that this results in increased pressure transmitted from the dilated ventricle to the overlying cerebrum.

Ito et al. reported a similar series of 11 cases with similar radiologic findings.[10] These authors noted that seven patients presented with seizures. Paroxysmal discharge was present in two patients, focal abnormality in three, and asymmetry in three. Hemiparesis, visual disturbance, and mental retardation were seen in five patients. These clinical manifestations again emphasize the frequency and severity of cerebral damage as the fundamental pathology in this condition.

Porencephaly

Porencephaly is a term with several different interpretations, anatomically and etiologically; in general, however, it is used to indicate cavitation of the brain, usually in communication with the ventricular system. Porencephaly may be congenital or acquired, and one cause of the acquired type is trauma. The infant brain is uniquely susceptible to porencephalic changes after several types of trauma; therefore, a frequent consequence of cerebral trauma in this age group is the later development of cavitation. (These changes are recognized much more frequently now than prior to CT scanning.)

The immature brain is particularly liable to cavitation, a liability which decreases progressively during the first few years of life. Whether this susceptibility is due to mechanical properties of the unmyelinated brain or to biologic fragility of the neurones is not clear, but it has been recognized for many years that perinatal, neonatal, and early infantile trauma are likely to result in porencephaly. The cyst is fluid-filled and occupies the cerebral white matter. It is commonly in communication with the ventricle and may appear in minimal form as a focal ventricular dilation or diverticulum.

Several types of trauma may lead to porencephaly. Penetrating injuries are rare in infancy. A more common mechanism is the shearing injury and hemorrhagic contusion from falls, direct impact, or shaking (Fig. 13.9). The initial area of injury undergoes reactive changes consisting of astroglial hypertrophy and microgial proliferation. After about one month the damaged tissue is replaced by a cavity with smooth gial walls.[11] Infrequently these cavities may be sufficiently loculated from the normal CSF pathways and undergo secondary enlargement. Under these circumstances fenestration of the cyst may be indicated to prevent further brain damage.

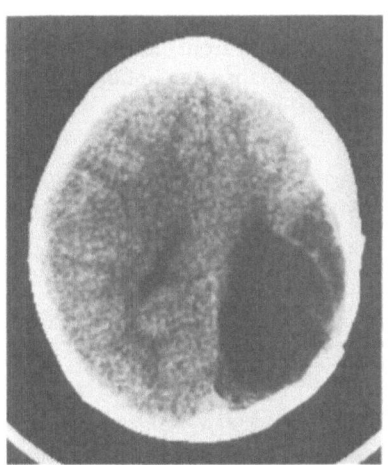 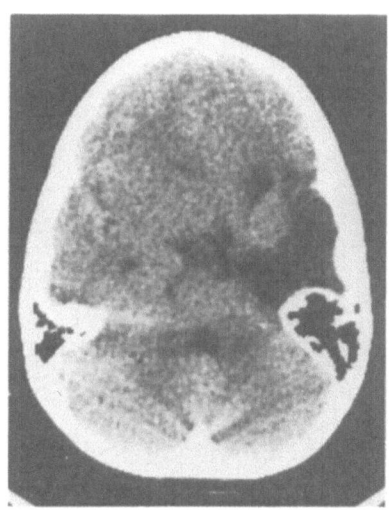

A   B

Figure 13.9. This 5-year-old has had right hemiplegia and seizures since an auto accident at 1 year of age. (**A**) Nonenhanced images show a large, multiseptated region of porencephaly involving the left temporal, parietal, and occipital lobes, seemingly in communication with the lateral ventricle. (**B**) The left temporal bone has altered its shape and position to help fill the void (Davidoff–Dyke–Masson effect).

A second cause of traumatic porencephaly is iatrogenic, occurring most frequently after repeated ventricular tapping through an open fontanel, especially in the presence of elevated intraventricular pressure. Again, it is apparent that the immature brain tissue has minimal resistance to separation and consequent cavitation when the ependymal ventricular lining has been violated. It seems unlikely that porencephalic cysts, usually in the frontal lobe, are the results of direct damage to the neural tissues from needle insertion (Fig. 13.10). Instead, it is probable that the punctured ependyma allows ventricular CSF, under elevated pressure, to enter the white matter and cause fiber separation.

A third type of cavitation may occur beneath a meningeal hematoma because of encephalomalacia and cystic degeneration of the brain tissue (Fig. 13.11). This may be due to the combined effects of direct trauma and possible vascular damage and infarction.

The clinical effects of porencephalic cysts depend greatly on the etiology and location of the cavity. Retardation of mental and motor development is sometimes a consequence, as well as focal neurologic deficit. Seizures are frequently seen in infants with porencephaly of traumatic origin.

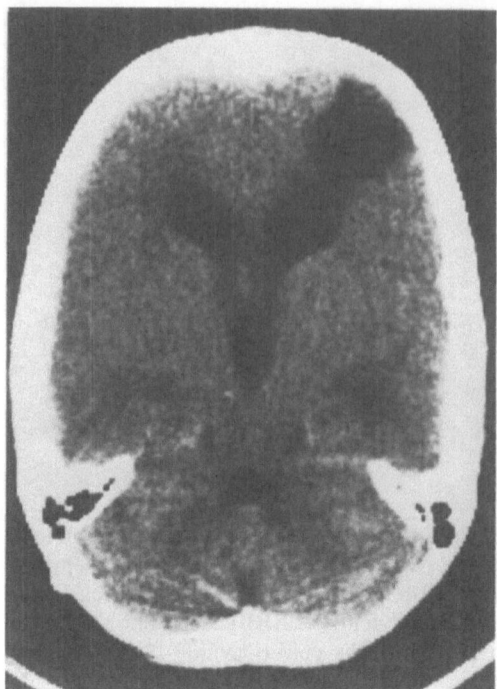

Figure 13.10. Eight-year-old child with left frontal poren-cephaly from multiple ventricular taps as an infant.

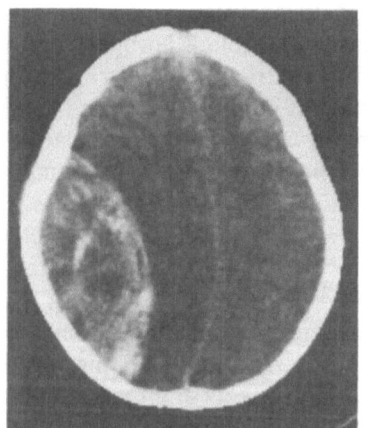

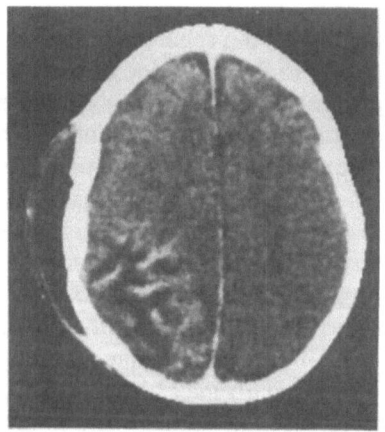

A   B

Figure 13.11. Seven-month-old infant fell down a flight of stairs and suffered right parietal fracture, rapid loss of consciousness, and respiratory arrest. (**A**) Non-enhanced axial images show a large lentiform epidural hematoma with adjacent brain edema causing right-to-left midline shift. (**B**) Four days later, contrast-enhanced CT shows gyral enhancement with central hypodensity in a parieto-occipital infarction.

Outcome

There is little information of statistical value available regarding the long-term effects of acute craniocerebral injury during infancy. It has been stated for many years that infants and children tolerate brain injury much better than adults. Recently, observations of survival after severe head injury have been reported, but no distinction has been made between infants and older children. For purposes of the present brief review of this material, therefore, both age groups will be considered together.

The possibility of death as well as permanent sequelae in the event of head injury is largely dependent on whether the brain damage is a direct result of the impact—with contusions, shearing, and intracerebral hemorrhage present—or a secondary result of a meningeal hematoma or a growing or depressed fracture. If the cerebral dysfunction is secondary, the likelihood of recovery is much better. As described earlier, encephalomalacia, presumably a result of infarction, may occur beneath an epidural hematoma, and microcephaly is not uncommon after chronic subdural hematoma in infancy. The mortality associated with acute subdural hemorrhage results from the associated brain injury or the unchecked pressure caused by the hematoma. Pagni reported 83% mortality in children.[21] Cerebral laceration and focal contusion are relatively uncommon in children, but associated mortality relates directly to the area of damage and the initial value of the patient on the Glasgow Coma Scale. Bruce et al. reported good recovery in all but one of 15 children who demonstrated a lucid interval, and good or moderate recovery in 76% of 34 children with no lucid interval. The mortality rate of all severely head-injured infants and children, as reported by Bruce et al., was approximately 6%.[1]

Long-term neuropsychologic damage following brain injury in infancy is presently under study, so only a few generalizations can be offered. Contrary to what might be expected, it appears that in many areas of function the immature brain has less plasticity than a more mature, developed brain. There are laboratory evidence and clinical observations to support this concept. The subject has been elegantly summarized by Levin et al.,[14] who state that the immature brain has demonstrated greater resilience to focal damage but decreased resilience to diffuse injury. Language function is the principal area of demonstrated plasticity in the immature brain. At present, however, there is limited quantitative data on the effect of brain injury in infancy on later intellectual and neuropsychologic parameters.

Brain trauma is always included in the list of causes of epilepsy, whether the trauma is sustained in the perinatal period, infancy, childhood, or later. The most complete statistics on this subject have been reported by Jennett.[12] No differences were noted between the incidence of early and late epilepsy in children (less than 16 years) and epilepsy following trauma in adulthood. The incidence of early epilepsy (occurring in the first week) was about 5% in all age groups. The majority of early seizures occur in the first 24 hours. Based on this consistency throughout the life span, it seems likely that these same figures would apply to brain trauma in infants.

In contrast, the incidence of late epilepsy (after 1 week) is lower following injury in infancy and childhood than after similar injury in adults. Jennett recorded an incidence of late epilepsy of about 19% after early epilepsy in the infancy period, with a total incidence of late epilepsy of about 3%.[12] The occurrence of early epilepsy is thus significantly predictable with respect to late seizures.

References

1. Bruce DA, Alavi A, Bilaniuk LT et al.: Diffuse cerebral swelling following head injuries in children: The syndrome of "malignant brain edema." *J Neurosurg* 1981;54:170–178.
2. Caffey J: The whiplash–shaken infant syndrome: Manual shaking by the extremities with whiplash-induced intracranial and intraocular bleedings, linked with residual permanent brain damage and mental retardation. *Pediatrics* 1974;54(4):396–403.
3. Collins WF, Pucci GR: Peritoneal drainage of subdural hematoma in infants. *J Ped* 1961;58:482–485.
4. Courville CB: Contrecoup injuries of the brain in infancy: Remarks on the mechanism of fatal traumatic lesions of early life. *Arch Surg* 1965;90:157–165.
5. Ellison PH, Tsai FY, Largent JA: Computed tomography in child abuse and cerebral contusion. *Pediatrics* 1978;62(2):151–154.
6. Gilles FH, Shillito J Jr: Infantile hydrocephalus: Retrocerebellar subdural hematoma. *J Ped* 1970;76(4):529–537.
7. Goldstein FP, Rosenghal SAE, Garancis JC, Sanford JL, Brackett CE Jr: Varieties of growing skull fractures in childhood. *J Neurosurg* 1970;33:25–28.
8. Gutierrez FA: Angiographic characteristics of certain subdural collections of fluid. *Child's Brain* 1977;3:48–61.
9. Gutierrez FA, Raimondi AJ: Acute subdural hematoma in infancy and childhood. *Child's Brain* 1975;1:269–290.
10. Ito H, Miwa T, Onodra Y: Growing skull fracture of childhood. *Child's Brain* 1977;3:116–126.
11. Jellinger K: The neuropathology of pediatric head injuries, in Shapiro K: *Pediatric Head Trauma*. Mt Kisco, NY, Futura Publishing Co Inc, 1983.
12. Jennett B: Trauma as a cause of epilepsy in childhood. *Dev Med Child Neurol* 1973;15:56–62.
13. Lende RA, Erickson TC: Growing fractures of childhood. *J Neurosurg* 1961;18:479–489.
14. Levin HS, Ersenberg HM, and Miner ME: Neurophysiologic findings in head injured children, in Shapiro K: *Pediatric Head Trauma*. Mt Kisco, NY, Futura Publishing Co Inc, 1983.
15. Lindenberg R, Freytag E: Morphology of brain lesions from blunt trauma in early infancy. *Arch Path* 1969;87:298–305.

16. Maki Y, Akimoto H, Enomoto T: Injuries of basal ganglia following head trauma in children. *Child's Brain* 1980;7:113–123.
17. Matson DD: *Neurosurgery of Infancy and Childhood*. Springfield, Ill, Charles C Thomas Publishers, 1969.
18. McClelland CQ, Rekate H, Kaufman B, Persse L: Cerebral injury in child abuse: A changing profile. *Child's Brain* 1980;7:225–235.
19. McLaurin RL, McLaurin KS: Calcified subdural hematoma in childhood. *J Neurosurg* 1966;24:648–655.
20. McLaurin RL, Isaacs E, Lewis HP: Results of nonoperative treatment on 15 cases of infantile subdural hematoma. *J Neurosurg* 1971;34:753–759.
21. Pagni CA, Signovoni G, Crotti F et al: Severe traumatic coma in infancy and childhood. *J Neurosurg Sci* 1975;19:120–128.
22. Till K: *Pediatric Neurosurgery*. Oxford, Blackwell Scientific Publications, 1975.

CHAPTER 14

Intracranial Hematomas

Maurice Choux, Gabriel Lena, and Lorenzo Genitori

Introduction

The nature and distribution of intracranial hematomas in children under 2
years of age are presented, with special attention being given to comparing
our observations with those already published. Pathogenesis and symptomatology are described and correlated with clinical management so as
to indicate appropriate and timely treatment.

Extradural Hematoma

According to the literature, posttraumatic extradural hematomas—the
origin of which may be diploic, arterial, or venous—in children are rare
(1.5 to 3% in large series of pediatric head injuries). Among 648 extradural
hematomas operated in Marseille, 185 were pediatric cases (26.5%)

Extradural hematomas in infants are considered as uncommon. In our
series of 185 extradural hematomas in children, 32 were under 2 years old
(17.3%).[7] McLaurin and Ford[26] had no infants in a series of 47 children
with extradural hematomas; McKissock et al.[25] found 6 infants in a series
of 125 cases; and Mazza et al.[28] 8 in a series of 62 cases. In addition,
Campbell,[4] Dechaume et al.,[9] Fenelon,[11] and Matson[27] found 11, 5, 7, and
16 cases, respectively. Extradural hematomas occurring in children under
the age of 1 are also rare: 3 among 40 pediatric cases for Hendrick and co-
workers,[18] and 12 among our series of 185 cases. The rarity of extradural
hematoma in infants may be explained by the dural adherences at the
level of the sutures, especially the coronal sutures, and the elasticity of
the skull at this age.

Extradural hematomas are extremely rare in the newborn. They are
generally discovered at autopsy. In 1978 Takagi et al.[36] presented 5 cases:
3 discovered among 134 autopsies and 2 treated surgically. (A complicated breech presentation or a forceps delivery may injure meningeal
arteries or venous sinuses, and a fracture may not always be present.)

Only 8 cases of epidural hematoma in neonates were reported in the literature review by GAMA[13] in 1958. Lebkowitz[22] attributes the formation of an extradural hematoma in the newborn to the marked degree of overlapping of the parietal bone and squamous portion of the temporal bone. The resulting edge can injure the dura and the vessels. For Campbell and Cohen[4] the main cause is the detachment of the dura from the inner table.

Takagi et al.,[36] studying the normal anatomical features of the skull and the dura in the newborn, explains the mechanism of extradural hematomas without a skull fracture. The authors point out the fibrovascular connections between the bone and the dura mater. The bleeding point may be the diplöe. A study of the cranial vault in infants shows the richness of the bone vascularization. In our series the bleeding point was the bone in 9 cases (29%). In 1 case (Fig. 14.1) with a large parietal fracture, an hematoma developed at the same time in the subcutaneous and epidural spaces through a large osseous diastasis. Aoki[2] has described the same unusual situation in a newborn baby.

In infants, rupture of a meningeal artery occurs less frequently than in adults. In our series, in 12 cases (39%) the bleeding point was the middle meningeal artery or its branches. In 8 cases (26%) it was the dura. Twice the bleeding was a wound of the dura, and in the other cases it was diffuse from the whole surface of the dura. Histological examination of the dura mater in infancy shows a dense vascularization, especially at the inner level.

Despite the tight adherences between the dura and the skull, the volume of an epidural hematoma in an infant may be great. In our experience the volume is usually more significant than in older children.[7] An epidural hematoma of more than 60 cc was present in 12 cases of our series. This

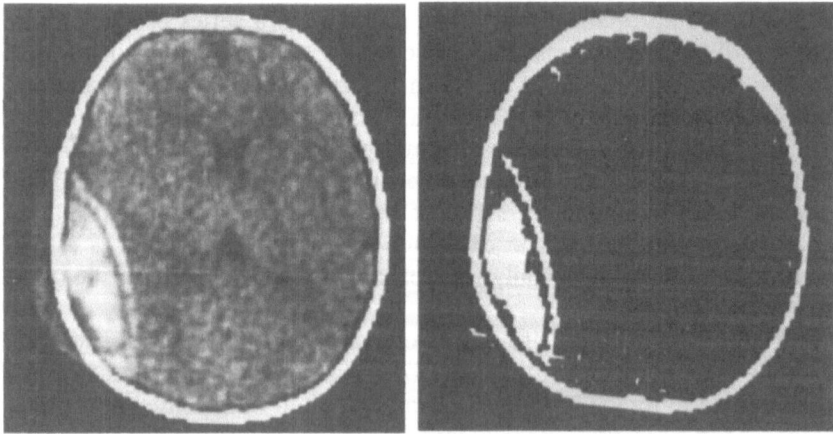

Figure 14.1. Subacute parietal extradural hematoma in a 12-month-old child, communicating with a cephalhematoma through a skull fracture.

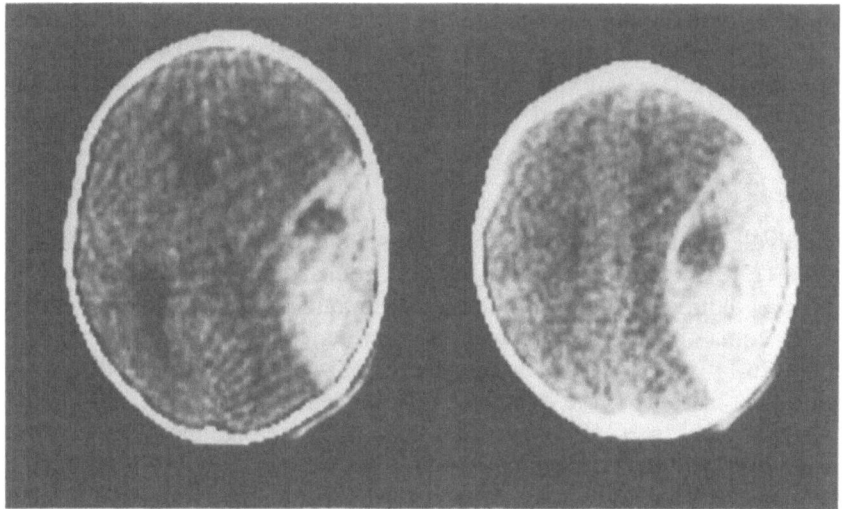

Figure 14.2. Huge extradural hematoma (150 cc in volume) in a 9-month-old baby.

volume accounts for the number of acute cases and the high incidence of anemia. The skull's elasticity and the disjunction of the sutures diminish the consequences of brain compression over a relatively long time period. Thus, acute anemia is not an exceptional occurrence in the evolution of an epidural hematoma in infancy (Fig. 14.2).

The anatomical site of epidural hematomas in infants is generally the same as in older children. One exception must be noted: the rarity of localized frontal extradural hematomas in children under 2 years old. There were no such cases in our series. In a series of 507 cases of extradural hematomas in children of all ages, a frontal localization is found in 20% of the cases. The localizations of hematomas in our 32 cases are shown in Figure 14.3. Despite the adhesion at the level of the suture, we noted 12

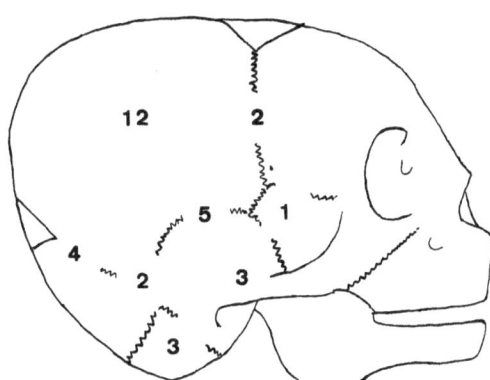

Figure 14.3. Localization of 32 cases of extradural hematomas in authors' series of 185 children.

extensive hematomas (1 frontotemporal, 3 parieto-occipital, 2 temporo-occipital, 4 temporoparietal and 2 parietotemporo-occipital). Bilateral epidural hematomas are exceptional in adults. Only one case in infants has been published (Saeki et al.[30]).

Clinical Findings

The evaluation of disturbances of consciousness is interesting, as in 7 cases (23%) in our series, the infants seemed entirely clear during the entire evolution of their hematoma. Six infants (19%) presented with an initial coma that persisted until surgery, ten (34%) became comatose, eight (26%) were confused without any comatose period, and 49% were not comatose during the evolution of their hematomas.

A true lucid interval was present in 60% of the patients. This interval lasted less than 6 hours in 7 cases, more than 1 day in 3, and more than 6 days in 2. A parietal hematoma in an 8-month-old child without any neurological deficit was discovered 21 days after the initial trauma.

In 14 cases, localizing signs were an hemiplegia or hemiparesis. These pyramidal signs occurred more frequently in infants (61%) than in older children (41%). Convulsions were observed in 3 cases. Bradycardia was infrequent (10%). In 9 cases anemia was present; 6 times it was severe.

Diagnosis

Plain x-rays of the skull showed a fracture in 26 cases (80%). In 2 cases secondary suture diastasis appeared a few days after trauma. Repeated plain x-rays of the skull were necessary to detect an evolving suture separation, which occurred in 20% of the cases.

Cerebral angiography previously, and now CT scans permit the diagnosis of extradural hematomas. In four cases an acute progression of the hematoma necessitated urgent surgical intervention without radiographical studies.

Surgery

The technique in nearly all cases in our series (30 cases) consisted of using a large bone flap that permits complete evacuation of the hematoma and hemostasis. Because of the frequency of osseous or dural origins of bleeding a large flap is required. In 3 acute cases, a burr hole was used but it subsequently became necessary to enlarge it.

Results

Three infants died; they were admitted in coma followed by an acute deterioration that lasted less than 8 hours. Twenty-one infants (68%) were normal without any sequelae. In 4 cases there were major sequelae (motor deficit or repeated convulsions).

Subdural Hematoma

Hematomas in the subdural space in infants are the most frequent post traumatic intracranial hematomas. The majority are diagnosed as post-traumatic, even if a history of trauma is unknown. Especially in infancy the trauma may be mild or ignored. A traumatic etiology may be suspected in cases of subcutaneous hematoma or skull fracture in an otherwise normal child.

Subdural hematomas in children under 2 years old must be separated from subdural hematomas in newborn resulting from birth trauma, and also from subdural hematomas in infants. One must distinguish among acute (the first 2 days), subacute (3 days to 3 weeks), and chronic (after 3 weeks) hematomas. This distinction is important because many acute hematomas are not diagnosed, and much of the literature on subdural hematomas deals with chronic hematomas. Despite the fact that a chronic subdural hematoma is the logical evolution of an untreated or ignored acute hematoma, we focus our study on acute or subacute subdural hematomas. It is clear that the incidence of classical chronic subdural effusion in infancy will diminish significantly when acute subdural hematomas are recognized and adequately treated.

The incidence of posttraumatic acute subdural hematoma is difficult to ascertain. Most series make no distinction between acute or chronic hematomas. In a series of children of all ages, the incidence rate is between 5.2% (Hendrick[18]) and 12% (Ingraham and Matson[19]). In our series of 6700 children with head trauma, subdural hematomas represent 4.3% of all cases. It is evident that subdural hematomas occur mostly in infants: 86% for Hendrick et al.,[18] 88.8% for Gutierrez and Raimondi,[15] 70% for Hayakawa,[17] and 73% for us. In the first 6 months, the rate of incidence is particularly high: 59.2% for Hendrick and 46% for us. Although series of acute subdural hematomas in children are rare in the literature, some have been reported: Suzuki et al.,[35] Sparacio et al.,[33] Gutierrez and Raimondi,[15] Alvarez-Garijo et al.,[1] and Hayakawa and Fujiwara[17] reported by 8, 6, 27, 7, and 27 cases, respectively.

Mechanism of Subdural Hematoma

If extradural hematomas generally have an arterial origin, subdural hematomas are more often due to a venous lesion. In the case of arterial bleeding the origins are cortical arteries, and the subdural hematoma is associated with cerebral contusion. In these cases the hematoma is of secondary importance, and the prognosis depends on the cerebral lesion.

When the subdural hematoma has a venous origin, however, one may distinguish three mechanisms:

1. tearing of bridging veins extending from the brain to the dura or the dural sinus (see Fig. 14.4);
2. laceration of the dura;
3. direct lesion of a sinus by a skull fracture or suture diastasis.

The common cause of subdural hematomas in infants is a tearing of bridging veins at the level of the sagittal sinus, which explains the incidence of interhemispheric or parasagittal subdural hematomas. This localization facilitates the diagnosis of such hematomas by the puncture of the fontanel. However, repeated punctures of the subdural space may be the cause of recurrent bleeding; that is, the needle itself may cause direct lesions of these bridging veins, especially in the case of a small fontanel. It should be noted that visualizing these interrupted veins by angiography or

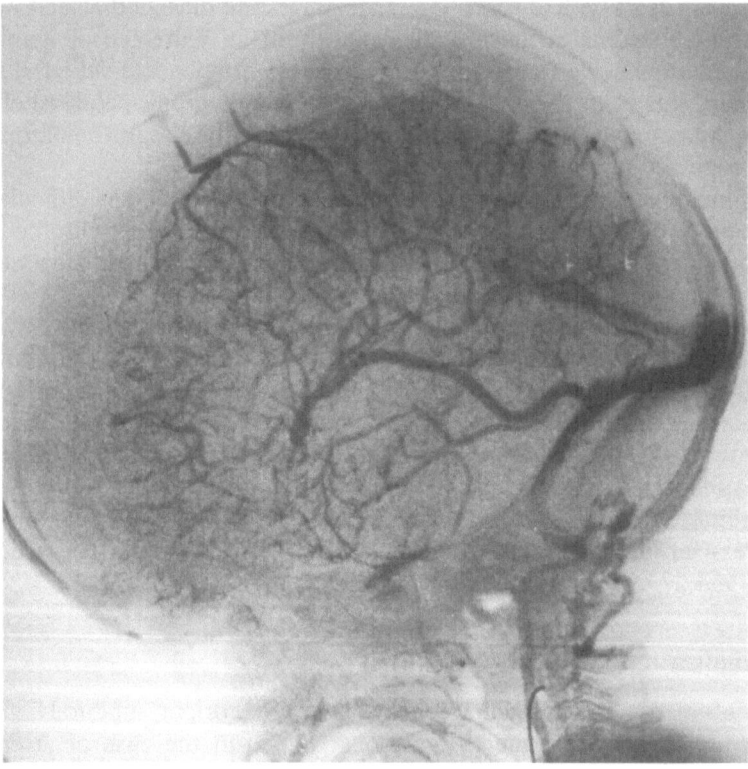

Figure 14.4. Angiography in a case of subdural hematoma showing bridging veins extending from the brain to the superior longitudinal sinus.

at the time of surgery is difficult. In cases of child abuse the mechanism of subdural hematoma may be repeated acceleration and deceleration injuries of the brain, which allow for the rupture of blood vessels. Guthkelch[14] and Caffey[3] have suggested that repeated shaking of the head of an infant may be responsible for acute subdural hematomas. Experimentally, in rhesus monkeys Ommaya and co-workers have demonstrated that rotational displacement of the head without significant head impact may produce acute subdural hematomas and severe contusions. With this mechanism the frequency of subdural hematomas without skull fractures can be explained.[12,23,38]

In an infant a laceration of the dura, with or without a skull fracture, may be the cause of a subdural hematoma. The lesion is a disruption of the different layers of the dura, generally at the level of the dural folds and near the tentorium. We have observed in two autopsy cases, localized laceration of the dura, without tears, and an attached clot at this level. We have previously demonstrated the significance of vascularization of the dura in neonates and small infants. Such a mechanism has been clearly demonstrated in newborn presenting with a fetal skull deformity. A direct lesion of the venous sinuses or bridging veins is possible in the case of a suture dysjunction or a pliable suture. Another mechanism particular to newborn is a skull lesion at the level of the posterior intraoccipital synchondrosis, with the separation of the basal and squamous parts of the occipital bone.

Subdural Hematoma in Newborn

In 1922 Capon[5] mentions that 2% of all stillborn neonates had subdural hemorrhages resulting from a difficult delivery. Craig[8] in 1938, Schipke et al.[31] in 1954, and Schwartz[32] in 1961 have documented subdural hematomas after birth trauma. Despite the improvement of obstetrical methods, the incidence of this complication remains significant in premature infants. In 1977, Larroche[21] in 700 autopsies found 11% who had subdural hemorrhages were preterm infants and 18% were term infants.

The causes of subdural hematomas in neonates are multiple, but breech delivery is a significant one. It is well recognized that subdural bleeding is more frequent in children of primiparous mothers. In the series of Takagi et al.,[37] 84% of posterior fossa subdural hematomas occurred in children of primiparous mothers. Subdural hematomas after birth trauma are generally located at the level of the cerebral convexity; they may be asymetrical, and unilateral subdural hematoma is not rare. A particular localization of such hematoma is the posterior fossa. Among 229 autopsied cases of intracranial hemorrhage in the newborn, Takagi et al.[37] found 23 cases (10%) of posterior fossa subdural hematoma.

The initial symptoms are an apparently asymptomatic interval of from 16 to 72 hours. Respiratory distress, convulsions, bulging of the fontanel, signs of intracranial hemorrhage with a state of shock, and anemia are the most usual symptoms.

Retinal hemorrhages are present in 30% to 50% of the cases. In a few cases of massive subdural bleeding, a comatous state may appear suddenly.

Skull x-rays may show a skull fracture in less than 30% to 40% of all cases. In contrast, splitting of the sutures is present in all cases (Fig. 14.5). Echography and CT scanning may allow the diagnosis especially in the initial period, when a subdural hematoma may be unilateral. Contusion, brain swelling, or a shift of midline structures may also be visualized. Supratentorial dilation of the ventricles may be present in cases of posterior fossa hematoma, either acutely or subsequently.

The treatment of subdural hematomas in newborn is controversial. Subdural taps may be both a method of diagnosis and a treatment. In acute hematomas, however, the tapping method at the level of the fontanel may not uncover temporal or occipital hematomas. An acute subdural hematoma may also be coagulated or liquefied. In acute cases or when the newborn is in bad condition, evacuation of some quantity of blood may help to pass a critical period. In other cases, continuous subdural external drainage is indicated. Sometimes burr holes or craniotomy are needed to evacuate a subdural clot.

Subdural Hematoma in Infants

Most subdural hematomas in children under 2 years old appear to be traumatic in origin. The head injury may be mild or ignored by the child's

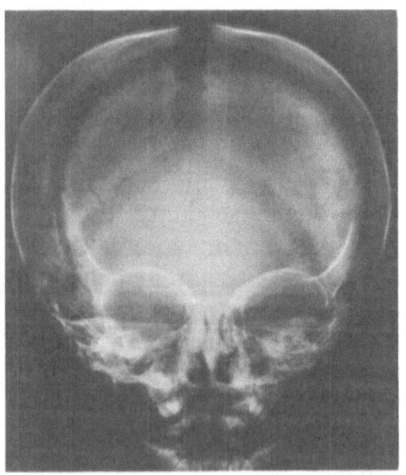 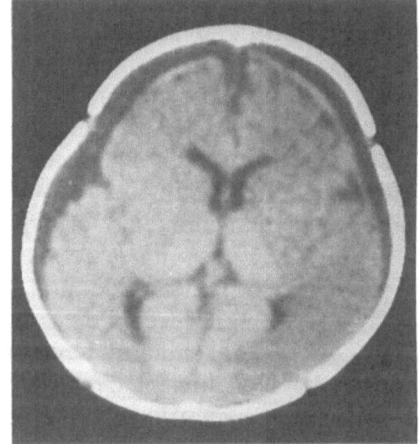

Figure 14.5. Acute bilateral subdural hematoma in a battered child with severe diastatic fracture of sagittal, coronal, and lambdoidal sutures.

family. Many traumas are the result of unobserved falls; repeated shaking of the baby may cause a subdural hematoma without evidence of external trauma. As stated earlier, this mechanism explains the absence of head impact and skull fracture in many subdural hematomas.[12,14,19,33]

Subdural hematomas are not uncommon in abused children. McClelland and co-workers[23] report 21 cases of head injury in battered children. Six of them were admitted with whiplash-shaken infant syndrome and 4 had evidence of acute subdural hematoma. In 1983 Hahn et al.[16] reported 77 cases; of these, 30 presented with subdural hematomas. If a subdural hematoma is a part of the battered child syndrome discussed by Kempe and Silverman[20] in 1962, its true incidence is variable: 28% for McHenry et al,[24] 29% for Hahn et al,[16] and 20% in our experience.

Clinically, acute or subacute subdural hematomas in infants are less dramatic than in neonates. Drowsiness is frequent but a comatose state is rare. Convulsions occur in more than 50% of the cases. Focal neurological signs may also be found. Retinal hemorrhage is present in 63% of the cases reported by Gutierriez and Raimondi,[15] and 55% for Hayakawa and Fujiwara.[17] In small children, hypovolemic shock may be present. Skull fracture is present in 41% of the cases reported by Gutierriez and Raimondi, 59% for Hayakawa and Fujiwara, and 45% for us. In contrast, depressed fracture associated with subdural hematoma is rare.

Ultrascanning and CT scanning are the proven method of identifying, locating, and determining the size of the hematoma as well as following up with the therapeutic management (Fig. 14.6 and Fig. 14.7).

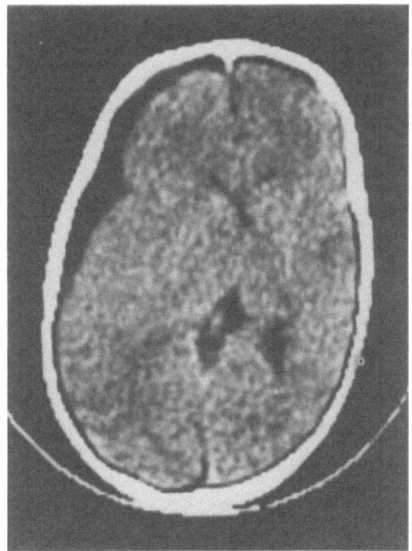

Figure 14.6. Acute left frontoparietal subdural hematoma with brain swelling.

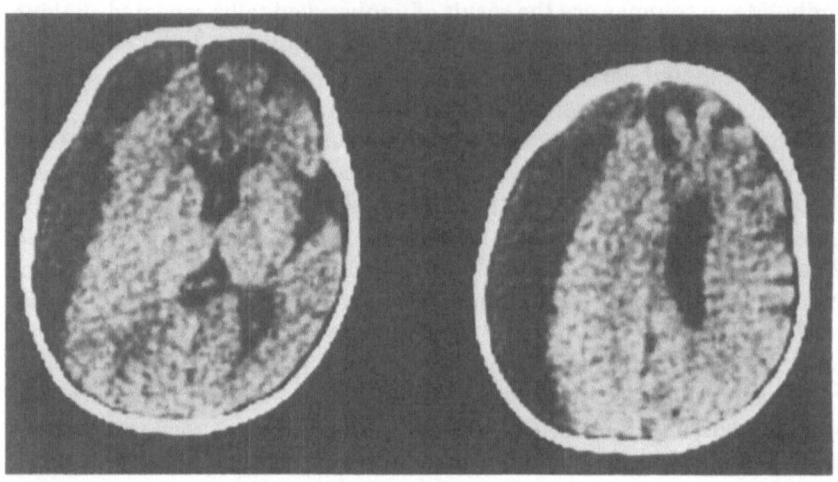

Figure 14.7. Subacute hemispheric subdural hematoma with a brain swelling.

Four methods of treatment may be used in cases of acute or subacute subdural hematoma:

1. subdural taps for diagnosis, but negative subdural taps are frequent in cases of basal or occipital hematomas;
2. a temporary external drainage of a subdural collection is useful in liquid hematomas;

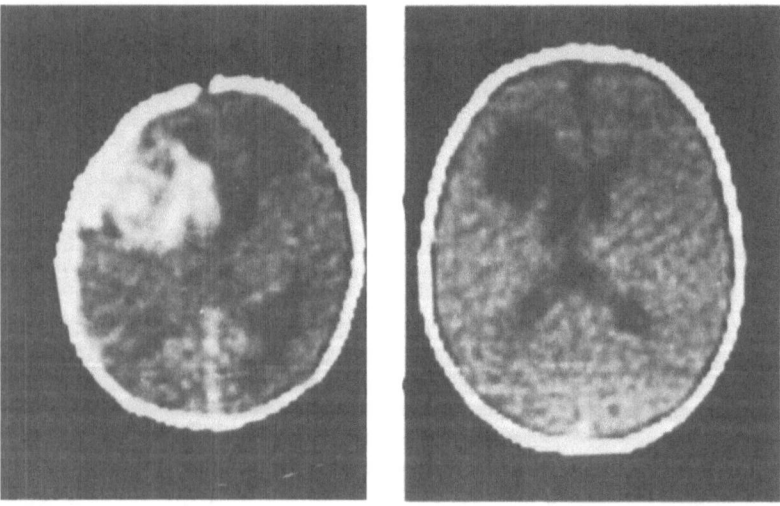

Figure 14.8. Intracerebral frontal hematoma in a newborn. Surgical evacuation, late CT-scan aspect.

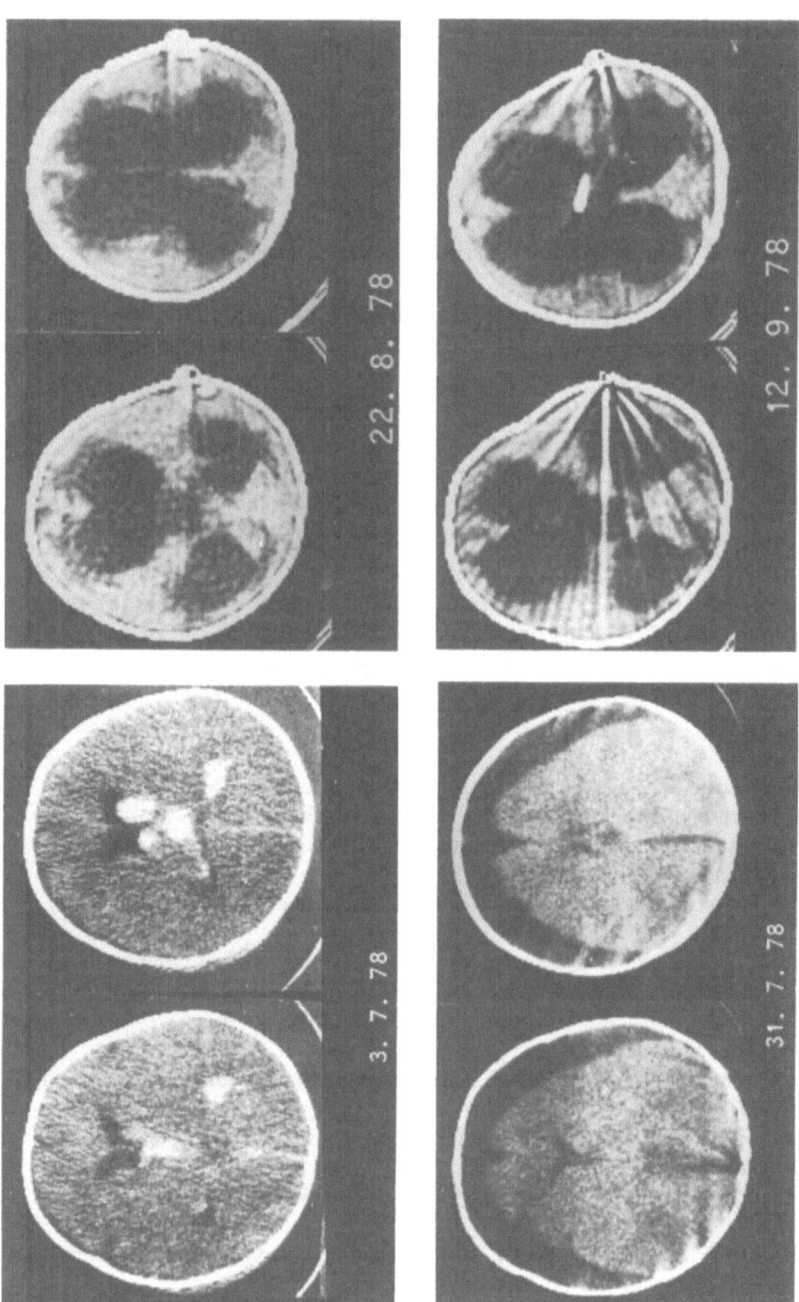

Figure 14.9. CT scan evolution of multiple intracerebral hematomas in a 14-month-old child. One month later bilateral subdural hematomas were discovered and treated by subdural drainage. Twenty days later the subdural hematoma disappeared, but bilateral dilation of the ventricles was present. The child was shunted, but the neurological evolution was bad.

3. an opening of the skull by burr hole or trephination is indicated to evacuate a subdural clot;
4. for a few authors an osteoplastic bone flap is recommended for removal of an extensive, solid clot.

In our experience, the majority of acute subdural hematomas may be evacuated by temporary subdural drainage, or a unilateral or bilateral trephination.

Intracerebral and Intracerebellar Hematomas

Posttraumatic intracerebral hematomas are rare in infants in comparison with older patients (Fig. 14.8). They are quite rare if we exclude intracerebral or intracerebellar hemorrhagic lesions in premature babies. The literature indicates the relative frequency of cerebellar hematomas in comparison with the rarity of supratentorial hematomas in obstetrical injuries.

Excluding the neonatal period, true posttraumatic intracerebral or intracerebellar hematomas are rare. Generally, brain swelling, laceration, or contusion are the major brain lesions. Small disseminated hematomas may be present. Very few surgical evacuations are needed in infancy.

The evolution of intracranial hematomas in infants is sometimes predictable. Repeated CT scans are needed to detect either an improvement or a worsening. An illustration of such evolution is shown in Figure 14.9.

References

1. Alvarez-Garijo JA, Gomila DT, Aytes AP, Mengual MV, Martin AA: Subdural hematomas in neonates. *Child's Brain* 1981;8:31–38.
2. Aoki N: Epidural hematoma communication with cephalohematoma in a neonate. *Neurosurgery* 1983;13:55–57.
3. Caffey J: On the theory and practice of shaking infants. *Am. J. Dis. Child.* 1972;124:161.
4. Campbell JB, Cohen J: Epidural hemorrhage and the skull of children. *Surg Gyn Obstet* 1951;92:257–280.
5. CAPON NB: Intracranial trauma in the new born. *Br J Obstet Gyn* 1922;29:572–580.
6. Carcassonne M, Choux M, Grisoli F: Extradural Hematomas in infant. *J Ped Surg* 1977;12:69–73.
7. Choux M, Grisoli F, Peragut JC: Extradural hematomas in children: 104 cases. *Child's Brain,* 1975;1:337–347.
8. Craig WS: Intracranial hemorrhage in the newborn. *Arch Dis Child* 1938;31:89.
9. Dechaume JP, Capuis JY, Bret P et al: L'hématome extra-dural du nourrisson. *Ann Chir Infant* (Paris) 1970;2:2–5.
10. Esparza J, Portillo JM, Mathos F, Lamas E: Extradural hemorrhage in the posterior fossa in the neonate. *Surg Neurol* 1982;17:341–343.

11. Fenelon J: L'hématome extradural. Thése, Université de Bordeaux, 1967.
12. Ferry PC, Tufts E, Ison JB: On shaking and subdural hematomas in infancy. *Child Neurol Soc Abstr* 1974;24:14.
13. Gama CH, Fenichel GM: Epidural hematoma of the newborn due to birth trauma. *Ped. Neurol.* 1985;1:52–53.
14. Guthkelch AN: Infantile subdural hematoma and its relationship to whiplash injuries. *Br Med J* 1971;1:430.
15. Gutierriez FA, Raimondi AJ: Acute subdural hematoma in infancy and childhood. *Child's Brain* 1975;1:269–290.
16. Hahn YS, Raimondi AJ, McLone DG, Yamanouchi Y: Traumatic mechanism of head injury in child abuse. *Child's Brain* 1983;10:229–241.
17. Hayakawa I, Fujiwara K: Acute traumatic subdural hematoma in children and its late results after surgery. *Child's Brain* (in preparation), 1984.
18. Hendrick EB, Harwood-Nash DCF, Hudson AR: Head injuries in children: A survey of 4465 consecutive cases at the hospital for thick children, Toronto, Canada. *Clin Neurosurg* 1964;2:46–65.
19. Ingraham FD, Matson DD: Subdural hematoma in infancy *J Ped*, 1944;24: 3–37.
20. Kempe CH, Silverman FN, Steele BF, Drogenmueller W, Silver HK: The battered child syndrome. *JAMA* 1962;181:17–24.
21. Larroche JC: Developmental pathology of the neonates. *Excerpta Medica (Amsterdam)*, 1977.
22. Lebkowitz LC: Extradural hemorrhage as a result of birth trauma. *Arch Ped* 1936;P3:404–407.
23. McClelland CQ, Rekate H, Kafman B, Persse L: Cerebral injury in child abuse: A changing profile. *Child's Brain* 1980;7:225–235.
24. McHenry T, Girdany BR, Elmer E: Unsuspected trauma with multiple skeletal injuries during infancy and childhood. *Pediatrics* 1963;31:903.
25. McKissock W, Taylor JC, Bloom WT, Till K: Extradural hematoma: Observations on 125 cases. *Lancet* 1960;2:167–172.
26. McLaurin RL, Ford LE: Extradural hematoma: Statistical survey of 47 cases. *J Neurosurg* 1964;21:364–371.
27. Matson DD: *Neurosurgery of Infancy and Childhood*, ed 2. Springfield, Ill, Charles C Thomas Publishers, 1969, pp 316–327.
28. Mazza C, Pasqualin A, Feriotti G, Da Pian R: Traumatic extradural hematomas in children: Experience with 62 cases. *Acta Neurochir.* 1982;65:67–80.
29. Ommaya AK, Faas F, Yarnell P: Whiplash injury and brain damage. *JAMA* 1968;204:285.
30. Saeki N, Hinokuma K, Vemura K, Makino H: Subacute bilateral epidural hematoma in an infant. *Surg Neurol* 1979;11:67–69.
31. Schipke R, Reige D, Scoville W: Acute subdural hemorrhage at birth. *Pediatrics* 1954;14:468–474.
32. Schwartz P: *Birth Injuries of the Newborn*. Basel, S Karger, 1961.
33. Sparacio RR, Khatib R, Cook AW: Acute subdural hematoma in infancy. *NYS J Med* 1971;71:212–213.
34. Sulama M, Vera P: An investigation into the occurence of perinatal subdural hematoma: Its diagnosis and treatment. *Acta Obstet Gynecol Scand* 1952;31:400–412.

35. Suzuki J, Aihara H, Suzuki S: Investigation of acute subdural hematoma in infancy. *Brain Nerve,* 1970;22:43–50.
36. Takagi T, Nagai R, Wakabayah S, Mizawa I, Hayashi K: Extradural hemorrhage in the newborn as a result of birth trauma. *Child's Brain,* 1978;4:306–318.
37. Takagi T, Fuluoka H, Wakabayashi S, Nagai H, Shibata HT: Posterior fossa subdural hemorrhage in the newborn as a result of birth trauma. *Child's Brain* 1982;9:102–113.
38. Till K: Subdural hematoma and effusion in infancy. *Br Med J:* 1968;400–402.

CHAPTER 15

Perinatal and Posttraumatic Seizures

N. Chiofalo, J. Madsen, and L. Basauri

Introduction

This chapter discusses traumatic perinatal seizures and crises following traumatic injuries during infancy. Because these are two completely different phenomena, they need to be analyzed separately. The newborn is not a small adult, not even a small child; newborn behave differently under both normal and pathological conditions.

Perinatal Seizures

Despite advanced obstetric technology birth trauma continues to be a well recognized cause of neonatal seizures (NNS), even though metabolic disturbances, especially hypocalcemia and hypoglycemia, are both significant causes of NNS.[27,33,41,42] However, in McInnery's series,[33] 95 patients with NNS, 30% of the cases, suffered difficulties at the time of birth, especially related to obstetric trauma. In Keen's series,[27] 14 out of 112 cases of NNS were recognized to be due to intracranial hemorrhage; 8 died in the neonatal period.

Often, there are no visible or recognizable signs of trauma in the neonate; consequently, the diagnosis may be delayed. This, obviously changes the prognosis. It is a well-known fact that during the first stages of life, there is a high resistance to seizures, which implies that conditions causing seizures must be severe. For this reason, prognosis is closely related to the etiological factors and to early and adequate treatment.

Incidence

Quantifying the incidence of seizures during the neonatal period is a difficult problem. Values have been quoted from 12.2 to 1.5 per 1,000 live births by Keen.[27] McInnery[33] found an incidence rate of 0.8% of all live births, and Tibbles[42] reported convulsions occurring once every 200 deliveries. Burke[3] noted a rate of 5.3 per 1,000; Craig,[8] 8 per 1000; and Brown[2] a higher incidence of 14.6 per 1000 live births. There is a consensus that the appearance of seizures resulting from obstetric trauma occurs more often as a complication of an intracerebral hemorrhage (ICH). In this condition, episodes may occur at a rate of from 20% to 44% (per our series[5]). The incidence rate is higher in preterm infants whose conditions are complicated by intraventricular and/or subependymal hemorrhage (IVH-SEH), although current thinking on this complication has changed in the last 15 years. The natural history of such hemorrhages can be traced by the use of computarized tomography and/or echotomography, which allow an exact, accurate, and noninvasive diagnosis. In premature infants, hemorrhage of the germinal plate can produce ICH or IVH, the latter being a constant finding in premature infants weighting less than 1500 gm. Studies of 45 neonates in this weight range demonstrated IVH in 43% of all cases[36]; it is the most frequent necropsy finding in neonates and premature babies.[12] In all cases of term infants, the cause of IVH is the rupture of the choroid plexus. In 87% of premature infants, it is the rupture of the germinal matrix.

Etiology

The etiology of NNS is not always clear. Twenty to 30% of its causes are unknown. It is generally accepted that hypocalcemia is the most frequent cause of NNS, with an incidence rate of about 20%; intracranial birth injury is the second most frequent cause. Often, factors are combined, and this can be a reason for error. In a traumatic delivery, serum calcium levels fall below normal values in the first 48 to 60 hours; therefore, convulsions in the first 72 hours of life may have independent causes that are secondary to the birth trauma, as we saw in some of the newborn we observed. The severity of IVH and SEH in low-weight infants increases the frequency of seizures during the postnatal period (to be discussed later).

Pathophysiology

The pathophysiologic aspects of seizures in newborn are generally unknown in terms of the fundamental mechanisms, but it is reasonable to suppose that a disturbance in energy resulting from hypoxemia, hypoglycemia, or ischemia may cause a failure of the potassium-sodium pump.

According to Volpe,[43] seizure phenomena in newborn differ considerably from those observed in older infants because of the critical neuroanatomical processes ocurring during the perinatal organizing period. Cortical organization of neurons and axonal and dendritic ramifications are as yet incompletely developed in the neonate; consequently, motor seizures are poorly defined. In contrast, the relatively well organized limbic structures and their connections to the diencephalon and brain stem may explain the frequent clinical manifestations of oral-buccal movements such as chewing and sucking, oculomotor signs, or apnea.

The mechanisms involved in IVH in premature babies are an increase of venous and capillary pressure with secondary failure of the left heart, which will lead to hypoxia, acidosis, and rupture of terminal veins.[7] Coagulation deficiencies are not a prominent factor.

Age

The age of onset of traumatic seizures shows two peaks; one in the first 48 hours of life and the second during the fifth to seventh days (120 to 168 hours). For the first period, the peak incidence of seizures is during the second day, and the most common etiologies are intracranial hemorrhage, cerebral contusion, or low birth weight complicated with IVH and SEH. Later onset in the second period may also be seen in the form of cerebral contusion when edema is the chief cause of convulsions, or when secondary metabolic disturbances are added to the trauma.

Type of Seizures

Perinatal seizures are one of the striking neurologic phenomena frequently faced as a medical emergency by the neonatologist. They are often difficult to recognize because they resemble normal movements of the newborn, and also because they may not impair consciousness. In their presentation, seizures in the neonatal period are independent from etiology, gestational age, or birth weight. However, tonic crises, even though they appear at any neonatal age, tend to be more frequent in premature babies.[32] According to Volpe,[43] seizures may be divided into minor and major categories. The first consists of paroxysmal episodes of grimacing, rowing, pedalling, or swimming; oral-bucal-lingual movements such as tasting, drooling, sucking, or swallowing; or paroxysmal movements of the eyes or eyelids, apnea, hyperpnea, dyspnea, pallor, or cyanosis. These crises usually occur without impairment of consciousness. Because of this, and because seizures can mimic normal movements of the newborn, their diagnosis can sometimes be missed. For this reason, seizures may evolve into status, thereby increasing the risk of mortality.

Minor seizures can occur in isolation in one or several forms, but they usually occur in combination with major crises. These latter belong to the motor type, especially those of the focal variety, and may be classified in terms of decreasing frequency and summarized as follows:

1. Tonic: usually generalized but may also be unilateral.
2. Focal-clonic: in the form of clonic twitchings and involving in a fixed manner only one region of the body (face or one extremity).

3. Multifocal clonic: involving a migration of the crises from one extremity to another, or from one side of the body to the other; usually assymetrical, and without a jacksonian sign.
4. Myoclonic: segmental or generalized.
5. Tonic-clonic: very rare in the newborn.

In an intensive-care unit in a children's hospital in Santiago, Chile, we conducted a retrospective analysis of 30 newborn with traumatic seizures and 15 followed prospectively (both by observation and TV monitoring). This analysis allowed us to reach conclusions similar to those of other authors. We have seen in the same child the simultaneous or progressive appearance of subtle crises—focal clonic or multifocal clonic—and erratic seizures; the child's state of consciousness could be very difficult to determinate. Tonic crises, rather frequent in the premature, are usually associated with brain-stem involvement (as proven by CT scan or necropsy). They may resemble decorticate or decerebrate positions. Cases like these prove the efficacy of the EEG to demonstrate electrical discharge. Myoclonic and tonic-clonic seizures have been exceptional in our series.

EEG Findings

To summarize the most frequent ictal or critical tracing patterns of the EEG is rather difficult. It can be said, however, that spikes, or more often slow spikes, are common ictal findings, as are also monomorphic delta waves with a range of 1 to 4 Hz.[13,15,16] A pattern of alpha-like rhythms between 6 and 10 cycles per second and an amplitude of 25 to 30 μV can be recorded more often in Rolandic and occipital leads. The electrical pattern may be a run of only one of the elements described, involving one or more areas but usually restricted to one. In other cases, with no strict relationship with brain damage, abnormalities can be a succession of different patterns varying in voltage and frequencies during the discharges and following the same topographical distribution.[14,19,34,35]

There have been seizures with different electrographic elements simultaneously recorded in different areas (Fig. 15.1). The burst-suppression pattern, critical or intercritical ("trace paroxistique" of French authors), may accompany a myoclonic seizure; over prolonged periods of flat or inactive EEG readings, discharges of asynchronous elements, spikes, and slow spikes or slow waves with variable voltage have been recorded. They are very similar to those observed in hypsarrythmia during sleep (Fig. 15.2). Clonic seizures generally have a fixed focus, whereas the multifocal clonic ones show a migration of focuses as well as multiple foci. Similar phenomena are observed with tonic seizures when they are occur in one or scattered parts of the body.

The importance of serial EEGs during the neonatal period has been demonstrated by the numerous ictal patterns incident to visible seizures.

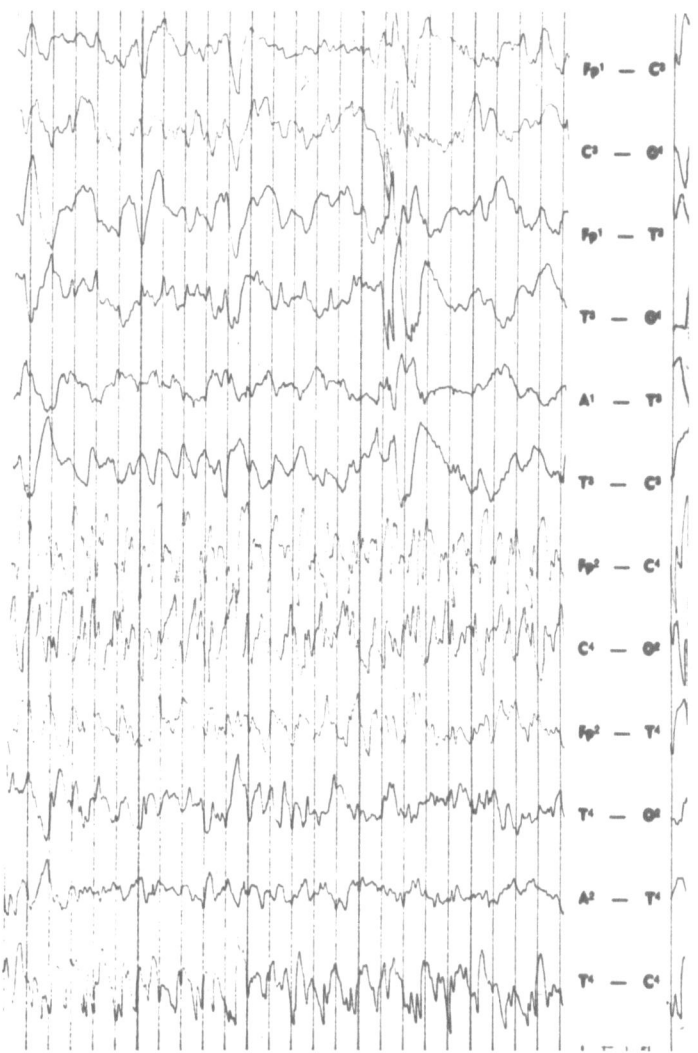

Figure 15.1. Hypsarrythmia-like pattern on left hemisphere. A "run" of slow spikes on right central area.

Frequently, underlying brain lesions in small babies cause only subclinical seizures.[20,30]

Interictal EEG

This EEG is intended to analyze the background activity that depends on gestational age. A fairly normal background in repeated EEGs indicates a good outcome, whereas the persistence of a serial abnormal background

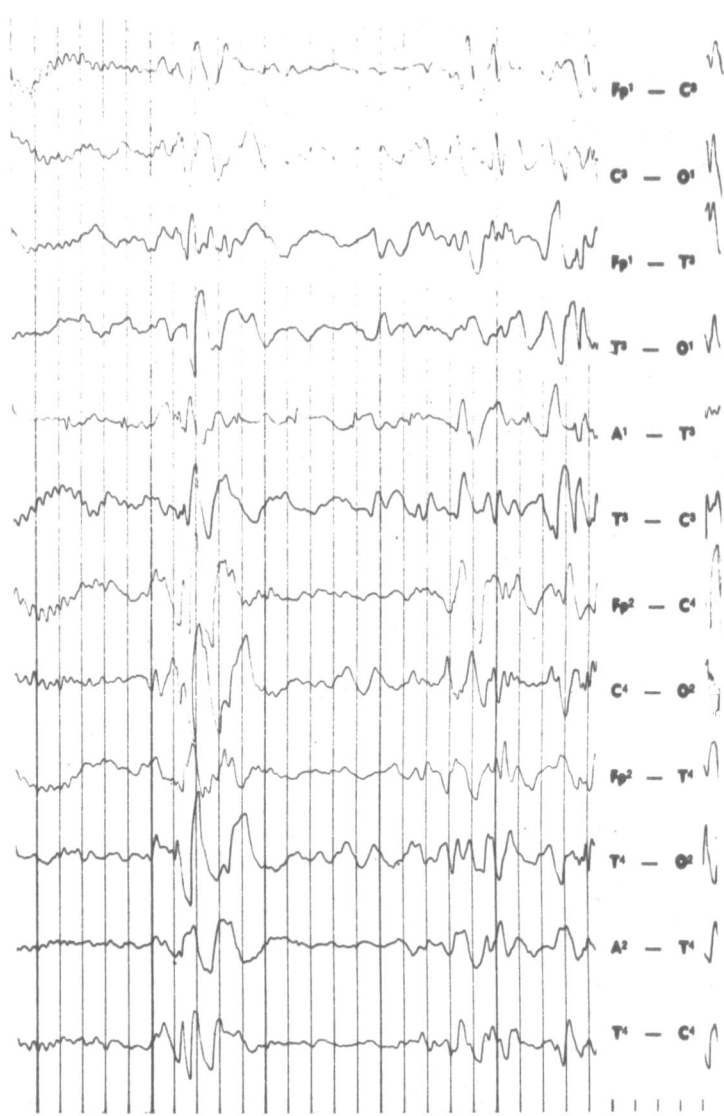

Figure 15.2. Burst suppression pattern.

points to severe brain damage. These abnormalities are the patterns maintaining flat or inactive rhythms, burst suppression, persistent asymmetries or asynchronies between both hemispheres, multifocal EEGs, and so on (Figs. 15.2–15.5).

In light of currently better prognoses of IVH, the usual finding of Rolandic sharp waves may be interpreted as a better outcome, but care must be

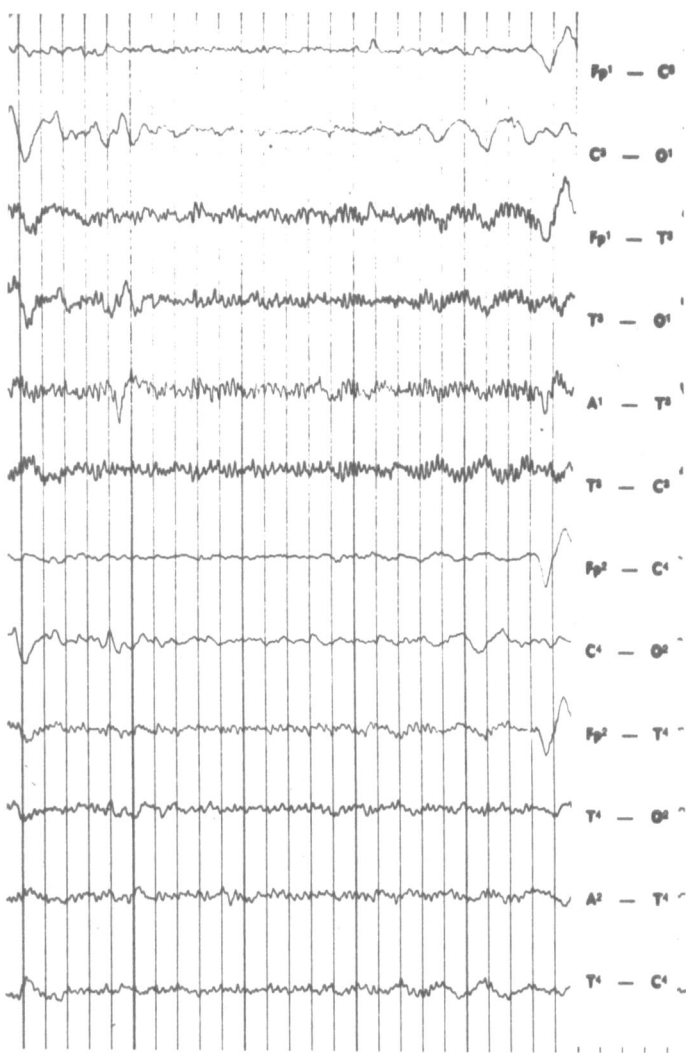

Figure 15.3. Alpha-like pattern on left hemisphere.

taken in that the background activity should progressively improve in serial EEGs.

Prognosis

Immediate and long-term prognoses of infants with perinatal seizures can be discussed from different points of view. First, the chance for long-term

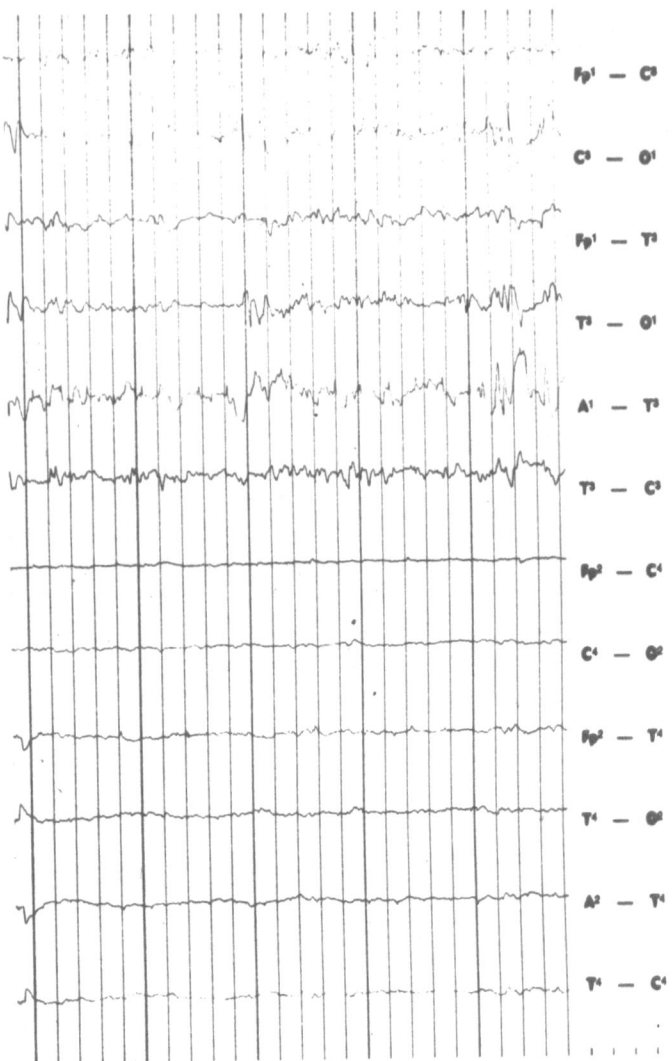

Figure 15.4. Hypsarrythmic pattern on left hemisphere. Hypovolted pattern on right hemisphere.

survival of a newborn suffering a traumatic birth (and especially the premature infant) has increased enormously over the last 15 years.[10,11,22,23,37]
Even when IVH is the main cause of death in the first 2 months of life, the
number of survivors and the quality of survival have improved dramatically. Seventy-eight per cent of all survivors of IVH have no clinical signs
or sequelae. Therefore, the incidence of seizure sequelae is currently
lower than reported earlier (i.e., as high as 85%, especially when associ-

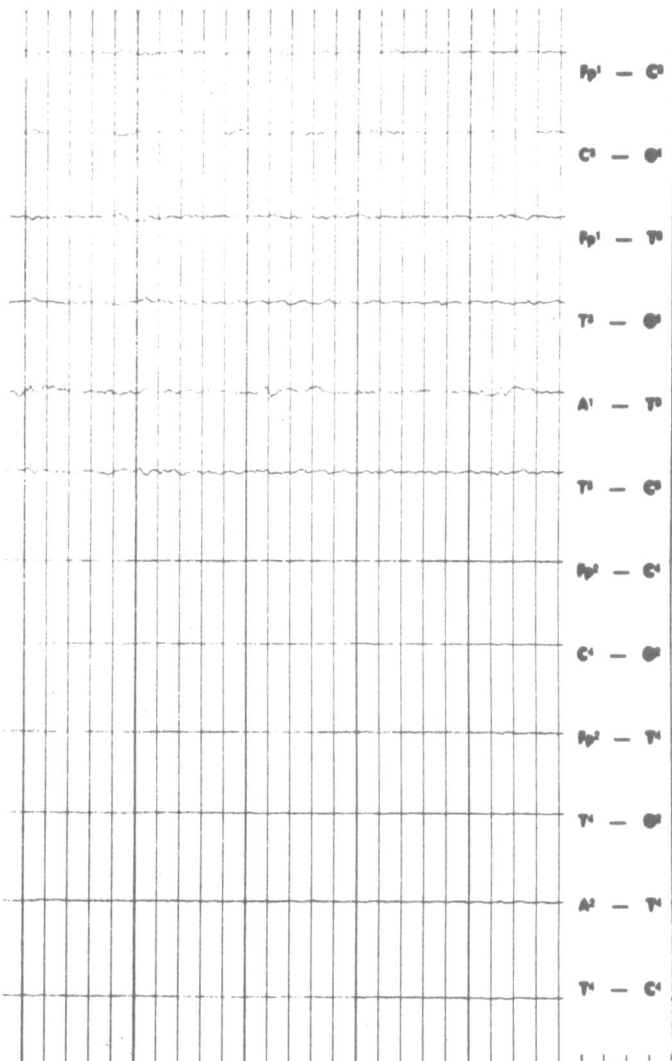

Figure 15.5. Flat or inactive EEG.

ated with SEH). The quantity of blood clots is prognostically important with regards to both mortality and survival sequelae, as are other suggested associated factors such as hypoxia, hyperoxemia, high peak pressure during mechanical ventilation, pulmonary interstitial emphysema, volume expansion, and hypercarbia.[21,24] Posthemorrhagic hydrocephalus that can be detected by systematic CT scans or echotomographic follow-up appear between 12 and 28 days after the trauma; the degree or amount of SEH/IVH does not affect the time of appearance.[18]

Usually, NNS starting longer after birth are associated with a higher survival rate. However, this condition is serious and can result in poor outcomes as well as neurological sequelae, especially when related to late-onset epilepsy. Prognosis also varies according to etiological factors. Convulsions secondary to cerebral contusion and subarachnoid hemorrhage have a good prognosis and are fairly easily controlled during the newborn period. However, noncomplicated trauma can sometimes lead to anoxia, infections, and postnatal asphyxia related to ventilatory insufficiency; these cases may be associated with a mortality rate of more than 50%, especially in low-birth-weight infants with NNS, if appropriate neonatal care is not immediate. Before the development of currently available techniques of neonatal care, mortality in such cases occurred within the first 2 years (most during the first two months) of life, and about 25% to 35% of the survivors were left with varying degrees of motor sequelae or mental deficiency. Only 15% to 25% were considered to develop normally.[1,3,8]

Prognosis related to the time of onset of seizures has often been emphasized in many of the published series. It is said that later onset in the newborn period has a better prognosis than when occurring in the first 3 days of life, probably because metabolic causes are included. However, we must remember the above-mentioned late onset of hydrocephalus as well as the observation that a comparison of autopsy findings with CT-scan lesions in low-birth-weight infants suggests that IVH and SEH appear approximately 40 hours after birth. For this reason, infants may begin to suffer seizures around 72 hours of life, which does not imply a better prognosis. Anticonvulsant medication in these cases has little effect on seizure activity and does not influence the ultimate outcome. Therefore, refractory therapeutic response indicates poor prognosis.

In contrast, infants who recover well from seizures after the first day of onset, who may be completely controlled within 5 days, usually have a positive long-term prognosis.[38] Not all seizures starting in the first 48 hours of life carry a poor prognosis. Cerebral contusion and subarachnoid hemorrhage cause early onset of seizures, but the outcome may be favorable.

According to Lombroso[32] and others, prognosis with EEGs seems to confirm certain facts: in term babies with seizures, the neurological outcome may be predicted in about 75% of the cases, according to EEG findings. Failure in 25% may be related to combinations of complications as well as an incorrect interpretation of the tracings, especially as related to maturational stages. Infants whose serial EEG readings are normal in the neonatal period usually remain normal at follow-up, or else suffer minor neurological sequelae. The importance of serial EEGs is shown in nonexceptional cases in which abnormalities of the first EEG pattern are transitory; the patterns may even return to normal before the patient has complete neurological or seizure recovery.

A normal EEG in preterm and term infants who suffer seizures only during their first or second days of life generally indicates a favorable prognosis.

Posttraumatic Epilepsy in Infants

Acute brain injuries in infants differ from those in adults just as they differ from those in the newborn. Pediatric injuries have their particular aspects, especially as they relate to the maturational stage at the time of trauma. Frequently, the intensity of the trauma has no direct correlation with either the symptomatology or the EEG findings. It is therefore often fruitless to try to predict end results on the basis of both clinical and EEG signs in infants with traumatic brain injuries immediately after their arrival in hospital. The responsibility of the specialist does not end when the acute phase is over. Modifications of the cerebral electrogenesis depend on numerous factors which may not be reliably established after the trauma. Serial observations long after the trauma may help to clarify some of these factors.

Thirty years ago, Kellaway[28] emphasized the importance of conducting longitudinal studies in order to understand the dynamics of the various effects of trauma on the electrical activity of the brain. An analysis of impact injuries to the infant head reveal that tension, compression, and bleeding are the basic physical factors of such injuries. An impact may cause compression and deformation of the skull even in the absence of fracture (occasionally elastic), but may also result in a depressed skull fracture over the impacted area, with the possibility of underlying damage. Pressure gradients through the brain may coexist and can produce concussion, cerebral contusion, cerebral hemorrhage, subdural hematoma, and/or laceration. If the brain injury has been followed by 3 of the above mentioned complications, one may predict early and long term prognosis and identify the sequelae.

It may be said that clinically and electrically, PTE cases are almost as complicated as those involving a more mature brain. For this reason, it is useful to discuss noncomplicated, closed-head trauma by analyzing the results of a randomized series of 143 children, ranging in age from 3 months to 5 years, which we reviewed in a prospective study.[5] In this sense children were not treated with prophylactic anticonvulsants, and the analysis was based on the EEG follow-up only. (The importance of preventive pharmacological treatment will be discussed later.) EEGs were performed during the first week after the trauma—80% during the first 3 days.

Table 15.1 details the immediate electrical abnormalities along with the correlated number of early transient convulsions (of varied types) that developed during the first week. Of the total number, 24 (17%) suffered

Table 15.1. Immediate EEG and seizure findings
following craniocerebral trauma.

EEG abnormalities	Number of cases	Early seizures
• Diffuse slow activity	28	2
• Slow monomorphic PO activity	24	4
• Paroxistic diffuse slow activity	63	10
• Focal slow activity or focal low voltage	24	5
• Diffuse spike activity (sym. or asym.)	4	3
Total	143	24

this early symptom. A follow-up of 92 of the total cases was performed for
a period ranging from 2 to 8 years after the head injury. The rules for
rhythm recovery in children have no strict correlation with the type of
initial abnormality, nor with the real severity of the trauma.

   The time required for recovery to a relatively stable level is somewhat
difficult to predict; but it is significant that, of the cases who recovered
completely from the clinical and EEG points of view, the highest percentage (75%) did so before the end of the first 6 months. The remaining did so
within 2 years. Forty-two cases (46%) belong to both groups, which nor-
malized their EEGs in the time shown in Figure 15.6.

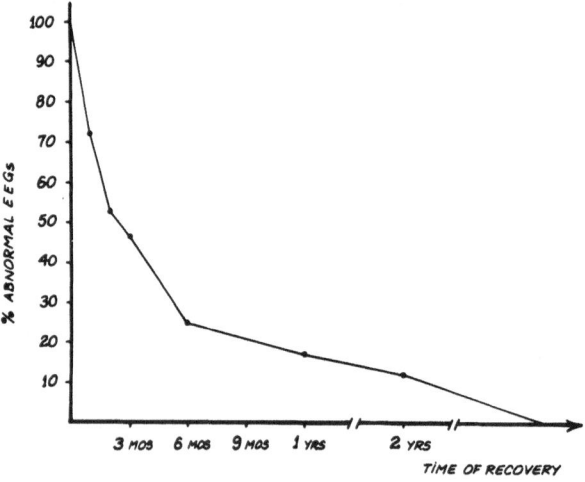

Figure 15.6. Time for EEG recovery from craniocerebral trauma.

An infant's EEG is not an accurate indicator of the coincidental damage resulting from the trauma, the time required for recovery, or the causes of recovery (whether or not it is complete). However, it seems that the ways in which the electrical abnormalities stabilize or modify negatively may suggest in some cases, the development of PTE. For the 50 infants in our series who continued to maintain EEG abnormalities, it is noteworthy that 12 (24%) had, at any moment of their evolution, some kind of delayed seizure, usually not related to the severity of their trauma. This figure coincides with the data of Young et al.,[45] who postulated that about 25% of patients under age 16 with acute intracranial trauma suffer posttraumatic seizures. We observed that the onset of seizures occurs in the first 3 months in 43% of cases and up to 1 year in 83%. In the remaining 17% it developed in a period of 2 years or more.

Although, as we have emphasized, there are not many predictable factors contributing to PTE in infants, the evolution of the EEGs that we observed have led us to some tentative conclusions regarding PTE as a sequela of head trauma. Patients who, immediately after trauma, show slow monomorphic discharges as a predominant abnormality that persists with no modification after 4 to 6 months may be more inclined to develop late epilepsy. Diffuse irregular slowness that changes into a paroxysmal activity may also indicate this possibility. Early slow or depressive focus, changing to focal or diffuse paroxysmal waves, and the appearance of spike activity at any location, may also indicate possible epileptic sequelae.

In contrast, slow posterior waves that may last for a long time—a common finding in children suffering head trauma—seem to have no precise prognostic value. This supports the still valuable statement of Cohn[6] that slow posterior waves are usually a nonspecific activity common to multiple encephalopathies, including subclinical responses to a variety of metabolic, toxic, and diverse agents affecting the child's brain.

We might add that certain clinical conditions of head trauma also appear to predict PTE. A closed fracture entails a risk of PTE of no more than 10%, whereas a compound injury entails a 20% risk of late epilepsy. If the dura is intact, the risk can be from 8% to 10%; if it is torn, the risk increases to up to 25%.

As to the prophylactic administration of anticonvulsants to prevent PTE in infants, there seems to be no doubt regarding their efficacy.[9,39,44,45] There are, however, differences of opinion regarding the manner in which drugs should be administered.[26,46,47] In our view, they should be given as early as possible—within the first few hours of the trauma so as to provide an immediate and sustained effect. Initially, the anticonvulsant can be administered intravenously according to body weight, followed by intramuscular maintenance doses until oral medication can be tolerated. Patients treated after the first 5 days of the trauma have a risk of PTE as high as 40%; those immediately treated have a much lower rate (6%).

In addition, despite the experience of some major head-injury centers in administering preventive anticonvulsants in relatively low doses,[39] several authors,[44,45] including the present authors,[4] agree on the maintenance of dosage adjustments based on serial plasma concentrations of the used drug to ensure a therapeutic level. The greatly reduced incidence of PTE in patients with high dosages suggest that effective action is provided only by an adequate dosage. (Compliance is another important factor; it must be enforced by the clinician.)

If these requirements are accurately followed (and here we are taking into account the fact that other current methodologies receive only scant attention in the literature), the incidence of seizures of late onset can range from 6% to 10% as opposed to 30% to 50% in patients not properly treated.

References

1. Ahvenainen EK; Intracranial hemorrhage and associated diseases in premature infants. *Ann Pediatr* 1972;80:37–42.
2. Brown JK, Cockburn F, Forfar JO: Clinical and chemical correlates in convulsions of the newborn. *Lancet* 1972;1:135.
3. Burke JB: The prognostic significance of neonatal convulsions. *Arch Dis Child* 1954;29:342–345.
4. Chiofalo N, Armengol V, Vidal P, Olivares O, Basauri L: Prophylactic antiepileptic treatment in severe head injury. Epilepsy International XIII Symposium, Vancouver, Canada, 1979.
5. Chiofalo N, Fuentes A, Basauri L, Madsen J, Ditzel L: Evolución electroclinica a distancia de la contusión cerebral traumática en el niño: Riesgo de la secuela epiléptica. *Rev Ped* 1980;51:253–256.
6. Cohn R: On the significance of biocciptal slow wave activity in the electroencephalograms of children. *Electroencephalogr Clin Neurophys* 1958;10:760.
7. Cole VA, Surbin GM, Olaffson A, Reynolds EDR, Rivers RPA, Smith JF: Pathogenesis of intraventricular hemorrhage in newborn infants. *Arch Dis Child* 1974;49:722–723.
8. Craig WA: Convulsive movements occurring in the first ten days of life. *Arch Dis Child* 1960;35:336.
9. D'Alessandro R, Ferrara R, Cortelli R, Temper P, Pazzaglia P, Sugaresi E: Post-traumatic epilepsy prediction and prophylaxis: Open problems (letter). *Arch Neurol* 1983;40:831.
10. D'Alessandro R, Tinuper P, Ferrara R, Cortelli P, Pazzaglie P, Sabattini L, Frank G, Lugaresi E: CT scan prediction of late post-traumatic epilepsy. *J Neurol Neurosurg Psych* 1982;45:1153–1155.
11. DiChiro G: CT features of premature and full term brain: The problematic borderline between normality and pathology related to perinatal hypoxic injury. *J Comput Assist Tomogr* 1983;4:434.
12. Donat JF, Okazaki H, Kleinberg F, Reagan TJ: Intraventricular hemorrhage in fullterm and premature infants. *Mayo Clin Proc* 1978;53:437–441.

13. Dreyfus-Brisac C, Samson-Dreyfus D, Fischgold H: Activité électrique cérebrale du prematuré et du nouveau-né. *Ann Pediatr* (Paris) 1955;31:1–7.
14. Dreyfus-Brisac C: The electroencephalogram of the premature infant. *World Neurol* 1962;3:5–15.
15. Dreyfus-Brisac C: The electroencephalogram of the premature and full-term newborn: Normal and abnormal development of waking and sleeping patterns, in Kellaway P, Petersen I (eds): *Clinical Electroencephalography*. New York, Grune & Stratton, 1964, p 186.
16. Dreyfus-Brisac C, Monod N: The EEG of fullterm newborns and premature infants, in Leiry G (ed): *Handbook of E.E.G. Clinical Neurophysiology*. Amsterdam, Elsevier Science Publishing Co Inc, 1975, pp 6–23.
17. Dubowitz LMS, Levine MI, Morante A, Palmer P, Dubpwitz, V: A correlation with real-time ultrasound. *J Ped* 1981;99:127–133.
18. Dykes FD, Ahmann PA, Kazzara A: Age of occurrence of severe posthemorrhagic hydrocephalus: Natural history. Program and Abstracts, Child Neurology Society. *Ann Neurol* 1982;12(2):225.
19. Ellingson RJ: The E.E.G. of premature and fullterm newborns, in Klass DW, Daly DD (eds): *Current Practice in Clinical Electroencephalography*. New York, Raven Press, Publishers, 1979, p 149.
20. Ellison PH, Franklin S, Jones G: Serial electroencephalography in the preterm infant as predictor of neurological sequelae. *Ann Neurol* 1982;12:213–214.
21. Fitzhardinge PM, Flodmark O, Fitz CR, Ashby S: The prognostic value of computed tomography of the brain in asphyxiated premature infants. *J Ped* 1982;100(3):476–481.
22. Flodmack O, Becker LE, Harwood-Nach DC et al.: Correlation between computed tomography and autopsy in premature and full-term neonates that have suffered perinatal asphyxia. *Radiology* 1980;137:93.
23. Flodmack O, Fitz CR, Harwood-Nash DC: CT diagnosis and short term prognosis of intracranial hemorrhage and hypoxic/ischemic brain damage in neonates. *J Comput Assist Tomogr* 1980;4:775.
24. Gray OP, Ackerman A, Fraser AJ: Intracranial hemorrhage and clotting defects in low-birth-weight infants. *Lancet* 1968;1:545–548.
25. Hack M, Fanaroff AA, Merkatz IR: The low-birth-weight infant evolution of a changing outlook. *N Engl J Med* 1979;301:1162–1165.
26. Johnson AL, Harris P, McQueen JK, Blackwood DH, Kalbag RM: Phenytoin prophylaxis for posttraumatic seizures (letter). *J Neurosurg* 1983;59(4):727–731.
27. Keen JH, Lee D: Sequelae of neonatal convulsions: Study of 112 children. *Arch Dis Child* 1973;48:542–546.
28. Kellaway P: Head injuries in children. *Electroencephalogr Clin Neurophys* 1955;7:492–498.
29. Keth HM: Convulsions in children under three years of age: A study of prognosis. *Mayo Clin Proc* 1964;39:895–907.
30. Knauss TA, Marshall RE: Seizures in a neonatal intensive care unit. *Dev Med Child Neurol* 1977;19:719–728.
31. Leech R, Kohnen O: Subependymal and intraventricular hemorrhages in the newborns. *Am J Pathol* 1974;77(3):465–475.
32. Lombroso CT: Convulsive disorders in newborns, in Thompson RA, Green

TR (eds): *Pediatric Neurology and Neurosurgery*. New York, Spectrum Publications, 1978, pp 202–239.

33. McInerny TK, Schubert WK: Prognosis of neonatal seizures. *Am J Dis Child* 1969;117:261–264.

34. Monod N, Dreyfus-Brisac C: Le trace paroxistique chez le nouveau-né. *Rev Neurol* (Paris) 1962;106:129–130.

35. Monod N, Pajot N, Guidesci S: The neonatal E.E.G.: Statistical studies and prognostic value in full-term and pre-term babies. *Electroencephalogr Clin Neurophys* 1972;32:529–544.

36. Papile LA, Burstein J, Burnstein R, Koffer H: Incidence and evolution of subependymal and introventricular hemorrhage: A study of infants with birth weights less than 1.500 gm. *J Ped* 1978;92(4)529–534.

37. Picard L, Claudon M, Roland J et al.: Cerebral computed tomography in premature infants with an attempt to staging developmental features. *J Comput Assist Tomogr* 1980;4:435.

38. Schub HS, Ahmann PA et al.: Prospective long-term follow-up of prematures with subependymal/intraventricular hemorrhage. *Ped Res* 1981;15:abstr. 1607, 1981.

39. Servit Z, Musil F: Prophylactic treatment of post-traumatic epilepsy: Results of a long-term follow-up in Czchoslovakia. *Epilepsia* 1981;22:315–320.

40. Shinnar S, Molteni R, Gammon K, D'Souza BJ, Altman J, Freeman, JM: Intraventricular hemorrhage in the premature infant: A changing outlook. *N Engl J Med* 1982;1464–1467.

41. Tharp BR, Cukier F, Monod N: The prognostic value of the electroencephalogram in premature infants. *Electroenceph Clin Neurophys* 1981;51:219–236.

42. Tibles JAR, Prichard JS: The prognostic value of the electroencephalogram in neonatal convulsions. *Pediatrics* 1965;5:778–787.

43. Volpe JJ: Neonatal seizures. *Clin Perinatol* 1977;4:43–63.

44. Wohns RNW, Wyler AR: Prophylactic phenitoin in severe head injuries. *J Neurosurg* 1979;51:507–509.

45. Young B, Rapp R, Brooks H, Madaus W, Norton JA: Posttraumatic epilepsy prophylaxis. *Epilepsia* 1979;20:671–681.

46. Young B, Rapp RP, Norton JA, Haak D, Walsh JW: Failure of prophylactically administered phenitoin to prevent post-traumatic seizures in children. *Child's Brain* 1983;10:185–192.

47. Young B, Rapp R, Norton JA, Haak D, Tibbs PA, Bean J: Failure of prophylactically administered phenitoin to prevent late post-traumatic seizures. *J Neurosurg* 1983;58:236–241.

CHAPTER 16

Posttraumatic Cerebral Vascular Injuries

Anthony J. Raimondi

Introduction

The range of vessels damaged from physical insult to the craniocerebrum is complete, though capillary damage (expressing itself clinically as cerebral contusion) in the newborn and venous damage in the infant (expressing itself clinically as subacute subdural hematoma) are the most commonly encountered. Because of the redundancy of the arteries within the basal cisterns and fissures, the long course of the cortical bridging veins within the subarachnoid spaces, and the location of the superior sagittal sinus beneath the metopic and sagittal sutures, these three vascular structures are particularly susceptible to the shearing forces that represent the characteristic pathogenesis of craniocerebral vascular damage in the fetus, newborn, and infant. This casts into sharp relief the significance of traumatic vascular pathology in these age categories.

In this chapter, the traumatic pathology of the vascular structures within the scalp, skull, pachymeninges, cerebral parenchyma, ventricles, and subarachnoid spaces are discussed. Because there are no vascular structures within the leptomeninges, damage to this structure is not herein considered. Moreover, because of the particular anatomical characteristics of the vault and base of the cranium, vascular injuries resulting from calvarial and basal structures are discussed separately. The significance of shearing injuries of the walls of the lateral and midline ventricular systems (which result in ependymal rupture) as the pathogenetic factor for intraventricular bleeding, as well as "central cavitation," are described mechanistically as forces responsible for the tearing of ependymal and subependymal arteries.

Little attention has been given to identification of the bleeding sources. The primary orientation of the surgeon has always been to identify the location of the collection of blood so as to remove it. Closed head injuries presenting as transient losses of consciousness are not studied neuroradiologically with angiography, and those patients remaining in coma and progressing to death or a vegetative state generally have such extensive parenchymal damage that a discrete vascular injury cannot be identified. Because serious head injuries almost invariably present as life threatening emergencies, little time is spent analyzing the details of vascular damage. This is unfortunate, as capillary, diploic, arterial, venous, and sinus bleeding differ greatly from one another and demand equally different surgical approaches.

The mechanics of vascular injury are the same as those for cerebral laceration: shearing forces, explosive forces, and cavitation. These physical insults and stresses are indirect, resulting from different densities of individual anatomical structures and different responses to acceleration and deceleration rates. The vertical course of the brain stem within the basal cisterns predisposes the midbrain and pons to shearing forces. The "floating" corpus callosum (between the large pericallosal cistern and the third ventricle) is similarly subject to shearing and cavitation forces. The open fontanels and sutures permit the cerebrum to flatten and expand beneath the skull as the menbranous bones separate from one another. This permits much greater stretching of vessels, which results in tears and stretch occlusion.

Age Categories

The nature of the injury varies almost directly with the age of the child. Perinatal injuries are incurred by the fetus in his or her passage through the birth canal; the newborn is susceptible to falls in the delivery room and nursery; the infant is subject to falls from the bassinet or high chair, and to automobile injuries; the toddler injures the craniocerebrum by falling while walking or running, being struck by an automobile, or bouncing around in the automobile as a passenger. All age categories within the first 2 years of life are subject to being battered. This does not appear to be more common in one cultural setting or another, though there are very real social influences.

Passage through the birth canal subjects the fetus to compressive craniocerebral injuries when uterine cervical dilation does not progress or there is a cephalopelvic disproportion. A precipitous delivery, in contrast, may result in the child's falling to the ground. Another very common cause for traumatic cerebral vascular injuries is forceps application; high application is associated with a higher incidence of damage and low application with a minimal incidence. The high and midforceps applications damage much more commonly the superficial temporal, middle meningeal, and vertebral arteries. The latter are almost invariably damaged at the craniovertebral junction, in their passage from the foramen transversarium, through the pachymeninges and leptomeninges, and into the subarachnoid spaces. Therefore, vertebral and basilar artery injuries are incurred, as are vertebral and posterior-inferior cerebellar artery injuries;

carotid, anterior cerebral, and middle cerebral artery injuries are the most uncommon, as are injuries to the deep venous structures. However, traumatic occlusion of the superior sagittal and transverse sinuses does occur.

Except for visible cutaneous evidence of injury (caput succedaneum, scalp or facial contusions), cerebrovascular damage suffered during the perinatal period is generally not clinically identified until much later. In fact, weeks, months, and years may pass before the true nature of neurologic dysfunction is identified. The so-called congenital giant aneurysm of the vertebro-basilar system is an example. The same applies to injuries that the newborn may suffer either in the delivery room or the nursery. Cerebral palsy, minimal brain damage, and so forth may result from this type of vascular injury.

For infants, falls from high chairs and bassinets are quite common, although rare when compared to automobile accidents. In the past several years, successful campaigns have been waged against the use of the high chair and bassinet, so that this cause for injury has decreased remarkably. Unfortunately, despite the fact that automobile accidents represent the most lethal noxae in the second and third trimesters of life, western society still has not been able to respond positively. By the time the child becomes a toddler, he or she begins to fall regularly. Fortunately, the child instinctively falls by dropping to the buttocks, so that head injuries from walking falls are rare. However, the exploratory instincts of a toddler and his or her lack of coordination combine to render the toddler particularly susceptible to falls from chairs, beds, tables, and windows. Also, because of their low stature and total unawareness of danger, toddlers suffer a high incidence of being struck by an automobile either in the streets in front of their homes, or, most tragic of all, while playing in the driveway of their homes. Their high degree of mobility and rapid psychomotor development are often responsible for their being allowed to play in the back seat of a car or station wagon while the vehicle is being driven by a parent.

The first 2 years of life are those in which the child is particularly vulnerable to senseless beatings by parents, siblings, sitters. The battered-child syndrome is well known. What is apparently not well known is that beatings inflict low-velocity acceleration injuries upon the child's head and craniovertebral junction—just the type that most commonly cause linear and eggshell skull fractures—explosive forces upon the membranous bones of the skull, and hyperextension-flexion injuries at the craniovertebral junction. These are common causes for diploic epidural hematoma, petrosphenoid fractures resulting in traumatic occlusion or rupture of the internal carotid arteries, and stretching tears of the vertebral artery in its course from the foramen transversarium of the atlas to the basilar artery. The explosive forces resulting from low-velocity acceleration head injuries split the metopic, coronal, lambdoidal, and sagittal sutures, thereby creating shearing forces that may either tear cortical bridging veins from the superior sagittal sinus or split the sinus itself for distances of 5 to 10 mm.

Anatomy

So as to present both the wide spectrum of vascular damages resulting from craniocerebral injury and an anatomoclinical correlation, two classifications will be discussed: anatomical compartments and bleeding sources.

The anatomical classification is predicated upon the existence of compartments, albeit potential rather than virtual, located between discrete anatomical structures. As an example, the highly mobile scalp overlying the mobile membranous bones provides a potential compartment into which a newborn or infant may bleed enough to present clinically with a picture of hypovolemic shock. Similarly, because of the extraordinarily loose adhesion of the outer layer of the dura to the membranous bones of the skull (with an exception, of course, along the suture line), diastatic fractures of the parietal or frontal bones often result in massive epidural-subgaleal hematomas that both elevate the scalp and compress the underlying brain. The very dense adhesion of the periosteum to the membranous bones limits subperiosteal hematomas to the area immediately surrounding linear or eggshell fractures. The amount of bleeding into the subperiosteal space is consequently of minimal clinical significance. Different from the subgaleal hematoma, it is exquisitely tender and very slow to resolve. The subgaleal hematoma results from tears of vessels located between the periosteum and the Galea; the subperiosteal hematoma results from bleeding from the outer table of the membranous bone; and the subgaleal-epidural hematoma results from diploic bleeding.

Collections of blood within the epidural space (with the exception of crushing and explosive injuries) do not cross the suture lines, as the outer layer of the dura, the suture, and the periosteum form an anatomical continuum between membranous bones. Tears in the middle meningeal artery (anterior, middle, posterior branches) do occur during the first 2 years of life. However, this form of vascular injury is not the most common, because tears in the superior sagittal and transverse sinuses represent the large majority of vascular injuries resulting in epidural hematomas. For this reason, newborn and infants generally suffer epidural hematomas located along the midsagittal plane, at the vertex, expanding over the parasagittal surfaces of both hemispheres. Also, tears in the transverse sinus result in epidural hematomas that extend from the supra- to the infratentorial compartments. Both of these—venous—epidural hematomas are treacherous in that the sinus is torn, thus (establishing an anatomical basis for air emboli). The repair of the sinus often necessitates reflecting flaps on either side of the midsagittal plane or across the anatomical line between the supra- and infratentorial compartments. This technique must also provide for repair of the sinus laceration.

Burst fractures, which are secondary to low velocity acceleration injuries, may strip the outer layer of the dura from the membranous skull, thereby causing bleeding from the inner table of the skull and resulting in well circumscribed epidural hematomas of very limited volume. This type of epidural hematoma is identical in its pathogenesis and extent to the subperiosteal hematoma.

The subdural compartment, especially over the convexity of the hemispheres, is commonly recognized to contain very large (acute or chronic) collections of blood. Though the bridging cortical veins are the most susceptible to damage from shearing forces (which generally tear them from the superior sagittal sinus), cerebral laceration and torn dural sinuses are not infrequently the pathogenic factors. Only rarely do cortical arteries tear, other than in association with compound craniocerebral injuries in which scalp, skull, meninges, and brain are lacerated.

Because of the absence of Pacchionian granules in the newborn and infant, the convexity, lateral, and basal bridging veins have lengthy courses within the subdural space. Because of the functional anatomy of the convexity bridging veins—one that brings the vein in an anterior direction as it exits from the subarachnoid space and then hooks it in a posterior direction (hairpin style) upon itself prior to turning anteriorly once more immediately upon entering the superior sagittal sinus—acceleration injuries most commonly result in tears of the bridging cortical vein from its insertion into the superior sagittal sinus. These are the most common injuries in the newborn and infant. Deceleration injuries, most common in late infancy and the toddler stage, result in tears of the bridging cortical vein from the cerebral convexity. Therefore, acute subdural hematomas, when removed, may present bleeding sources at either the dural sinus or the cerebral convexity. The fact that a child has been injured in an automobile accident (either struck by or within the vehicle) should suggest a deceleration injury, whereas battered children suffer acceleration injuries. The same general mechanistic and pathogenic principles apply to bridging veins entering the cavernous sinus (sphenoparietal system) and the transverse sinus at the sigmoid sinus (vein of Labbé).

Subarachnoid bleeding is an expression of either a regional cerebral contusion or, very rarely, torn arteries. The regional cerebral contusion results either from deceleration injuries or contrecoup acceleration injuries that damage cortical vessels. Shearing and stretching forces may rend or tear the vertebral, posterior inferior cerebellar, or middle cerebral arteries, permitting an outpouring of arterial blood into the basal cisterns. When the opening in these major vessels of the base of the brain is small, the subarachnoid hemorrhage may not be significant enough to announce itself clinically. Instead, there is a leakage of blood and a false aneurysm forms around the rent in the artery. Over time, these false aneurysms increase dramatically in size, developing into giant aneurysms or aneurysmal tumors. The author doubts that the reported "congenital" aneurysms of the vertebral, posterior inferior cerebellar, and middle cerebral systems are anything other than posttraumatic (false) aneurysms. The fact that these aneurysms are most common in the vertebral basilar system is in support of their posttraumatic nature because of the high incidence of extension flexion movement (and injuries!) at the craniovertebral junction during passage through the birth canal.

Intraventricular hemorrhages (IVHs), other than those occurring in the premature, extremely low-birth-weight newborn (IVH in association with respiratory distress syndrome), may be venous, arterial, or chorioidal in genesis. These result from shearing forces across the lamina terminalis, foramina of Monro and/or brain stem-cerebral hemisphere junctions. These forces, either direct or indirect (i.e., cavitation), tear the cerebral parenchyma and those vessels within it at the ependymal surface. Discrete bleeding into the lateral and/or midline ventrical systems may result. The very selective anatomical limitation of bleeding into the ventricular system, whether lateral or midline, is indicative of extraventricular hemorrhage. Posttraumatic occlusive vascular disease, less dramatic and consequently much less often diagnosed, is clinically obvious only when the carotid or middle cerebral systems are involved. Occlusion of a single vertebral or anterior cerebral artery in the newborn and infant is clinically silent. Posttraumatic occlusion of the anteromedial and anterolateral perforating systems, independent of occlusion of the internal carotid, may well occur. However, it has not been reported, and the author has never documented a case. Similarly, posttraumatic occlusion of the posterolateral and posteromedial perforating system as isolated entities does not occur. Basilar fractures, sincipital in this age category, do cause occlusion of the internal carotid arteries within the cavernous sinuses and the basilar artery distal to the anterior-inferior cerebellar artery. When fractures extend across the body of the sphenoid, both internal carotid arteries may become stenosed and occluded superior to the cavernous sinuses and unilateral or bilateral caroticocavernous fistulae may occur.

The pathogenesis of traumatic vascular damage, whether hemorrhagic or occlusive, rests primarily within shearing forces. Indeed, as already discussed, direct injury may be inflicted upon individual vessels. This is rare, however. Because of the high degree of mobility of the scalp on the skull, and of individual membranous bones of the skull upon one another and over the dura, tearing of subgaleal vessels and subgaleal hematoma may result. The hypermobility of the membranous bones of the calvarium, which permits molding of the skull for passage through the birth canal, causes shearing forces to occur between skull and dura in instances of sudden impact. These forces may tear the pachymeninges from the inner table of the skull or lacerate the dural sinuses, both of which result in epidural hematomas. The same forces, if severe enough, may result in the tearing of bridging cortical veins, subarachnoid arteries, and basal dural sinuses.

The brain of the newborn and infants is not yet myelinated and is itself subject to shearing forces at the cortical, subcortical, parenchymal-ventricular, interhemispheral–corpus callosum, and cerebral hemisphere–brain stem levels. The resulting cerebral lacerations and/or cavitation can damage parenchymal and vascular structures and can cause petechial hemorrhages, contusions, intraventricular bleeding, and intracerebral hematomas. Consequently, when the craniocerebral injury is of such a nature and severity as to produce shearing forces, the presence or absence of intracranial mass lesions (such as epidural, subdural, or intracerebral hematomas) are epiphenomenae that are of no clinical significance. That is, the underlying brain damage is itself so severe that removal of the intracranial clots will not alter the clinical course.

In summary, posttraumatic intracranial vascular injury may result in discrete, localized hemorrhages or occlusion. If the hemorrhages occur in potential anatomical spaces (subgaleal, subdural, etc.) and are pathogenetic, their removal may be curative. If the vascular damage results in the formation of a false aneurysm or an aneurysmal tumor, these must be treated surgically as soon as identified because they invariably increase in size and cause brain-stem compression or hemispheral destruction. If the injury causes vascular occlusion, however, no treatment exists. Cerebral laceration is a defined traumatic condition that may exist alone or in association with other forms of intracranial vascular damage. Although its anatomical variants can be described, there is no clinical pathological correlation permitting either prognosis or treatment.

CHAPTER 17

Posttraumatic Hydrocephalus in the Neonate and Infant

Thomas G. Luerssen, Leslie N. Sutton, Derek A. Bruce, and Luis Schut

Introduction

This chapter presents a review of the diagnosis and management of post-traumatic ventricular enlargement in the very young child. Although it is well known that ventricular enlargement can occur after head trauma, the etiology of this phenomenon, its therapy, and its prognosis are quite variable. A discussion of this type of hydrocephalus should consider those processes which cause a permanent or transient disruption of normal cerebrospinal fluid (CSF) dynamics as well as those which cause secondary ventricular enlargement as a result of cortical (neuronal) loss. The management of the very young child who develops ventricular enlargement after a head injury must be individualized, giving consideration to the mechanism of the initial injury, the initial clinical findings and radiographic studies, the subsequent clinical course, and the results of follow-up radiographic studies and ancillary tests.

Incidence

The reported incidence rate of posttraumatic hydrocephalus in several series of patients of all ages varies widely from 8% to 72%[6,10], largely because of the variation in the definition of posttraumatic hydrocephalus. Hydrocephalus requiring shunting is remarkably uncommon after a head injury. In series of adult patients, this incidence rate has ranged between 1% and 4%.[9,10]

No data concerning the frequency of hydrocephalus following head trauma are available for the pediatric age group in general or for neonates and infants in particular. At our institution, just less than 5% of all head-injured children less than 2 years old have developed progressive hydrocephalus requiring the insertion of a shunt; this percentage is quite similar to that reported for the adult age group. These data exclude a significantly larger population of neonates and infants who develop ventricular enlargement as a result of neonatal intraventricular hemorrhage, which is occasionally, although infrequently, of traumatic origin.

Pathophysiology

Most of the CSF is formed within the lateral ventricles. From there it flows through the paired foramina of Monro into the III ventricle and proceeds caudally through the aqueduct of Sylvius into the IV ventricle. At this point, the CSF becomes subarachnoid by passing through the foramina of Lushka and Magendie to enter the basal cisterns. Subsequently, the flow of CSF divides to course rostrally over the cerebral hemispheres and caudally into the posterior spinal canal and lumber cistern, where it turns to ascend along the ventral aspect of the spinal canal and re-enter the basal cisterns.[13]

The majority of CSF is absorbed through the arachnoidal villi that penetrate the major dural (venous) sinuses in the cranium and, to a lesser extent, the epidural veins along the spinal nerve roots. Under normal conditions, the absorption of CSF is equal to the rate of production: about 0.35 ml per minute.[4] However, it is apparent that under certain physiologic conditions, these absorptive mechanisms are not functioning at full capacity; therefore, the system can accommodate some pathologic obstructions in the distal CSF pathways without the occurrence of any clinical symptoms or radiographic signs of hydrocephalus.[3]

Within this complex system, the occurrence of hydrocephalus (with the singular exception of the ventricular enlargement that occurs as a result of cortical atrophy or porencephaly), can be considered to be due to a defect in CSF absorption. However, the lesions that cause this defect can occur at any location in the CSF pathway. They frequently cause pathological changes at several levels, all of which act in concert to cause symptomatic hydrocephalus. For instance, an intraventricular hemorrhage that initially causes an obstruction to CSF flow through the ventricular system can also result in leptomeningeal fibrosis with or without obliteration of the intracellular channels of the arachnoidal villi, thereby causing a distal absorptive block. These entities have been termed "obstructive" and "communicating" hydrocephalus, respectively. (With the advent of computer assisted tomography, these general terms seem to be less important than in the past, but they are ingrained in current teaching and should not be totally discarded.) With improved diagnostic techniques and current therapy it is no longer as useful as it once was to categorize hydrocephalus as simply obstructive or communicating. It does seem useful, however, to establish a conceptual approximation of the level of the defect in CSF circulation, because it may have some influence on both the selection of diagnostic studies and management options. Accordingly, intraventricular or aqueductal obstruction can result in significant ventricular enlargement, with accompanying compression of the cortical mantle. The hydrocephalus resulting from a distal absorptive block is usually associated with much less ventricular enlargement in the radiographic studies.

Finally, it is important to emphasize that there is no correlation between the degree of ventricular enlargement demonstrated on radiographic studies and the attendant intracranial pressure (ICP). Children can develop very high CSF pressures with small ventricles, whereas children with extreme hydrocephalus resulting from aqueductal or intraventricular obstructions may actually demonstrate relatively low intracranial pressure.

Clinical Evaluation

The hallmark of hydrocephalus in the child under 2 years old is an excessive rate of cranial enlargement. The compensation provided by sutural diastasis and the open fontanels is such that other overt symptoms of elevated ICP are either not seen or are delayed in presentation until these compensatory mechanisms are exhausted. Therefore, it is incumbent upon the physician who is caring for a young child with a head injury to obtain frequent measurements of head circumference during the posttraumatic period. A series of measurements is more important than any single measurement, even if the initial value were indicative of macrocephaly. Progressive enlargement of the cranial vault at a rate above that predicted for normal growth is indicative of an ongoing process that requires further investigation. In addition to progressive macrocephaly, very young children can exhibit irritability, changes in appetite or behavior, or intermittent lethargy. Later, other characteristic signs of increased ICP appear, including sixth nerve palsies or Parinaud's syndrome.[12]

In contrast to term infants, children who are born prematurely may not exhibit any outward signs of hydrocephalus despite significant ventricular enlargement. In these children the traditional criteria of enlarging head circumference, separating sutures, and a bulging fontanel may not appear for several days or even weeks after the onset of hydrocephalus. The reason for this can be directly ascribed to the developmental state of the brain. Children of this age have been shown to exhibit a paucity of cerebral myelin as well as a relative excess of water in the periventricular white matter. In the face of progressive ventricular enlargement, much less force is required to compress the cortical mantle than to overcome the restrictions of the dura or skull.[23] Accordingly, an enlarging head circumference is usually considered to be a late sign of hydrocephalus in the premature population. The early clinical signs of hydrocephalus in children of this age may be the onset of apneic spells, intermittent bradycardia, or a change in ventilatory parameters, all of which represent a significant threat to life. Therefore, it has been our routine to screen intermittently with cranial ultrasound *any* infant considered at risk for the development of hydrocephalus even if the child is asymptomatic.

In the older infant with closed fontanels, the only early clinical indication of symptomatic hydrocephalus may be a plateau in, or reversal of, what otherwise seems to be a gratifying neurologic recovery. A significant change in a child's behavior, especially one for the worse, should not be discounted. It is reasonable to study these children in order to exclude the onset of hydrocephalus, which, if found, may be expeditiously treated and therefore not interfere with the continuing recovery. Again, it should be recalled that overt signs of increased ICP occur only late in the course of hydrocephalus.

Acute hydrocephalus is infrequent after significant head trauma, but if it occurs, the intracranial pressure may elevate so rapidly as to overwhelm the previously described compensatory mechanisms that function so well for slowly progressive infantile hydrocephalus. An open fontanel does not protect against a rapid rise in intracranial pressure, nor does palpation of the fontanel provide a reliable assessment of the magnitude of the intracranial pressure. Very small children who are symptomatic from elevated intracranial pressure are extremely difficult to evaluate and follow clinically; therefore, direct monitoring of ICP may be necessary in order to manage appropriately such patients.

The clinical diagnosis of progressive acquired hydrocephalus generally requires radiologic confirmation. Computer assisted tomography is the diagnostic study of choice, at least for the initial evaluation. B-mode ultrasound may be recommended as the initial screening procedure for hydrocephalus that frequently occurs after neonatal intraventricular hemorrhage. It is also preferable for very small infants who are in critical condition and for whom a move to a CT scanner is contraindicated. B-mode ultrasound can delineate the ventricular system supratentorially as well as the location and configuration of both intraventricular or intracerebral hemorrhages.[7] However, computer assisted tomography is probably better for demonstrating the anatomy of the posterior fossa and the subarachnoid spaces, as well as the bony anatomy of the cranial vault. Furthermore, tomography is more sensitive than ultrasound for detecting subtle changes in ventricular size or configuration. Once baseline information has been obtained by tomography and there is no radiographic evidence of an acutely evolving process in the brain parenchyma or extracerebral spaces, one can be comfortable using ultrasound to monitor any changes in ventricular size over the long term. The use of B-mode ultrasound of the brain is limited somewhat by the age of the child (i.e., because of the progressively diminishing fontanel window in the growing infant).

Occasionally, computer assisted tomographic studies will aid in management. The appearance of enlarged IV ventricle and subarachnoid cisterns is good indirect evidence that the absorptive defect is at the most distal end of the CSF pathway. Thus, lumbar punctures would be safe for diagnosis and therapy, as would consideration of placing a shunt into the lumbar cistern.

Although computer assisted tomography remains the most sensitive technique available to study the anatomical changes that occur following significant head trauma, preliminary work with magnetic resonance imaging of the brain suggests that this technique may be more sensitive for the study of progressive hydrocephalus with its attendant transependymal shifts of CSF. As magnetic resonance units are refined and become more readily available, this imaging modality may augment or supplant CT scanning as the best way to study CSF dynamics in pediatric patients.

In the older infant whose sutures have fused, it will occasionally be necessary to pursue other diagnostic studies. The most important diagnostic information one can add to a radiographic study demonstrating ventriculomegaly of any magnitude is a determination of CSF pressure. In the acute phase, this information may already have been provided by an intracranial pressure monitor. Elevations in intracranial pressure that occur 10 days to 2 weeks after what appears to be successful therapy for the acute injury are not infrequently due to hydrocephalus. The ventricular enlargement may be very subtle and may occur with the appearance of extracerebral CSF on a tomograph. In the absence of direct ICP monitoring, the CSF pressure may be measured by lumbar puncture, a procedure that can be recommended only after one has excluded the presence of a mass lesion or aqueductal block. However, isolated single measurements of CSF pressure may not provide an accurate reflection of the chronic situation, especially when one is dealing with slowly progressive hydrocephalus. Thus, even if the CSF pressure seems low at the time of lumbar puncture, the removal of some CSF may result in clinical improvement. This would be indirect evidence that permanent CSF diversion may be beneficial. Only rarely does it seem necessary to pursue extensive studies of CSF dynamics, absorbtion by ventricular or cisternal infusions, or the installation of radioisotope.

Finally, one may occasionally see children who appear to be exhibiting early ventricular enlargement a few days after a severe diffuse brain injury. However, when serial CT scans are studied carefully, it becomes apparent that the ventricular system was initially effaced by the brain swelling and the ventricular enlargement occurring on the scan is a result of the ventricular system's return to normal size as the brain swelling subsides. In most situations, this radiographic change is preceded by clinical improvement. This "early ventricular enlargement" does not necessarily herald the onset of progressive symptomatic hydrocephalus.

Etiology

For the purposes of this discussion, posttraumatic hydrocephalus can be conveniently divided into that which occurs acutely following the injury and that which develops sometime later, either weeks or months after the traumatic event. The concept of delayed ventriculomegaly encompasses not only progressive hydrocephalus but also posttraumatic cerebral atrophy and the traumatic porencephalies. These forms of hydrocephalus may occasionally share similar etiologies, and certainly acute hydrocephalus can evolve into chronic hydrocephalus; but each has individual clinical considerations and a somewhat different management approach.

When hydrocephalus occurs within hours after head trauma, it is usually due to obstruction of the ventricular outflow pathways by intraventricular or extraventricular hematomas or secondary mass effects. In the older infant, the occurrence of severe enough intracranial hemorrhage to cause obstructive phenomena is rare.[26] There are isolated case reports of acute hydrocephalus occurring in young children after head injury, which has been ascribed to direct obstruction of the basal cisterns by subarachnoid blood.[18] A child with acute hydrocephalus may look well early after the injury, only to undergo rapid neurologic deterioration several hours later as a result of acutely elevated intracranial pressure. Even if initial CT scans are unremarkable, if the patient is deteriorating neurologically the studies should be repeated in order to rule out acute hydrocephalus or the development of a delayed traumatic intracerebral hematoma.

In the neonatal age group, significant intracranial hemorrhage is not uncommon. Volpe has divided this phenomenon into four groups by locus of occurrence: subdural, subarachnoid, intracerebellar, and periventricular-intraventricular.[22] All of these lesions have been associated with the subsequent development of hydrocephalus, and all have been noted to occur after birth trauma.

Subdural hemorrhage in the neonatal age group is almost always due to birth trauma. Fortunately, it is the least commonly occurring type of intracranial hemorrhage, a fact attributable mostly to improved obstetrical techniques. Subdural hemorrhage occurs as a consequence of head molding and is therefore associated with cephalopelvic disproportion, prolonged labor, unusual presentations at delivery, and the use of forceps. This lesion is usually a result of a disruption of the tentorium or falx cerebri. It is occasionally seen in association with occipital osteodiastasis resulting from cranial molding or forceps compression. Depending on its magnitude and location, subdural hemorrhage can result in ventricular enlargement. If the subdural hemorrhage occurs over the cerebral convexities, the ventricular enlargement, if it occurs, is almost always delayed in presentation. However, when the hemorrhage occurs in the region of the tentorium or posterior fossa, there is a high incidence of acute hydrocephalus because of aqueductal, IV ventricular, or incisural obstruction (Fig. 17.1). The neurologic symptoms occurring with this lesion are usually due to direct compression of the hematoma upon the neural structures of the posterior fossa and not to the ventricular dilation. There-

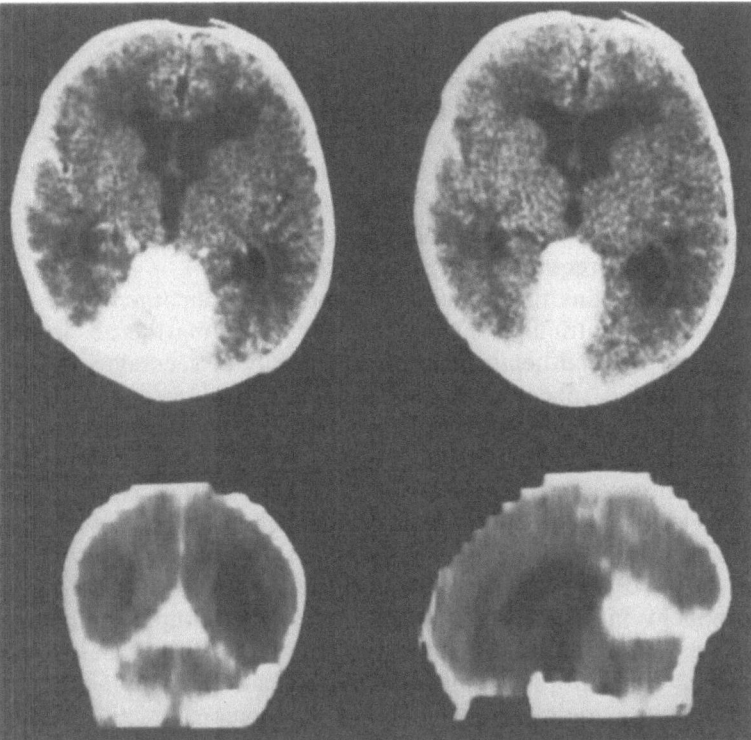

Figure 17.1. Several hours after a birth complicated by a precipitous delivery, this male infant was noted to have a bulging fontanel and suture diastasis. The CT scan demonstrated acute obstructive hydrocephalus secondary to a hemorrhage within the dural leaves of the tentorium and falx. The child was treated conservatively. During the first week the fontanel became softer, the ventricular system diminished in size, and CSF circulation was restored. The head circumference grew at the expected rate over the next several months. The child is developing normally.

fore, therapy should be directed to ventricular decompression and to rapid removal of the posterior fossa mass.

Primary subarachnoid hemorrhage occurring as an isolated entity is probably very frequent after birth but rarely causes complications. In the term infant, it is usually due to birth trauma with the same predisposing factors described with subdural hemorrhage. In the premature infant, hypoxia has been implicated as the primary etiology.[22] Hydrocephalus, if it occurs, is usually delayed in presentation.

Intracerebellar hemorrhage in the neonate may be traumatic or spontaneous; the latter is usually associated with the sequelae of hypoxia. These lesions can result in acute obstructive hydrocephalus but, as with posterior fossa subdural hematomas, the major clinical consideration is brain-stem compression, and therapy should be directed primarily at the lesion in the posterior fossa.

Neonatal intraventricular hemorrhage is the most common form of intracranial hemorrhage occurring in the neonatal age group. It is seen in up to 45% of premature newborn weighing less than 1500 grams. The pathogenesis of this particular lesion is extremely complex and has been reviewed by Volpe and others.[1,20,21] Large intraventricular or periventricular hemorrhages are quite frequently associated with acute ventricular dilation that may require rather urgent treatment.

Any of the lesions that cause acute ventricular enlargement can also cause delayed ventricular enlargement by preventing the absorption of CSF. An intracranial hemorrhage that primarily or secondarily involves the subarachnoid space can subsequently result in chronic progressive hydrocephalus. Subarachnoid blood has been shown to cause obliterative basal arachnoiditis and occlusion of the intercellular spaces of the arachnoid villi. In general, the greater the magnitude of the hemorrhage, the more likely the development of symptomatic, chronic, progressive hydrocephalus.

Lorber and Bhat have reviewed the occurrence of post-hemorrhagic hydrocephalus in infants.[11] The major cause of intracranial hemorrhage in their series was birth injury, accounting for 60% of their cases of hydrocephalus. A small proportion of patients were battered, and in the remainder no definite etiology was found. The vast majority of these children became symptomatic within the first 6 months of life. Every patient exhibited abnormal cranial enlargement. Other important symptoms were seizures and what these authors categorized as "acute severe illness." Over half of the children who exhibited symptoms other than cranial enlargement died. The overall outcome of their patients was influenced by the extent of the initial injury and their mode of therapy; however, one half of the surviving children exhibited normal development and intelligence.

In the older child, chronic hydrocephalus is probably also due to intracranial hemorrhage, even if the blood is not seen on initial radiographic studies. These children usually demonstrate the delayed onset of drowsiness, behavior change, hypertonic extremities, or visual disturbances. In general, the CT scans show ventricular enlargement, although sometimes to only a minimal degree, suggesting a distal CSF absorptive block (Fig. 17.2).

The most common cause of delayed ventricular enlargement after head injury is cortical atrophy. In a large series of adult patients, up to 78% developed some degree of ventriculomegaly on follow-up CT scans obtained as early as 2 weeks after the injury.[10] Cortical atrophy can be focal or diffuse, and the resulting cortical loss is associated with corresponding dilation of the ventricular system. Therefore, patients with intracerebral hematomas or localized cerebral infarctions can be expected to develop a focal ventricular enlargement into or around the area of the insult.

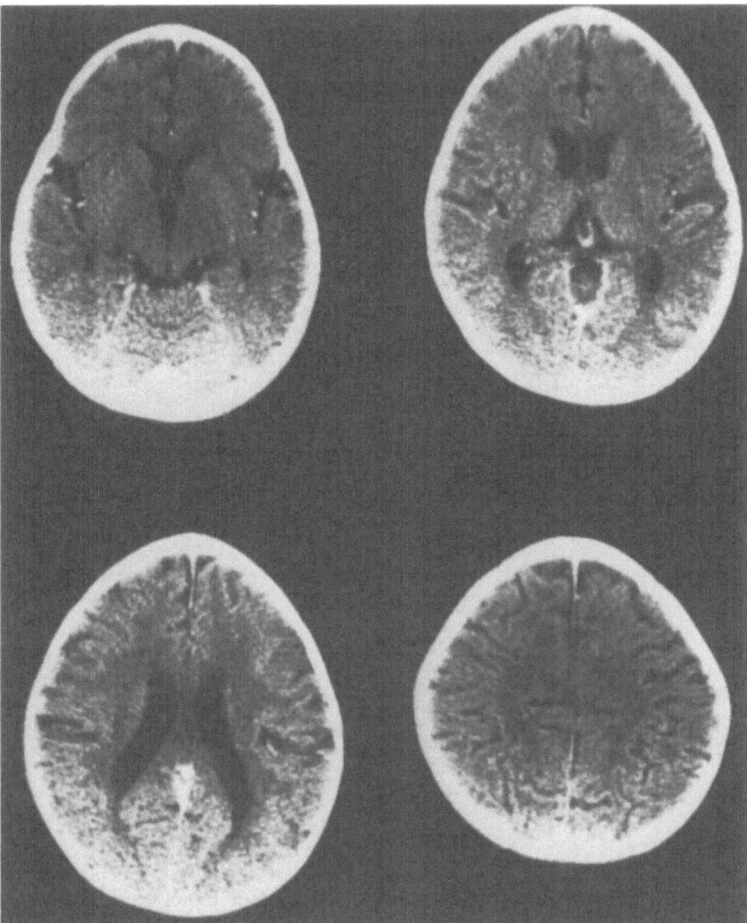

Figure 17.2. This 20-month-old female was seen 2 months after a closed head injury from which she initially appeared to have recovered full neurologic function. While she was undergoing physical rehabilitation for long bone fractures, her parents noted a marked change in her behavior. On examination she was found to have chronic papilledema. The CT scan demonstrated mild ventricular enlargement and distention of the subarachnoid cisterns. A lumbar puncture was performed; it indicated CSF pressure of 320 mm of water. A lumboperitoneal shunt was inserted, resulting in complete resolution of her symptoms.

One of the most common causes of infantile posttraumatic cortical atrophy at our hospital is the diffuse axonal injury seen as a result of shaking. These infants characteristically present with an altered level of consciousness, seizures, retinal hemorrhages, and a bulging fontanel. CT scan shows punctate hemorrhages in the white matter and evidence of subarachnoid or intraventricular bleeding.[25] After recovery from the acute

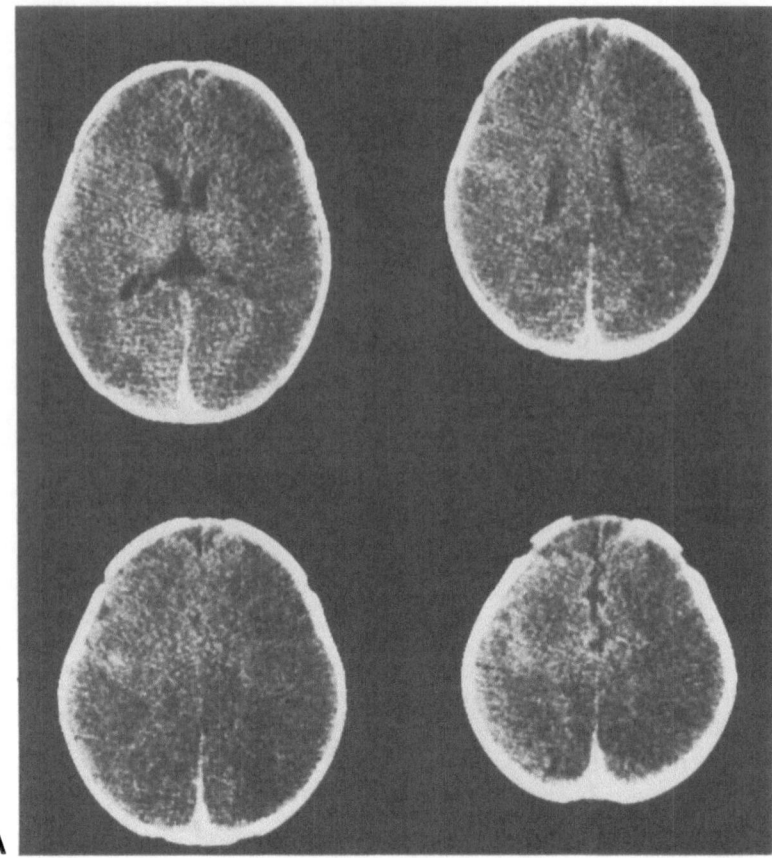

A

Figure 17.3. A 3-month-old female was admitted after experiencing a series of generalized seizures. A history of a shaking injury was obtained. On examination the fontanel was bulging and the infant exhibited bilateral retinal hemorrhages. The initial CT scan (**A**—above) shows subarachnoid hemorrhage, multiple punctate hemorrhages throughout the cerebral white matter, and generalized brain swelling. The intracranial pressure was monitored during the first 48 hours after the injury and was readily controlled with medical and ventilatory therapy. The next CT scan (**B**—p. 251) was performed 12 days later. It demonstrated significant ventricular enlargement. The fontanel was sunken. Several weeks later, the head circumference had not changed, and the last CT scan (**C**—p. 252) showed further progression of the ventricular enlargement, which is clearly due to profound cortical atrophy. She remains developmentally delayed.

injury, the fontanel softens and head growth ceases. This corresponds to the finding of progressive enlargement of the ventricles, sulci, and subarachnoid cisterns (Fig. 17.3).

Occasionally, cortical atrophy may be mistaken for progressive hydrocephalus. It is important to remember that global anoxic or metabolic insults have been associated with lesions known to cause progressive

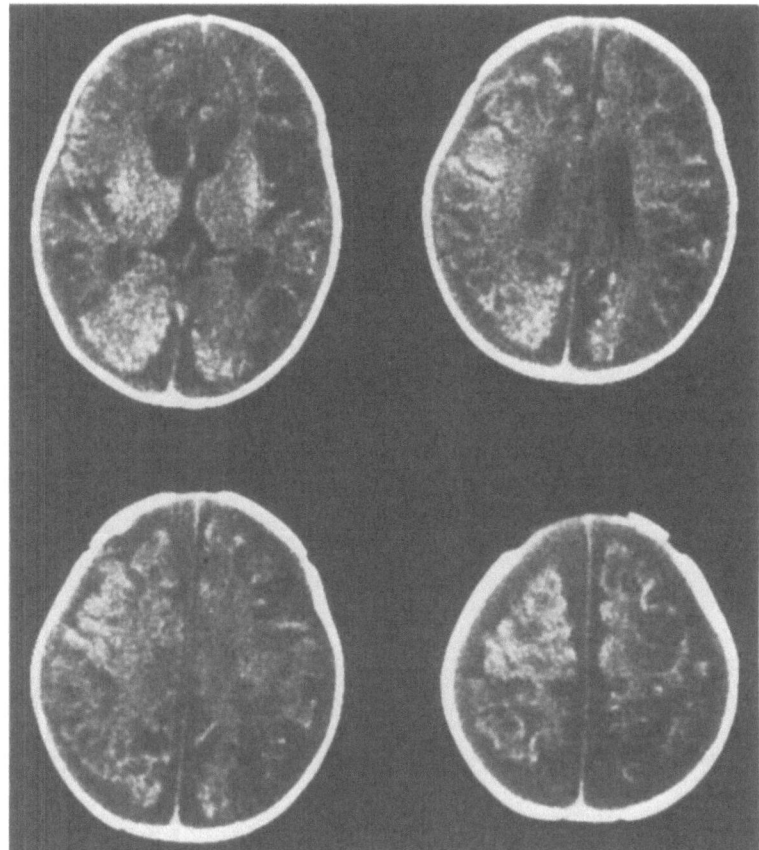

B

Figure 17.3B

hydrocephalus—specifically, neonatal subarachnoid or intraventricular hemorrhage. Delayed ventricular enlargement which occurs in these patients is quite frequently due to atrophy resulting from a global insult, not to obstruction of CSF pathways by the hemorrhage.[5] The clinical picture permits one to distinguish between them: there are no signs of progressive head enlargement or elevated CSF pressure. Children suffering cortical atrophy should not be expected to respond to CSF diversion.

Management

The management of posttraumatic hydrocephalus is dictated largely by the urgency of the clinical situation. Any small child who is deteriorating neurologically from what appears to be acute hydrocephalus should undergo ventricular decompression as soon as possible. Fortunately, when

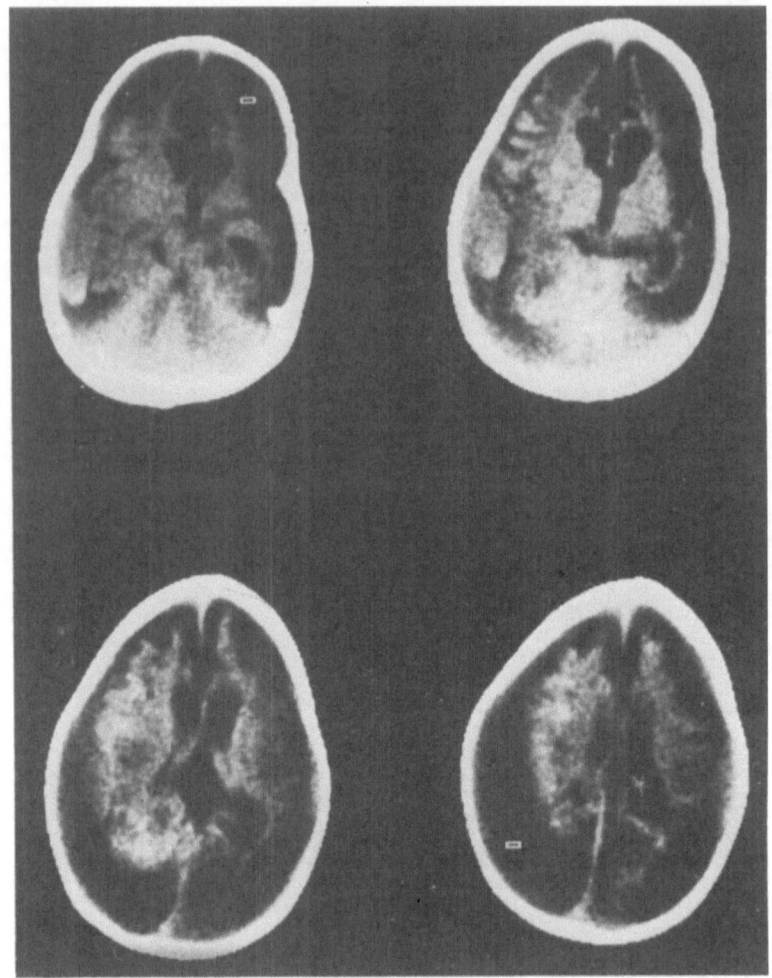

C

Figure 17.3C

dealing with newborn and infants the ventriculaı system is easy to puncture by way of the anterior fontanel. Following a sterile preparation, a
medium gauge spinal needle is introduced through the skin of the lateral
portion of the anterior fontanel and aimed toward the inner canthus of the
ipsilateral eye. The needle is carefully advanced, and penetration of the
dura is usually felt, at which point the stylet may be withdrawn and the
subdural space may be sampled for either CSF or blood. The stylet is then
replaced, and the needle is advanced carefully into the frontal horn of the
lateral ventricle. At this point, the stylet is again withdrawn and increments of CSF may be removed.

Ventricular puncture with a needle should be performed only as an
emergency procedure and should not be routinely repeated as a means of

therapy. It has been shown that repeated penetration of the brain with a needle can result in porencephalic changes at the puncture site.[16] If indicated, adequate temporary ventricular drainage can be accomplished simply by inserting a teflon venous catheter through the lateral fontanel, in the same manner as a ventricular puncture, and securing this catheter by way of a suture and a brace to prevent movement. The advantage of this technique is that it may be performed readily, at the bedside, and with minimal possibility of morbidity. However, there is a relatively high rate of occlusion of the catheter with blood or debris, which necessitates its removal or replacement. Furthermore, there is a significant risk of infection if the catheter is left in place for more than a few days.

For longer periods, the proximal portion of a shunt or ventricular reservoir system may be implanted subcutaneously and then periodically drained by percutaneous needling of the reservoir. These systems are probably less prone to infection but involve more of an operative procedure to place.

Several devices have been invented strictly for the purpose of external ventricular drainage. Most of these consist of a silastic ventricular catheter introduced into the ventricle through either a twist drill or a burr hole. The distal portion of the system is then passed through a subcutaneous tunnel and brought out through a separate incision. Most systems include a series of stopcocks or injection ports interposed between the ventricular end and the collecting apparatus, thereby providing ready access for sampling CSF, monitoring ICP, and, if necessary, injecting medications retrograde into the ventricles. These systems may be left in place for relatively long periods of time with minimal possibility of morbidity, other than as already described above in the discussion of insertion of teflon venous catheters. Although the insertion of these types of systems involves somewhat more of an operative procedure, they can nonetheless be placed at the bedside under local anesthesia, and the extremely low complication rate probably warrants the extra time and effort involved.

In the intermediate phase, or if the hydrocephalus seems to be slowly progressive, several therapeutic options are available. Serial lumbar punctures may be performed for the purpose of draining spinal fluid but only if the CSF pathways communicate freely with the lumbar cistern. Serial lumbar punctures are relatively safe, although they become progressively more difficult as multiple punctures are performed. In the older child with mild ventriculomegaly and the occurrence of extracerebral CSF collections, a series of lumbar punctures may be all that is necessary to carry the patient through a transient period of decreased CSF absorption.

Several drugs have been shown to be effective in decreasing CSF production and may aid in the management of slowly progressive hydrocephalus. Acetazolamide has been shown to cause up to a 50% reduction in the rate of CSF production.[15] Furosemide has also been shown to decrease CSF production (by an unknown mechanism), although to a lesser extent than acetazolamide.[2,14] There is some evidence that corticosteroids may reduce the rate of CSF formation,[24] although other investigators have found that CSF production is not affected by corticosteroid administration.[19] Naturally, there are complications associated with the long-term use of all of these drugs; therefore, medical management of progressive hydrocephalus with drugs should be undertaken only as a temporary measure.

The treatment of choice for chronic progressive hydrocephalus is permanent CSF diversion. This involves the placement of a shunt system from the lateral ventricles or lumbar subarachnoid space either into the peritoneal cavity or the jugular vein. The choice of the shunt system is generally dictated by the individual surgeon's experience and clinical considerations, including the amount of CSF produced and the availability of access for the distal catheter. In general, peritoneal shunts have been shown to cause less morbidity and to require less revisions than jugular shunts.[8] Furthermore, infection of atrial shunts is associated with septicemia, endocarditis, and nephritis. The techniques for placing and revising ventriculoperitoneal or ventriculojugular shunts have been described previously.[17]

A shunt from the lumbar subarachnoid cistern to the peritoneum occasionally may be recommended, especially if the ventricular system is not markedly dilated. These systems can be used only in patients whose CSF fluid pathways communicate freely with the lumbar cistern. Lumboperitoneal shunts have the same general advantages and complications as ventriculoperitoneal shunts. However, these systems offer the additional advantage of avoiding the penetration of the cerebral cortex. Experience with lumboperitoneal shunting is limited, and the use of this system should be restricted to specialized situations.

Once a shunt system has been placed, it is incumbent upon the physicians caring for the child to reassess continuously the shunt function and the neurologic development of the child. Shunt-dependent children rarely outgrow the need for a shunt. Shunt malfunctions may be expressed as overt symptoms of elevated ICP or by very subtle changes in behavior patterns, vision, or school work. The child recovering from a head injury should probably undergo relatively detailed neuropsychological testing at predetermined intervals in order to document recovery or to detect subtle changes that may require further investigations.

Outcome

In general, the occurrence of hydrocephalus after head injury should be considered to be a single part of a multifaceted disease process. However, appropriate management of symptomatic hydrocephalus should allow complete expression of neurologic potential during the recovery phase.

Initially, the goal of management is to maintain adequate cerebral perfusion by adequate control of ICP throughout the acute phase of the injury. Over the long term, the neurologic outcome is directly related to the mechanism and severity of the cerebral injury and does not correlate statistically with the presence or absence of progressive hydrocephalus. In the case of cortical atrophy, this also appears to be the case. Minimal ventricular dilation has not been statistically associated with poor outcome in large series of patients of all ages.[10] Extensive ventricular enlargement as a result of profound cortical atrophy has been associated with poor neurologic outcome, but this finding appears to be strictly a function of the initial underlying cerebral insult.

References

1. Ahmann PA, Lazarra A, Dykes FD, Brann AW, Schwartz JF: Intraventricular hemorrhage in the high risk infant: Incidence and outcome. *Ann Neurol* 1980;7:118–124.
2. Buhrley LE, Reed DJ: The effect of furosemide in sodium-22 uptake into cerebrospinal fluid and brain. *Exp Brain Res* 1972;14:503–510.
3. Cutler RPW, Page L, Galicich J, Watters GV: Formation and absorption of cerebrospinal fluid in man. *Brain* 1968;91:707–720.
4. Cutler RPW, Spertell RB: Cerebrospinal fluid—a selective review. *Ann Neurol* 1982;11:1–10.
5. Flodmark O, Scotti G, Harwood-Nash DC: Clinical significance of ventriculomegaly in children with or without intracranial hemorrhage: An 18 month follow-up study. *J Comput Assist Tomogr* 1981;5:663–673.
6. French BN, Dublin AB: The value of computerized tomography in the management of 1000 consecutive head injuries. *Surg Neurol* 1977;7:171–183.
7. Horbar JD, Walters CL, Philip AGS, Lucey JF: Ultrasound detection of changing ventricular size in post hemorrhagic hydrocephalus. *Pediatrics* 1980;66:674–678.
8. Keucher TR, Mealey J: Long-term results after ventriculoatrial and ventriculoperitoneal shunting for infantile hydrocephalus. *J Neurosurg* 1979;50:179–186.
9. Kishore PRS, Lipper MH, Miller JD: Girevendulis DP, Becker DP, Vines FS: Post-traumatic hydrocephalus in patients with severe head injury. *Neuroradiology* 1978;16:261–265.
10. Levin HS, Meyers CA, Grossman RG, Sarwar M: Ventricular enlargement after closed head injury. *Arch Neurol* 1981;38:623–629.
11. Lorber J, Bhat US: Posthaemorrhagic hydrocephalus. *Arch Dis Child* 1974;49:751–762.
12. Milhorat TH: *Hydrocephalus and the Cerebrospinal Fluid.* Baltimore, Williams & Wilkins Co, 1972.
13. Milhorat TH: The third circulation revisited. *J Neurosurg* 1975;42:628–645.
14. Reed DJ: The effects of furosemide on cerebrospinal fluid flow. *Arch Int Pharmacodyn* 1969;178:324–330.
15. Rubin RC, Henderson ES, Ommaya AK, Walker MD, Rall DP: The produc-

tion of cerebrospinal fluid in man and its modification by acetazolamide. *J Neurosurg* 1966;25:430–436.

16. Salmon JH: Puncture porencephaly: Pathogenesis and prevention. *Am J Dis Child* 1967;114:72–79.
17. Schut L, Sutton LN: Technics of shunting in the pediatric age group, in Ransohoff J (ed): Modern Technics in Surgery—Neurosurgery, Mt. Kisko, New York, Futura Publishing Co, Inc, 1983, ch 28, pp 1–11.
18. Takagi H, Tamaki Y, Morii S, Ohwada T: Rapid enlargement of ventricles within seven hours after head injury. *Surg Neurol* 1981;16:103–105.
19. Vela AR, Carey BE, Thompson BM: Further data on the acute effect of intravenous steroids on canine CSF secretion and absorption. *J Neurosurg* 1979;50:477–482.
20. Volpe JJ: Neonatal intracranial hemorrhage—pathophysiology, neuropathology, and clinical features. *Clin Perinatology* 1977;4:77–102.
21. Volpe JJ: Neonatal intraventricular hemorrhage. *N Engl J Med* 1981;304:886–891.
22. Volpe JJ: *Neurology of the Newborn*. Philadelphia, Saunders and Co, 1981.
23. Volpe JJ, Pasternak JF, Allen WC: Ventricular dilatation preceeding rapid head growth following neonatal intracranial hemorrhage. *Am J Dis Child* 1977;131:1212–1215.
24. Weiss MH, Nulsen FE: The effect of glucocorticoids on CSF flow in dogs. *J Neurosurg* 1970;32:452–458.
25. Zimmerman RA, Bilaniuk LT, Gennarelli TA: Computed tomography of shearing injuries of the cerebral white matter. *Radiology* 1978;127:393–396.
26. Zimmerman RA, Bilaniuk LT: Radiology of craniocerebral trauma, in Shapiro K (ed): *Pediatric Head Trauma*. Mt. Kisko, New York, Futura Publishing Co Inc, 1983.

CHAPTER 18

Outcomes of Craniocerebral Trauma in Infants

Harold J. Hoffman and Chopeow Taecholarn

Introduction

The brain of the infant differs greatly from that of the older child or adult because of its lack of myelination. Myelin confers both strength and elasticity on the brain; thus, when the infant's brain is subjected to stress, the white matter readily tears. Such tears can underlie the intact dura and skull and may lead to the production of cavities that frequently contain blood and eventually become smooth-walled glial scars. Only when myelination has sufficiently progressed—that is, when the infant is beyond 6 months old—do areas of contusion in the brain appear that are similar to those seen in the older child or adult.

We reviewed severe head injuries in neonates and infants less than 1 year old who were in our hospital during the period January 1976 to December 1980 (inclusively). For purposes of our study, severe head injury is defined as a head injury requiring operative intervention, having an intracranial hematoma, or having physical or mental sequelae (including, for example, seizures, hydrocephalus, and leptomeningeal cysts), or any combination of these factors. Altogether, 120 patients were available for review. Twenty-six of these sustained their head injuries as a result of birth trauma; 15, as a result of child abuse; and 13, as a result of a motor vehicle accident. Two infants were hit by flying objects, 42 were injured as a result of a fall, and 12 fell down a flight of stairs, usually in a baby walker. Ten patients were admitted with no history of trauma and only suggestive evidence of child abuse. Sixty-two of our patients were males, and 58 were females. (See Table 18.1 for the etiology of head injuries in our series.) All patients had a follow-up of at least 3 years in order to allow for an adequate assessment of outcome.

Birth Trauma

Depressed skull fractures, which were found in 11 infants, were the most common type of head injury seen in patients injured at birth. The area of depression was always of the "ping-pong ball" type and was never asso-

Table 18.1. Etiology of severe head injury in series of 120 infants.*

Etiology	No. of patients
Birth trauma	26
Child abuse	15
Possible child abuse	10
Motor vehicle accident	13
Fall	42
Fall down stairs (baby walker)	12
Hit by flying object	2
Total	120

* HSC: Jan 1976–Dec 1980.

ciated with any significant intracranial pathology. The fractures were easily elevated and the children were left without any deficit. Fifteen patients, however, sustained some form of intracranial hematoma; 1 patient had an extradural hematoma, 7 had subdural hematomas, 6 had intracerebral hematomas (4 of these associated with a subdural hematoma), and 1 had a cerebellar hematoma. Also, one patient had an isolated intracerebellar hematoma. (See Table 18.2 for a summary of injuries associated with birth trauma in our series.)

Depressed Skull Fractures

The most common cause of a depressed skull fracture in this series of infants was a fall—from the arms of a parent or babysitter, from a couch or changing table, or down a flight of stairs in a baby walker. One patient sustained a significant head injury in a motor vehicle accident; 1 was hit by a flying baseball, and 11 sustained depressed fractures as a result of birth trauma.

Table 18.2. Injuries associated with birth trauma.

Injury	No. of patients
Depressed skull fracture	11
Extradural hematoma	1
Subdural hematoma	7
Intracerebral hematoma	1
Intracerebral and subdural hematoma	4
Intracerebral and intracerebellar hematoma	1
Intracerebellar hematoma	1
Total	26

Table 18.3. Etiology of depressed skull fractures.

Etiology	No. of patients
Birth trauma	11
Fall	26
Motor vehicle accident	1
Flying baseball	1
Total	39

As a group, these patients did well. Thirty-seven of the 39 patients are normal. Two children had trouble with seizures; 1 of these became seizure-free and is now normal, whereas the other went on to develop temporal lobe epilepsy and has a persistent neurologic deficit. This particular child had an epidural hematoma in association with the depressed fracture. He sustained his depressed fracture as the result of a motor vehicle accident and is left with a residual hemiparesis and delayed speech development. (See Table 18.3 for the etiology of depressed skull fractures in our series.)

Intracranial Hematomas

Sixty-four patients had some form of intracranial hematoma (see Table 18.4). Thirty-seven of these had a supratentorial subdural hematoma. Two of these latter patients died, 15 of the survivors are normal, and 20 are left with a significant deficit. Three have hydrocephalus; 2 of these have normal intelligence, and one is retarded. Eight patients, 4 of whom are otherwise normal, are troubled with persistent seizures. Three patients are severely impaired by delayed physical and mental development; 2 have a mild motor weakness associated with a speech deficit; 1 patient

Table 18.4. Intracranial hematomas.

Type	No. of patients
Supratentorial subdural hematoma	37
Posterior fossa subdural hematoma	3
Combined compartment subdural hematoma	2
Intracerebral hematoma	7
Intracerebral and intracerebellar hematoma	1
Intracerebral and subdural hematoma	7
Intracerebellar hematoma	1
Extradural hematoma	6
Total	64

displays only retardation; 1 patient has optic atrophy and poor vision; and 3 patients have significant neuropsychological disturbances, including hyperactivity and aggressive behavior.

Five patients had a post-traumatic posterior fossa subdural hematoma; and in 2 of these, the hematoma extended into the supratentorial compartment. All have recovered fully and are neurologically and intellectually normal.

Seven patients had an isolated intracerebral hematoma. Three of these patients are now perfectly normal; 2 are retarded both physically and mentally; 1 has epilepsy; and 1 has shunted hydrocephalus and an homonymous hemianopia.

Seven patients with an intracerebral hematoma had an associated subdural hematoma. Four of these patients are perfectly normal, 2 are physically and mentally retarded, and 1 has shunted hydrocephalus but is otherwise well.

One patient with an intracerebellar hematoma in association with his intracerebral hematoma has been left with a seizure disorder but is otherwise well. One patient with a discrete intracerebellar hematoma is significantly handicapped with seizures and spastic quadriplegia.

Six patients had extradural hematomas. Five of these are normal, and 1 has a residual hemiparesis and speech deficit.

Cerebral Contusion

Ten patients had significant cerebral contusion associated with cerebral edema. Five of these patients died, 4 are troubled with seizures, and 1 is retarded.

Hydrocephalus

Hydrocephalus developed in 6 of these 120 patients as a direct consequence of the injury. In 4 patients, the hydrocephalus followed a subdural hematoma. One patient developed hydrocephalus after treatment of a combined intracerebral and subdural hematoma, and one after treatment of an intracerebral hematoma.

Epilepsy

Twenty-seven of the 120 patients developed seizures at some point in their clinical course. Eleven patients developed seizures within the first 24 hours of their injury; 9 of these went on to have no further seizure problems. Two, however, continue to have a persistent seizure problem. Eight patients with early seizures harbored subdural hematomas.

Sixteen patients began their seizures beyond 24 hours after the injury. Eight of these are now seizure-free and off anticonvulsants, and 8 remain on anticonvulsants; 2 of them have their seizure problem under full control.

Growing Skull Fractures

Four patients developed growing skull fractures. These developed within 6 months of their skull fracture. They were all managed with duraplasty and acrylic cranioplasty. All of these patients have made a full recovery and are normal.

Meningitis

Three patients developed purulent meningitis, probably as the result of a basal skull fracture. The offending organisms were H-influenza B, pneumococcus, and a coliform bacillus. The child with the coliform meningitis died, but the other 2 children have made a full recovery.

Mortality

During the period of time that these 120 patients were under review, 744 patients under 1 year old with head injuries were admitted to our institution. Most of these patients had minor head injuries and did well. Of the 120 with severe head injuries, there were a total of 7 deaths, 5 occurring in the group with cerebral contusion and 2 in those patients with a subdural

Table 18.5. Outcomes: severe head injury.

Outcome	No. of patients
Hydrocephalus	6
Epilepsy (otherwise well)	7
Significant neurologic deficit	4
Significant neurologic and intellectual deficit	8
Mental retardation	2
Behavior disorder	2
Death	7
Normal	84
Total	120

hematoma. Three among the remaining 624 head-injured infants died of nonneurological causes. One patient with a mild head injury aspirated and died of pulmonary complications, and 2 with multiple injuries died of shock and pulmonary problems.

Summary

Head injuries in infants are a major cause for concern. The infant with a significant head injury is prone to major sequelae. Of the 120 severely injured infants in our series, 7 have died, 6 have hydrocephalus, 7 have poorly controlled seizures, and 16 are handicapped by intellectual, neurological, and emotional sequelae. Despite these problems, 84 patients have made a full recovery (see Table 18.5).

CHAPTER 19

Rehabilitation Medicine Following Severe Head Injury in Infants and Children

G. Kaiser, A. Rüdeberg, I. Fankhauser, and C. Zumbühl

Introduction

The aim of rehabilitation following severe head injury is to avoid complications from the trauma and to enable independence and social integration. Normal development is an additional goal in childhood, especially in the newborn and infant. At this age the cerebrum exhibits a remarkable increment of volume and maturation.[8] Many functions, such as speech, are not developed. Moreover, the younger the child, the less known is the premorbid personality; that is, the child's presumed level of development before the trauma is unknown.

In contrast to children, infants are not genuinely "accident prone." Their traumas seem more likely to be a result of inadequate supervision, which in turn may be a function of the unhappy psychological condition of the mother.[34] Thus, on the one hand a newborn or infant cannot be "thrown back" in development to the same extent as an older child (e.g., into dementia); but on the other hand, the younger the child, the more psychomotor development is delayed following trauma. The cerebrum is more vulnerable before age 2 than after; at this stage of considerable brain growth, malnutrition can cause gross lesions (reduced volume of the cerebellum) and microscopic lesions (reduced number of synapses).[8] (However, localized lesions of the brain can be concealed because other body parts take charge of its function; that is, functional representation is plastic.)[13,34]

Therefore, rehabilitation begun in infancy needs to be pursued until the end of development; at the very least, follow-up after head trauma is needed from infancy to adolescence to check whether rehabilitation is necessary.

Incidence, Extent, and Outcome of Severe Head Injury in Infants

Knowing how to appraise damage in infants is of great importance for the successful application of rehabilitation measures. The incidence of hospital referrals for newborn and infants, as reported in the literature, varies greatly. Hendrick et al.[17] reported an incidence for infants of up to 25% of all head-injured children who were hospitalized; birth trauma amounted to 6% of all such children. Since 1962 the composition of these patients has changed, probably independent of the hospital, by virtue of the decreasing number of traumatic birth injuries and the increasing number of road accidents. In our clinic the rate of incidence of head injured children up to 2 years old was less than 10%; that of neonates, less than 1% (referred from 1978 to 1982). But the percentage of severely injured infants was 43% as compared to 21.5% in children up to 16 years old.[20] One-fourth of the neonates as well as of infants up to 2 years old died as a result of their head injuries.

In infancy, therefore, a higher number of severely injured patients has to be expected. In addition, in this age group quite different circumstances of accident are encountered (e.g., the battered-child syndrome with recurring use of force, direct blows to the head, whiplash-shaken infant syndrome, etc.[14] Battering occurs in from one-third to one-half of all head injured infants, and up to 85% of all abused children are less than 2 years old.[15] Along with birth trauma and child abuse, falls from furniture and home and road accidents (within or out of a baby carriage) are also common causes of injury.

Altogether, the prognosis of those patients up to 2 years old is less favorable than that of school-aged children.[1,13,32] In contrast to the older child (with a 24-hour limit of coma), in the infant posttraumatic unconsciousness of more than 1 hour means that a severe head injury has already occurred. The majority of these infants exhibit diminished intelligence, and only 50% pass regular school tests later on. Moderate to severe residual neurological and psycho-organic signs—such as diminished general intelligence, divergent performance on subtests and/or disorders of visual motor function, and disturbances of emotion and behavior—nearly always follow a coma lasting from 24 hours to 7 days.[24] If the coma turns into an apallic syndrome, total recovery is impossible; younger children probably have bad outcomes and remain totally dependent or in a permanent vegetative state.[25] As Gros et al.[13] have stated, infants exhibit the same course after long-lasting coma as after encephalopathies: for example, slow psychomotor development with an increasing gap between developmental and chronological age.

Transient and permanent disturbances of perception are difficult to recognize (Fig. 19.1) but can interfere substantially with normal intellectual development. The same is true for neuropsychological findings (e.g.,

Figure 19.1. Thirteen-month-old boy with cerebral contusion and polytrauma suffering from a clouded consciousness during first two weeks and a cortical blindness lasting a month. The child does not find his way about the new environment and situation. Twenty-four hours following head injury, the child exhibits whinning temper and defective responsiveness.

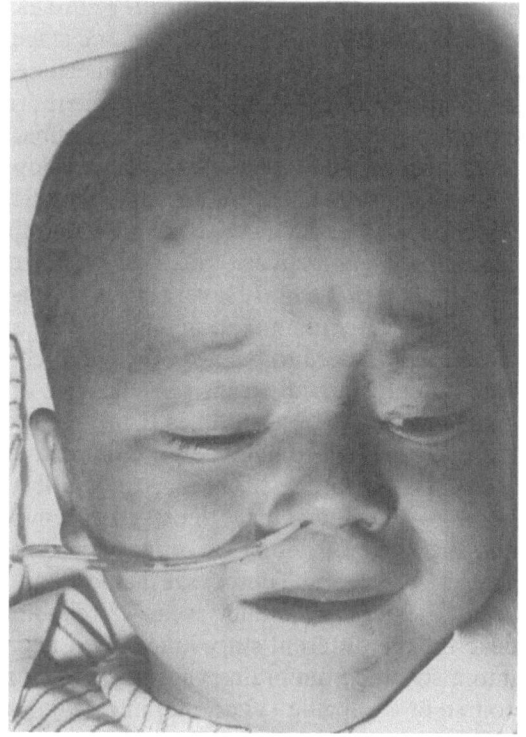

delayed development of speech) but even more difficult to prove. As in older children, infants may develop diencephalic, brain stem and cerebellar signs, such as arterial hypertension, obesity, diabetes insipitus, or sleep disorders.[6,13,25,27]

After head injury, particularly in infants, the following so-called late complications must be taken into account: posttraumatic epilepsy, posttraumatic hydrocephalus, and/or growing skull fracture. In infants, convulsions during the first two posttraumatic weeks seem to occur less often than in older children, but posttraumatic epilepsy is more frequent.[4] In general the incidence of posttraumatic epilepsy is between 5% and 10% and up to 25% to 30% in childhood.[18,33]

Natural History Following Severe Head Injury

In order to undertake successfully rehabilitation of severely head injured children, it is important to know the different stages and patterns that can be observed in the patient following the injury. Depending on the different stages, the level of consciousness, psychic condition, patterns of posture and motion, and vegetative functions are essentially involved. Moreover, there is a continuous change from one stage to the other, and the level of consciousness and psychic condition can be evaluated only with difficulty in infants (by observing eye movement, reaction to surroundings, and limitation of movements). The best possible pattern of movement is equal to the age-dependent psychomotor development.

Lange-Cosack and Tepfer[23] have identified three stages of severe head injury: coma, clouded consciousness, and the so-called transit syndrome. The duration and severity of these stages depend on the severity of the head injury. In the most severe cases, coma occurs from 1 week up to 100 weeks after the trauma. Head injuries with an initial coma of 1 to 7 days or more may proceed to a stage of clouded consciousness lasting between 1 and 2 months and a "transit syndrome" of from 3 months to 2 years in duration. In any case, it takes from 3 to 6 months (up to 2 to 3 years or more) for a child to achieve psychic recovery or a constant condition.[22]

The classification of the posttraumatic course proposed by Gerstenbrand[30]—the acute stage, the stage of remission, the stage of integration, and the stage of defect—overlaps to some extent the classifications of Lange-Cosack and Tepfer (see Table 19.1). The Gerstenbrand stages are used to establish distinct areas of rehabilitation. It may be difficult to describe the different stages, however, because the acute stage may turn into a so-called midbrain syndrome and change immediately (or over the course of an apallic syndrome) into one of the above-mentioned stages.

During the acute stage, the level of consciousness renders an experience of and a reaction to the actual situation impossible. The patterns of posture and motion and the vegetative functions (e.g., respiration, circulation, micturition, and defecation) are abnormal or damaged. During the midbrain syndrome the spasticity of the extensor muscles are of special significance. The apallic syndrome exhibits a beginning flexion posture and spontaneous or reactive mass contractions of the limbs.[11,31] The alternating cycles of sleep and waking state (open eyes) are at the beginning not combined with an ability to experience and react (coma vigil, Fig. 19.2). Later on there is a capacity to experience (first on an emotional level) unless there is a clear reaction to the surroundings. This dissocia-

Table 19.1. Stages following head injury.

Stage	Condition
Acute stage	Coma
Stage of remission ⎫	
⎬	Clouded consciousness
	"Transit syndrome"
Stage of integration ⎭	
Stage of defect	Total recovery/
	constant condition

Source: References, 23, 30.

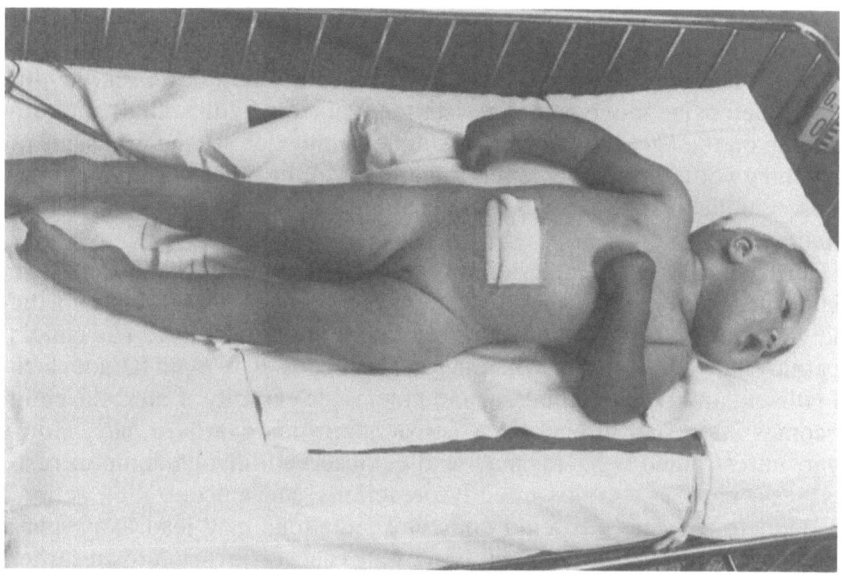

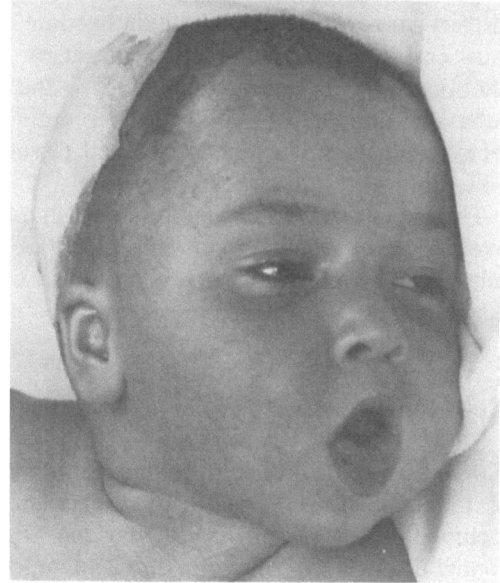

Figure 19.2. Twenty-month-old girl with cerebral contusion, subdural hygroma, and polytrauma. Four and one-half weeks following head injury, the child presents a well-developed apallic syndrome (open eyes without ability to experience react, and spasticity of the legs).

tion of the capacity to experience and the capacity to react may cause the examiner to assess mistakenly the child as comatose. The danger of misinterpretation of the level of consciousness already exists during the acute stage and, later on, during the stage of remission. It may lead to an inappropriate reaction to the environment and, therefore, induce a psychoreactive pseudocoma vigil, or "sleeping beauty syndrome."[35]

During the stage of remission, the infants' consciousness is still clouded; the infant starts to fix and to follow the surroundings with the eyes. Psychotic pictures and motor restlessness may be observed. Intended defensive movements, assisted movements by the child, and (depending on the age) the obeying of simple commands are the first signs of beginning voluntary movements. In contrast to the other vegetative functions, the sleep/waking cycle, micturition, and defecation may still be affected.

During the stage of integration, consciousness is re-established. The child finds his or her way—depending on the age—increasingly in the individual environment and begins relating to place and time. The child's apathic, slackened, and/or whining temper is caused by rapid fatigue, lack of pulsion, and reduced thinking and mnemonic capacity. Later, the child becomes interested in his or her surroundings and starts to play. However, unrestrained behavior may also be observed, involving motor restlessness, paroxia, surplus affective reactions, and uncontrolled action. Inadequate responses to environmental situations may lead to psychoreactive disorders (e.g., enuresis). In every case a regression to an earlier stage of behavior and activity occurs. During the stage of integration, an already known paresis and ataxia become more distinctly visible (in certain cases, extrapyramidal signs also). The above-mentioned psychoorganic signs additionally involve the child's emotional and social behavior, and the possibility of perceptive and neuropsychological defects (such as amaurosis or delayed development of speech) has to be taken into account.

The beginning of the stage of defect can be determined only retrospectively. This may not be possible until the child has successfully started school (and, at the latest, before the end of adolescence); assessment of development is not possible earlier.

Rehabilitation

Rehabilitation is of the entire injured individual.[27] Therefore, *all* sequelae of trauma need to be treated, and the patient's entire environment must be included in his or her care. Regular check-ups (CT scans, EEGs, psychological tests, etc.), follow-ups (for example, after recovery of consciousness), and evaluation of the success of rehabilitation are all necessary. During regular conferences of the rehabilitation team, intermediate and long-term goals are fixed, treatment schedules set up, and rehabilitative measures coordinated. Treatment schedules depend on the patient's age, the severity of the signs, and the posttraumatic stage.[22] Rehabilitation must begin in the Intensive Care Unit during the acute stage of the head injury; similarly, the patient's environment must immediately be tailored to promote rehabilitation. At all points, the facts of the patient's rapid fatigue and lessened capacity for strain must be considered. (Remission may amount to only 10 minutes and to 20 to 40 minutes during the stage of integration.)[30] The course and the measures of rehabilitation have to be recorded precisely; a diary may be useful for the parents.

Aims of Rehabilitation

The two major aims of rehabilitation of a child who suffers severe head injury may be defined as follows:

1. To provide a physical and psychical development that is as normal as possible.
2. If impossible because of permanent deficits, to provide for the best possible independence and social incorporation for the child.

Because the infant is at the beginning of his or her development, in this age group the first aim is uppermost. Later on, the second has to be considered, as the measures of rehabilitation following severe head injury must be extended to encompass the choice of occupation and training for the young adult. In addition, all relatives of the injured child, especially the parents, and all persons dealing with rehabilitation measures must be brought into a balanced relation to the injured child. Overprotection as well as overstrain have to be avoided,[32] and what the child is able to do must be checked repeatedly.

Indication for Rehabilitation

The indication for measures of rehabilitation for children depends on the severity of the head injury, insofar as sequelae of trauma become obvious or must be expected. Rehabilitation is always indicated in infants up to 2 years old if the coma lasts more than 1 hour. In case of doubt, the severity of the injury has to be evaluated repeatedly if and when rehabilitation becomes necessary. As listed in Table 19.2, the following conditions (in-

Table 19.2. Indications for rehabilitation.

Posttraumatic coma less than 1 hour in duration
Polytrauma with or without shock or
   respiratory insufficiency
Battered-child syndrome
Subdural and/or intracerebral hematoma
Complicated compound depressed fracture
Pretraumatic cerebral lesions
Unfavorable social situation;
   abnormal reaction to head injury

dependent of the length of the coma) may require rehabilitation measures, and infants must therefore be checked for them:

1. Preexisting cerebral lesions.
2. Unfavorable social integration or abnormal reactions of the family following head injury.
3. Battered child syndrome.
4. Polytrauma with or without shock and respiratory insufficiency.
5. Subdural or intracerebral hematoma.
6. Compound depressed fracture with dural tears and contusion.
7. Posttraumatic epilepsy.

Organization of Rehabilitation

In the relevant literature it is often claimed that, after the acute stage of head injury, the child should be treated in a rehabilitation clinic with an experienced staff.[30] This is often impossible for several reasons. First, a qualified rehabilitation clinic may not be available. (This is especially the case for infants with head injuries.) Second, an available rehabilitation clinic may be crowded (i.e., there may be a waiting period for new patients). Finally, because of the sequelae of trauma (e.g., polytrauma or complications of initial treatment), transfer to a rehabilitation clinic may not be indicated even beyond the acute stage. Therefore, the place of rehabilitation must be adjusted to local conditions. (The same may be valid with regard to rehabilitation on an in- or out-patient basis.)

This difficulty can be overcome by adequate organization of rehabilitation staff (Fig. 19.3). Each center to which children are referred during the acute stage of head injury should have a rehabilitation specialist who orders, coordinates and leads all rehabilitation measures. She or he oversees a team of different specialists such as physiotherapists, hospital psychologists, educational therapists, speech and occupational therapists, hospital teachers, and social workers. These specialists may perhaps already be available as a team for other kinds of patients (e.g., those with

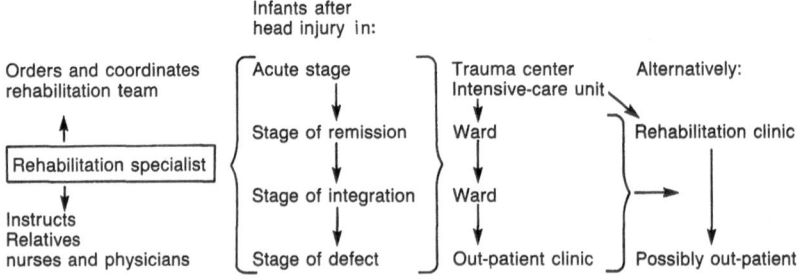

Figure 19.3. Organization of rehabilitation staff.

cerebral palsy). After such a team has been initiated into its new function, it can substitute for an actual rehabilitation staff (as occurs successfully in the rehabilitation of our youngest out-patients). The nurses and all surgeons and physicians (pediatric neurosurgeons and surgeons, pediatricians, and neuropediatricians) involved, as well as the relatives of the patient, must be integrated into the measures of rehabilitation. This can be achieved by offering conferences on the individual case, by lectures and, if necessary, by the employment of a rehabilitation assistant. In this way rehabilitation may also be practicable in the trauma center even during the stages of remission and integration. Of course, the child should be transferred from the Intensive Care Unit to the ward as quickly as possible and should by no means be separated from other children, as stimulation by the environment is an important part of recovery.

Stimulating the Level of Consciousness, Perception, and the Vegetative Functions

According to Will,[37] the rapidity and extent of a child's recovery of damaged brain functions can be enhanced with the following measures:

1. Adapting the child step by step to the environment, which is perceived as something new by the patient.
2. Stimulating the child by a continuously changing and stressful environment.
3. Supporting the stimulating effects of the environment and the regeneration of damaged neurons (nerve growth factors and enzymes) by drugs.

Applying the second measure, Le Winn and Dimancescu[26] have developed the so-called environment enrichment program. When this program was applied in the first 12 to 24 hours following head injury in a child, the authors observed a better recovery from the coma than in control subjects. According to their program, short stimuli (for instance, shining a flashlight or ringing a hand bell) are applied repeatedly during the day six times an hour for five minutes. By involving the parents and relatives (or using audio-visual methods such as tape recordings of voices familiar to the child, as well as bringing his or her favorite toys), not only is the level of consciousness and sensory perception stimulated by familiar things, but also the awakening child's fears about the unfamiliar environment are lessened if the personal world of memory is aroused.[10] In addition, the danger of a reactive akinetic mutism is diminished.[35] As soon as possible, the mother should care for the child in the same way as she did before the injury—by washing him or her and changing diapers (so as to give familiar tactile, acoustic, and visual impressions).[10] Nurses and physiotherapists should handle the child as if he or she were awake or at least capable of experience (i.e., with tender and quiet touches and accompanying words appropriate to the age of the child).[35]

Food intake is the first of the vegetative functions that must be rehabilitated. During the acute stage (depending on the injury), the physiotherapist or speech therapist should stimulate the muscles of the mouth to close the lips and later promote the intake of mashed food by training the patient to eat and swallow (e.g., through sensitization of the gingiva to enhance and coordinate the motility of the mouth and the tongue, or the use of oral stereotype patterns).[22] In addition, mouth hygiene and the danger of hypognathia have to be considered. During the stage of remission and integration, the induction of regular micturition and defecation becomes necessary (and, depending on the age, the education of cleanliness).

Physiotherapy

The goals of physiotherapy are to avoid contractures, to regulate muscle tone, to assist in functional improvement or recovery from paralysis, and to promote normal psychomotor development to the extent possible. The latter is supported in our clinic by Bobath's theory.[5] In different centers other neurophysiological methods are used, such as those of Doman et al.,[8] Kabati,[19] or Vojta.[36] Their use depends on the experience of the physiotherapists and on the individual case.

During the acute stage, abnormal positions of the extremities and of the spine as well as contracture of the joints must be avoided. To this end, regular passive therapy and regular change of position are undertaken. Care must be taken so that severe vegetative reactions and, later, para-articular calcifications do not occur. Changes of position help to regulate the muscle tone and to avoid secondary lesions of the extremities (for instance, the danger of dislocating the hip as a result of continuous hypertonia). Later on, the program may be completed by nursing the infant in a supine position in a hammock or by the so-called *mise en charge* position.[10] In addition, management of respiratory function is needed by vibromassage, clasping, and so forth.

During the stage of remission and integration, active physical therapy is increasingly possible. Every attempted movement referring to a certain function has to be supported, and lost movements must be learned again. Aided by the already mentioned neurophysiological techniques of treatment, psychomotor development is stimulated according to the child's developmental age. Pathological movements are hindered by appropriate measures; simultaneously, normal automatic movements are stimulated.

The psychomotor progress determines the organization of the rehabilitation program. Children who are not yet ambulatory are put on the floor and learn to move forward by crawling. Sensitivity may be stimulated by a brush massage and the sense of touch promoted by aiding the child in touching his or her own body with his or her own hands.

From the beginning the parents must be progressively integrated into the physiotherapy program. The active cooperation of the parents makes relating to the patient easier; at the same time, the parents' anxiety as well as their possible sense of guilt can be overcome. During these post-traumatic stages, the teamwork of physiotherapists, clinical psychologists, and speech and educational therapists is very important. A schedule of daily routines with stages of therapy and rest assists the child in finding normal rhythms of sleep and waking and thereby in cooperating better during the waking state. As rehabilitation progresses the program of therapy is increasingly extended through, for example, exercises in a therapeutic bath (to help neutralize gravitation).

As soon as the child reaches the stage of defect, previous advances should be improved (e.g., a better gait should be promoted). In certain cases the physiotherapist must be content with the present result, and in all cases a recurrence of abnormal patterns of movement must be avoided.

As soon as the child is treated as an out-patient, regular follow-ups by the rehabilitation specialist and the physiotherapist become necessary—initially monthly and later on every 3 to 6 months. Otherwise the occurrence of pathological patterns of movement may be missed. Even after a long time, assistance of the parents or re-initiation of physical therapy may become necessary.

The Role of the Clinical Psychologist and Pediatric Psychiatrist

These professionals' functions concern the injured child, the family, and finally all persons involved in the patient's rehabilitation. The infant or child must have a battery of different psychological tests to evaluate intellectual performance and emotional and social behavior after the injury. For infants only simple tests can be used (alone with careful observation)—for instance, the Denver development screening test. Later on the following have to be tested in all pediatric cases: specified intellectual as well as neuropsychological performance (e.g., aphasia), visual perception, power of concentration, mnemonic performance, and control of emotion (using, for example, Wechsler intelligence test for children and the Bender gestalt test). If the patient's general intelligence is nearly normal, a greater variability can be observed in the subtests than in normal individuals.[24] Such partial defects often concern the visuomotor performance. The recognition of different spatial structures and the ability to perform movements guided by the eye is thus an important condition for cognitive development, and for the acquisition of reading and writing skills.[28] The results of such psychological tests permit the parents to adapt the timing of the child's schooling and to choose an educational system suited to the child's intellectual performance, emotional behavior, and psychoorganic defect and able to support or even to treat the child (e.g., through training of cerebral performance.)[22,30,32]

The parents' reactions to their child's head injury must be observed and directed so that neither overprotectiveness nor overstrain occur. Pre-existing structural facts of the family must be discovered and, if possible, improved by the social worker; children belonging to already troubled families are especially prone to severe psychiatric disorders following head injury.[34]

In addition, the clinical psychologist and/or pediatric psychiatrist must ensure that *all* persons involved in rehabilitation are brought into a balanced relation to the injured child. Demands upon the injured child's intellectual performance should be moderate; possible abnormal reactions of the child to the environment should be known; and insight into the psychoorganic defects, should be cultivated in all persons involved in caring for the child.

The Role of Nurses and Physicians

Nurses in the intensive care unit and on the ward must observe, during the rehabilitation of head injured children, several points. During the acute and remission stages, the care of the skin is very important because of the danger of pressure ulcers. Frequent changes of position, synthetic coats, water-filled pillows, and physical methods of skin care (e.g., rubbing with ice packs followed by the application of a hair dryer). During the stage of remission, nurses contribute to the physiotherapy program and to the training of food intake, micturition, and defecation. If the patient is restless, the attentive nurse often recognizes a simple cause (e.g. a dry mouth).

Surgeons and physicians must be cautious in their statements concerning the prognosis and should transmit to parents only such information as is in agreement with the prognosis of emergency, intensive care, and rehabilitation specialists.

Early Intervention Programs (Educational Therapy)

The major goal of an early intervention program is to reestablish the prerequisite for a nearly normal development of intellect and personality in a very young child with brain trauma. An important feature of such a program is the use of special educators (educational therapists), trained in specific pedagogical techniques, who can conduct a home-based, parent-oriented, educational program. Although physiotherapy must always be started immediately after brain trauma, the start of early special educational therapy requires a stage of diagnostic evaluation.

In the child with a recent brain trauma who has reached the stage of remission, the various aspects of the patient's psychomotor development should be examined. The following aspects must be considered: gross motor development, fine motor development, behavior profile, speech, social behavior, and cognitive function (see Table 19.3). If a deficit is found, the child will be introduced into a program of observation or possibly, according to the developmental age, into an immediate early intervention program.

The aim of the observation period is to record the individual dynamics of recovery in the various skills mentioned above, to follow the course of further "normal" development of the child, and to register how the latter differs from the development of the healthy child. During the remission phase such examinations have to be done once a week. In the stage of deficit, once the diagnosis has been established, these observations have to be performed at intervals of 6 weeks to 3 months. The prolonged observation time serves to permit an individual diagnosis and to prevent a too rapid, sterotypical categorization that could lead to the choice of an erroneous program of intervention.

Until the child has reached the age of $1\frac{1}{2}$ years, the examination may be performed by a neuropediatrician or by a pediatric rehabilitation specialist. Thereafter, the examination should be done by a pediatric psychologist. From the first month of life until the age of about 12 months, physiotherapy will suffice as early intervention program, as the acquisition of motor skills dominates development at this age. From 12 to 18 months of developmental age, a special educational program should be introduced. This program has to be adequate for every type of defect—that is, if possible the child should have a specialized educator with experience

Table 19.3. Developmental diagnosis in the early infancy.

Tests	Criteria	Results
Denver developmental screening test (pediatrician/neuropediatrician)	Gross motor area Fine motor area Adaptation Language/speech Social contact	Rapid separate evaluation of developmental age
Gesell developmental schedules (neuropediatrician/rehabilitation pediatrician)	Gross motor area Fine motor area Adpative behavior Speech behavior Social behavior	Global developmental quotient
Münchener funktionelle entwicklungsdiagnostik (neuropediatrician/rehabilitation pediatrician)	Gross motor area Fine motor area Perception Speech Social behavior	Separate developmental age in 5 areas
Bayley scales of infant development, 0–2 years (child psychologist)	Mental skills Motor skills Test behavior	Separate developmental quotient

Source: References 2, 9, 16, 21, 29.

relevant to the deficit. It is thus important to make use of specialists in perception deficits, in occupational therapy, and in behavior abnormalities.

These treatments should be repeated at weekly intervals at the beginning and, if possible, they should be organized in the child's home. The special educator will thus introduce the therapeutic techniques to the parents, giving them advice on pedagogical techniques and therapeutical materials. As soon as the therapy has been well established, the frequency of treatment can be reduced to twice a month.

The application of early intervention programs requires a regular check-up (once to twice a year by a neuropediatrician or psychologist). Thus, retardation of development, learning deficits, or behavior disorders will be recognized and additional treatment (e.g., psychomotor therapy, prolongation of logopedic treatment, treatment of dyslexia, help with choice of educational system and starting school) instituted during the pre-school age. All these measures have to be organized and supported by the rehabilitation team, aided by social workers who help the parents practically and improve the information exchange between the medical team, paramedical personnel, and school administrators.

The older the child, the more necessary are additional rehabilitation specialists, as well as speech and occupational therapists and regular teachers. (With infant patients, these specialists' functions are often performed by physiotherapists and educational therapists.)

Drug Therapy for Infants and Young Children

Drug therapy may be an important aid during the rehabilitation of very young children. There are three possibilities of treatment, depending on the target signs. If, on the one hand, cortical functions (disorders of learning processes or perception) are involved, drugs such as Piracetam or Pyritinol may be used; they are claimed to improve the cerebral metabolism. On the other hand, if subcortical signs must be treated (hyperactivity, disorders of attention, impulsiveness, fear, and depressed states), Methylphenidat (which has a paradoxical effect) or Imipramin and Desipramin may be used. In addition, Diazepam (which combats restlessness, breath-holding attacks, and spasticity of the muscles) and Levodopa (which combats rigor, tremor, etc.) may be indicated. Finally, drugs such as Thioridazin which can improve disturbed social behavior, may be considered.

Rehabilitation on an Out-Patient Basis

Infants and toddlers should, if possible, be treated as in-patients during the stages of remission and integration. The moment when rehabilitation may take place on an out-patient basis depends on the following circumstances: course after the head injury, success of the rehabilitation measures, situation of the family, local organization of the rehabilitation clinic, distance of the family from the rehabilitation center, and availability of rehabilitation specialists at the place of residence. In addition, the number of rehabilitation measures and therapeutic sessions involved plays an important role. In the literature, the length of rehabilitation for in-patients up to 12 months old is estimated at between 1½ to 3 years and, following an apallic syndrome, at between 1 and 4 years.[30]

The rehabilitation of out-patients requires a competent coordinator or rehabilitation specialist. He or she organizes regular follow-ups, if possible together with the surgeons and physicians of the acute stage. They serve not only to check the successes or pitfalls of rehabilitation measures and to fix further measures, but also to study the results of treatment during the acute stage (such as neurointensive care).

Prognosis of Rehabilitation

There is general agreement that the final outcome following severe head injury is better with prompt than with delayed rehabilitation (or none at all), except in about one-third of all apallic patients who cannot be rehabilitated.[25] Because we think a random study rehabilitation measures would be unethical, we have examined studies comparing older groups of head-injured children without sufficient rehabilitation with groups that had adequate rehabilitation. For instance, from 1975 to 1976 Gobiet[12] found that 90% of all head injured children were educable individuals following rehabilitation as compared to 75% of an older group that had inadequate rehabilitation. In addition, our experience—that either a delayed or a prematurely begun rehabilitation program yields unfavorable results— argues in favor of the usefulness of timely and adequate rehabilitation.

References

1. Auriach A, Gros C, Dimeglio E: Les séquelles des traumatismes crâniens graves de l'enfant: Expérience vécue dans un centre spécialisé pour enfants. *Cahiers Rééd Réadapt* 1974;9:112–122.
2. Bayley N: Bayley scales of infant development. New York, Psychological Corporation, 1969.
3. Berger M, Gerstenbrand F: Aufgabe der ambulanten Nachbehandlung des Schädel-Hirn-Traumas beim Kind. *Z Kinderchir* 1981;33(suppl):266–271.
4. Black P, Shepard RH, Walker AE: Outcome of head trauma: Age and post-traumatic seizures, in Outcome of severe damage to the central nervous system. *Ciba Foundation Symposium 34.* New York Elsevier Excerpta Medica, 1975, pp 215–226.
5. Bobath K, Bobath B: Motor development in the different type of cerebral palsy. London, Heinemann, 1975.

6. Brink JD, Imbus C, Woo-Sam J: Physical recovery after severe closed head trauma in children and adolescents. *J Ped* 1980;97:721–727.
7. Dobbing J: Nutrition et développement cérébral. *Documents scientifiques Guigoz* 1980;108:2–13.
8. Doman RJ, Doman G, Spitz EB, Zucman E, Delacato C: Children with severe brain injures: Neúrological organisation in terms of mobility. *JAMA* 1960;174:257–262.
9. Frankenburg WK, Dodds JB: The Denver Developmental Screening Test. *J Ped* 1967;71:181–191.
10. Friderich J: Ueber die Rehabilitation nach schwerem Schädel-Hirn Trauma im Kindesalter. *Ther Umsch* 1981;38:323–327.
11. Gerstenbrand F: Das traumatische appalische Syndrom. Klinik, Morphologie, Pathophysiologie und Behandlung. Vienna, Springer-Verlag Wein, 1967.
12. Gobiet W: Advances in management of severe head injuries in childhood. *Acta Neurochir* (Wein) 1977;39:201–210.
13. Gros C, Baldy-Molinier M, Gros-Massoubre A, Masquefa C: L'avenir éloigné des comas traumatiques de l'enfant. *Neurochirurgie* 1969;15:35–50.
14. Guthkelch AN: Infantile subdural hematoma and its relationship to whiplash injury. *Br Med J* 1971;2:430–431.
15. Haha YS, Raimondi AJ, McLone DG, Yamanouchi Y: Traumatic mechanisms of head injury in child abuse. *Child's Brain* 1983;10:229–241.
16. Hellbrügge T et al.: Münchner funktionelle Entwicklungs-diagnostik, Lebensjahr 1. München, 1978.
17. Hendrick EB, Harwood-Hash DCF, Hudson AR: Head injuries in children: A survey of 4465 consecutive cases at the Hospital for Sick Children, Toronto, Canada. Clin Neurosurg, 1963;11:46–65.
18. Jennett B: Trauma as a cause of epilepsy in childhood. *Dev Med Child Neurol* 1973;15:56–62.
19. Kabat H: Proprioceptive facilitation in therapeutic exercise, in *Therapeutic Exercise* Licht S (ed): ed 2.
20. Kaiser G, Pfenninger J: Effect of neurointensive care upon outcome following severe head injury in childhood—a preliminary report. *Neuropediatrics* (in press).
21. Knobloch H, Pasamanick B: The developmental screening inventory, in Knobloch H, Pasamanick B (eds): *Gesell and Amatruda's Developmental Diagnosis*, ed 3. New York, Harper & Row Publishers Inc, 1974.
22. Lange-Cosack H: Rehabilitation nach Hirntraumen im Kindesalter. *Rehabilitation* 1972;11:74–80.
23. Lange-Cosack H, Tepfer G: Das Hirntrauma im Kindes und Jugendalter. *Schriftenreihe Neurologie* 12. (Vienna, Springer-Verlag, 1973.
24. Lange-Cosack H, Wider B, Schlesener HJ, Grumme T, Kubicki S: Spätfolgen nach Schädelhirntraumen im Säuglings und Kleinkindalter, Lebensjahr 1–5. *Neuropädiatrie* 1979;10:105–127.
25. Lange-Cosack H, Riebel U, Grumme T, Schlesener HJ: Possibilities and limitations of rehabilitation after traumatic apallic syndrome in children and adolescents. *Neuro-pediatrics* 1981;12:337–365.
26. Le Winn EB, Dimancescu MD: Environmental deprivation and enrichment in coma. *Lancet* 1978;2(8081):156–157.

27. Markus E: Die Rehabilitation des Kindes nach schwerem Schädel-Hirn-Trauma. *Z Kinderchir* 1981;33(suppl):297–301.
28. Michel M: Diagnostik und Therapie der zentralen Wahrnehmungsstörungen bei Kindern nach Schädel-Hirn-Trauma. ·*Z Kinderchir* 1981;33(suppl):302–304.
29. Osofsky JD (ed): *Handbook of Infant Development*. New York, John Wiley & Sons Inc., 1979.
30. Piorreck S: Praktische Erfahrungen in der Rehabilitation von Kindern nach schwerem Schädel-Hirn-Trauma. *Z Kinderchir* 1981;33:221–228.
31. Plum F, Posner JB: Diagnosis of stupor and coma, in *Contemporary Neurology Series*, ed 2. Philadelphia, Davis, 1972.
32. Remschmidt H: Psychosoziale Folgen nach Schädel-Hirn-Traumen im Kindesalter. *Monatsschr Kinderheilkd* 1979;127:436–440.
33. Roche M, Dieterich E: Posttraumatische Epilepsie im Kindesalter. *Z Kinderchir* 1981;33(suppl):236–238.
34. Shaffer D, Chadwick O, Rutter M: Psychiatric outcome of localized head injury in children, in Outcome of severe damage to the central nervous system. *Ciba Foundation Symposium* 34. New York, Elsevier Excerpta Medica 1975.
35. Todorow S: Recovery of children after severe head injury. Psychoreactive Superimpositions. *Scand J Rehab* Med 1975;7:93–96.
36. Vojta V: Die cerebralen Bewegungsstörungen im Säuglingsalter. Stuttgart, Ferdinand Enke Verlag, 1974.
37. Will BE: Methods for promoting functional recovery following brain damage, in Berenberg SR (ed): *Brain—Fetal and Infant: Current Research on Normal and Abnormal Development*. The Hague, Martinus Nijhoff Medical Division, 1977.

Index